HEALING
HOTELS
OF THE WORLD

EDITED BY
ANNE BIGING &
DR. ELISABETH IXMEIER

teNeues

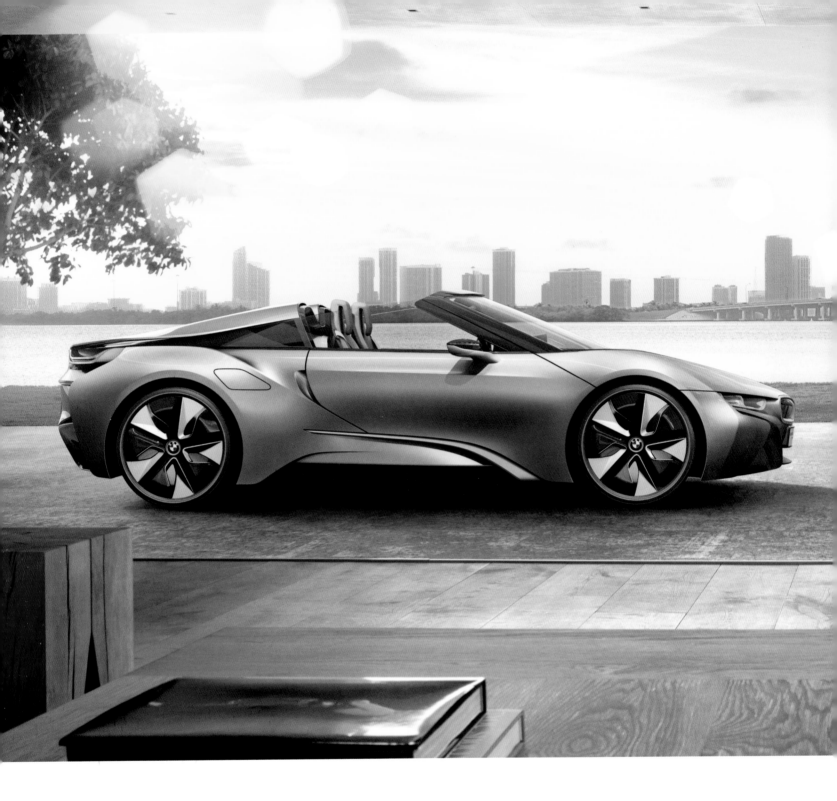

OVERINDULGE
RESPONSIBLY.

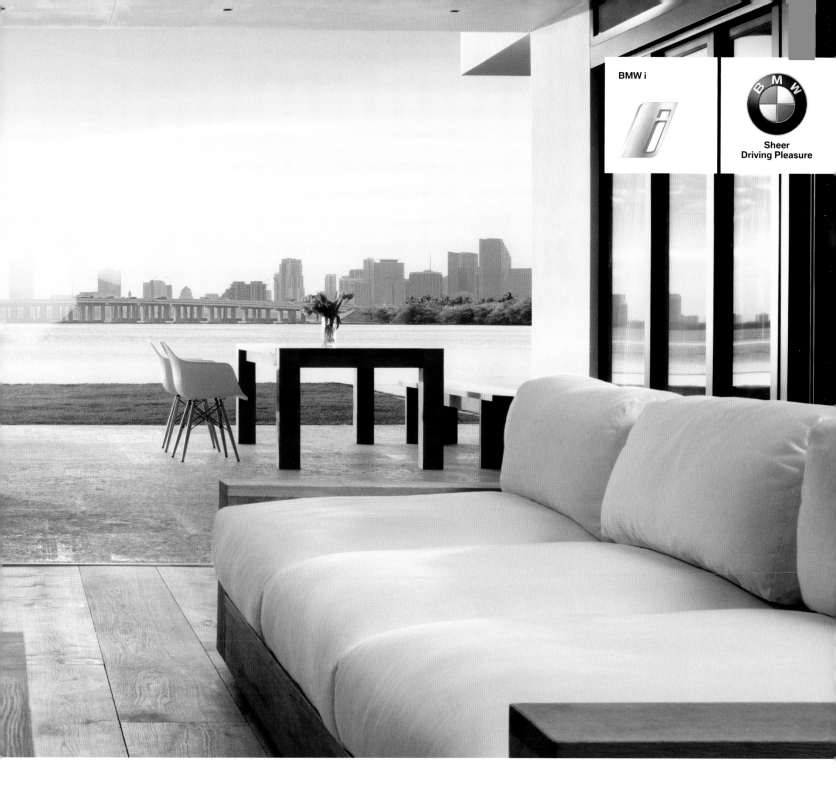

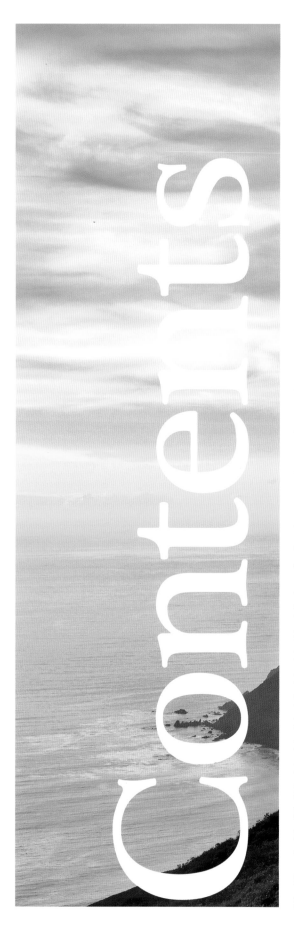

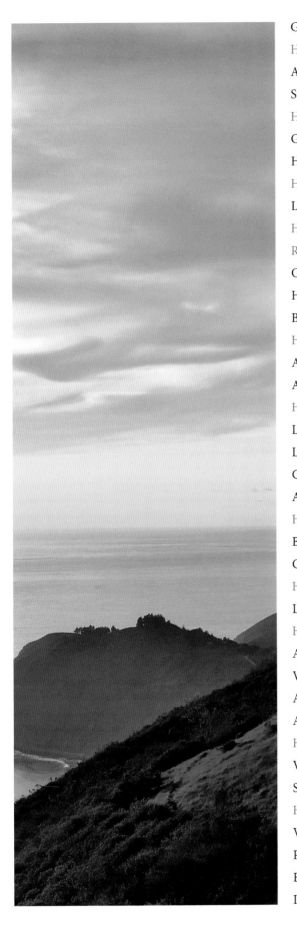

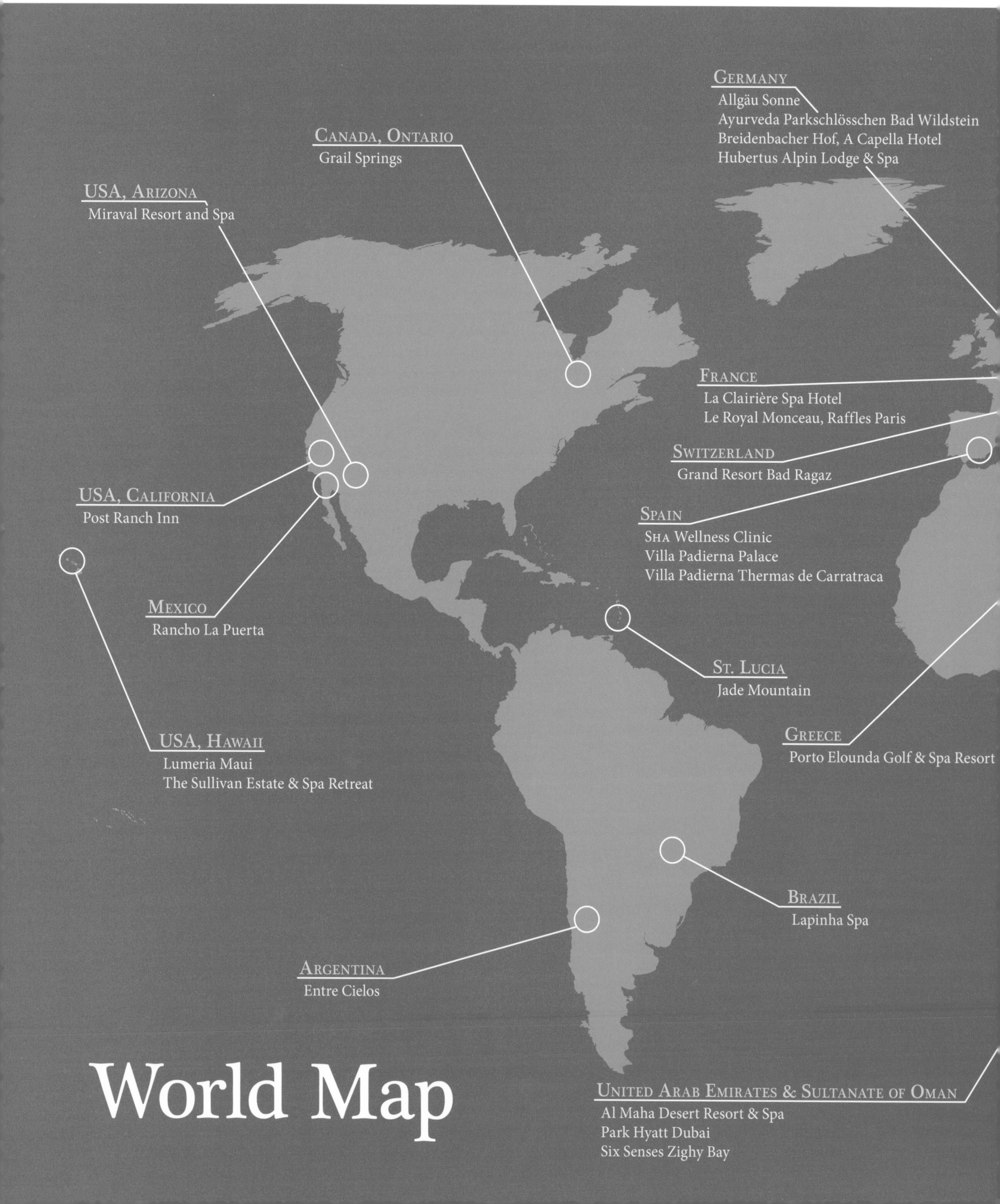

GERMANY
Allgäu Sonne
Ayurveda Parkschlösschen Bad Wildstein
Breidenbacher Hof, A Capella Hotel
Hubertus Alpin Lodge & Spa

CANADA, ONTARIO
Grail Springs

USA, ARIZONA
Miraval Resort and Spa

FRANCE
La Clairière Spa Hotel
Le Royal Monceau, Raffles Paris

SWITZERLAND
Grand Resort Bad Ragaz

SPAIN
SHA Wellness Clinic
Villa Padierna Palace
Villa Padierna Thermas de Carratraca

USA, CALIFORNIA
Post Ranch Inn

MEXICO
Rancho La Puerta

ST. LUCIA
Jade Mountain

GREECE
Porto Elounda Golf & Spa Resort

USA, HAWAII
Lumeria Maui
The Sullivan Estate & Spa Retreat

BRAZIL
Lapinha Spa

ARGENTINA
Entre Cielos

World Map

UNITED ARAB EMIRATES & SULTANATE OF OMAN
Al Maha Desert Resort & Spa
Park Hyatt Dubai
Six Senses Zighy Bay

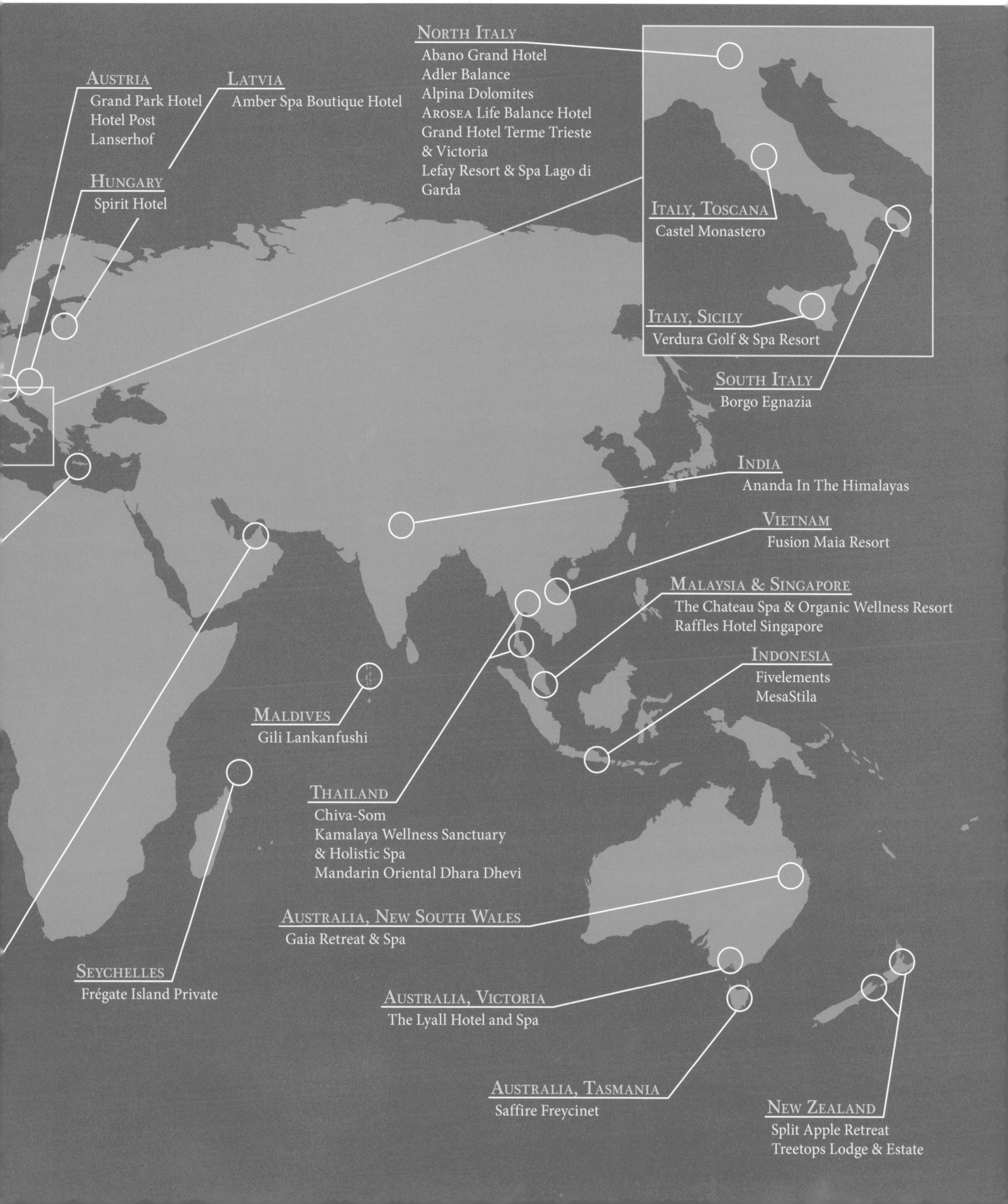

NORTH ITALY
Abano Grand Hotel
Adler Balance
Alpina Dolomites
AROSEA Life Balance Hotel
Grand Hotel Terme Trieste
& Victoria
Lefay Resort & Spa Lago di
Garda

ITALY, TOSCANA
Castel Monastero

ITALY, SICILY
Verdura Golf & Spa Resort

SOUTH ITALY
Borgo Egnazia

AUSTRIA
Grand Park Hotel
Hotel Post
Lanserhof

LATVIA
Amber Spa Boutique Hotel

HUNGARY
Spirit Hotel

INDIA
Ananda In The Himalayas

VIETNAM
Fusion Maia Resort

MALAYSIA & SINGAPORE
The Chateau Spa & Organic Wellness Resort
Raffles Hotel Singapore

INDONESIA
Fivelements
MesaStila

MALDIVES
Gili Lankanfushi

THAILAND
Chiva-Som
Kamalaya Wellness Sanctuary
& Holistic Spa
Mandarin Oriental Dhara Dhevi

AUSTRALIA, NEW SOUTH WALES
Gaia Retreat & Spa

SEYCHELLES
Frégate Island Private

AUSTRALIA, VICTORIA
The Lyall Hotel and Spa

AUSTRALIA, TASMANIA
Saffire Freycinet

NEW ZEALAND
Split Apple Retreat
Treetops Lodge & Estate

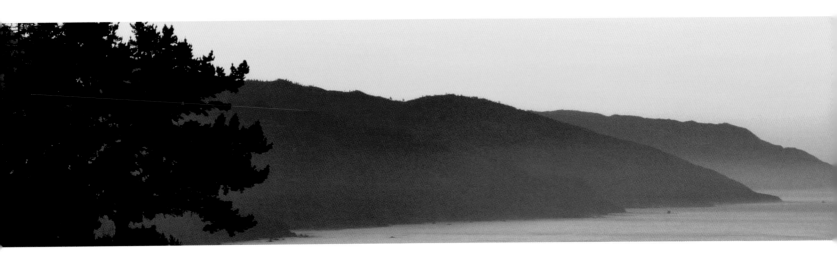

Healing Hotels of the World

supports the William J. Clinton Foundation

After leaving the White House, President Clinton established the William J. Clinton Foundation with the mission to improve global health, strengthen economies, promote health and wellness, and protect the environment by fostering partnerships among governments, businesses, nongovernmental organizations (NGOs), and private citizens to turn good intentions into measurable results.

Since 2001, President Clinton's vision and leadership have resulted in more than 4.5 million people benefiting from lifesaving HIV/AIDS treatment; more than 15,000 U.S. schools building healthier learning environments; more than 10,000 jobs created and businesses strengthened; 23,000 farmers improving food security and livelihoods; and more than 2,000 tons of carbon dioxide being reduced through commercial and residential retrofits in the U.S.

In 2012, President Clinton expanded the focus of his Foundation's work to address the priority of health and wellness for all generations in the United States through the Clinton Health Matters Initiative (CHMI). CHMI works to activate individuals, communities, and organizations to make health and wellness a priority, with the goal of improving the quality of life for all Americans. Additionally, President Clinton has redefined the way we think about giving and philanthropy through his Clinton Global Initiative (CGI), whose members have made nearly 2,300 commitments which have already improved the lives of more than 400 million people in more than 180 countries.

By purchasing this book you are contributing to healthier futures around the world.

Healing Hotels of the World

unterstützt die William J. Clinton Foundation

Nach seiner Amtszeit im Weißen Haus gründete Präsident Clinton die William J. Clinton Foundation. Die Stiftung setzt sich weltweit für die Themen Gesundheit, Stärkung der Wirtschaft und Umweltschutz ein. Dazu werden Partnerschaften zwischen Regierungen, Wirtschaft, Nichtregierungsorganisationen (NGOs) und Bürgern angestrebt, um gute Absichten in messbare Ergebnisse zu überführen.

Mehr als 4,5 Millionen Menschen haben seit 2001 durch Präsident Clintons Initiative lebenserhaltende HIV/AIDS-Behandlungen erhalten; mehr als 15 000 amerikanische Schulen profitieren von einem gesünderen Lernumfeld; über 10 000 Arbeitsstellen wurden geschaffen und die Existenzgrundlage von 23 000 landwirtschaftlichen Betrieben verbessert. Zudem hat man durch private und wirtschaftliche Sanierungen in den USA eine Emissionsreduzierung von 2 000 Tonnen Kohlendioxid erreicht.

2012 hat Präsident Clinton seine Stiftung um die Clinton Health Matters Intiative (CHMI) erweitert. Diese Initiative setzt einen Schwerpunkt auf Gesundheit für alle Altersgruppen. Zusätzlich hat Präsident Clinton durch die Clinton Global Initiative (CGI) eine neue Dimension der Philanthropie entwickelt. Die Mitglieder haben sich verpflichtet, die Lebensumstände von über 400 Millionen Menschen in mehr als 180 Ländern zu verbessern.

Durch den Kauf dieses Buches investieren Sie in eine gesündere Zukunft für alle.

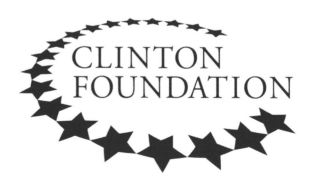

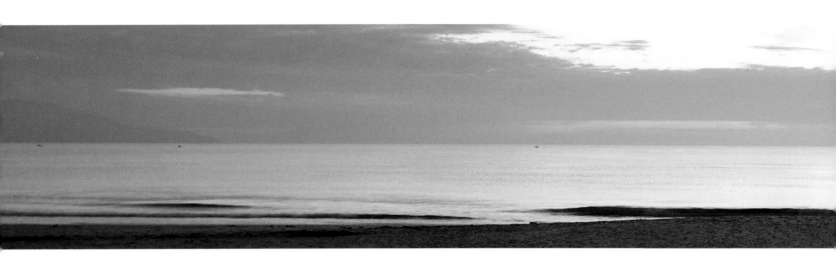

Introduction

"It is our vision that guests of a Healing Hotel become whole again in body, mind, and soul, freeing them to enjoy the sacredness and abundance of life."

The search for happiness, contentment, and well-being is as old as humanity itself. We have long known that the source of this precious state of abundance and well-being lies within ourselves. We each hold the key in our own hands.

In today's complex world, we face the daily challenges of life whilst keeping our eyes on the ultimate goal: finding happiness! With a holistic understanding of life, we take responsibility for our circumstances, our sense of life, and our health.

There are many different ways in which we can approach this goal. For some, it is tranquility and for others the sensual impressions of nature that enable us to experience the moment with complete mindfulness. There may also be times when it is good to engage in lifestyle coaching to identify the barriers keeping happiness at bay. Often we also need support on the physical level in the form of movement, diet, massage, conventional or alternative medical consultations, and holistic healing methods.

Healing Hotels of the World bring together hotels and resorts around the world that offer best-in-world holistic health programs. Most of these special hideaways are located in places where nature helps us find our way back to ourselves; rediscovering our feelings and hearts. Counseling and therapeutic programs help get our bodies back on track and stimulate their power of self-healing. We return home feeling healthier and refreshed, with a new sense of life and new vitality. The effects are long-lasting, since we have learned how to lead a healthier and therefore happier life, even in the everyday world.

Living a healthy and fulfilled life means understanding that we are complex beings in whom mind and body are interconnected. It also means recognizing that we live in an interconnected world, one in which we take responsibility for our communities, nature, and the planet.

We offer our thanks to those wonderful visionaries who established these hotels and resorts, working together with their staff to create unique retreats and experiences. They give us more pleasure in life, inner growth, and peace within ourselves—and thus in the world all around us.

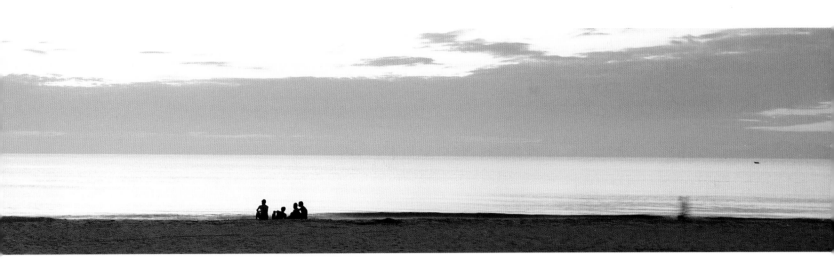

Einleitung

„Es ist unsere Vision, dass die Gäste eines Healing Hotels ihr eigenes Wohlbefinden
und damit die Bedeutung und Fülle des Lebens wiederentdecken."

Die Suche nach Glück, Zufriedenheit und Wohlbefinden ist so alt wie die Menschheit selbst. Wir wissen
längst, dass die Quelle zu diesem kostbaren Zustand der Fülle und des Wohlfühlens in uns selbst liegt.
Wir halten den Schlüssel in unserer Hand.

In der komplexen Gegenwart erfahren wir täglich die Herausforderung, uns selbst nicht zu verlieren
und unser wichtigstes Ziel im Auge zu behalten: Wir wollen glücklich sein! Mit einem ganzheitlichen
Lebensverständnis übernehmen wir Verantwortung für unsere Lebensumstände, unser Lebensgefühl,
unsere Gesundheit.

Wir können uns dabei in unterschiedlicher Form unterstützen lassen. Für den einen ist es die Stille, für
andere sind es die sinnlichen Eindrücke der Natur, die uns den Moment ganz bewusst erfahren lassen.
Es können aber auch Gespräche sein, die uns die eigene Realität spiegeln, sodass wir verstehen, wo Blockaden
in unserem Leben liegen. Oft brauchen wir auch auf der körperlichen Ebene Unterstützung in Form
von Bewegung, Ernährung, Massagen, schulmedizinischen oder alternativen Untersuchungen und
ganzheitlichen Heilmethoden.

Healing Hotels of the World vereint Hotels und Resorts weltweit, die ganzheitliche Gesundheitsangebote
auf höchstem Niveau anbieten. Die meisten dieser Refugien befinden sich an Orten, an denen uns die
Natur unterstützt, zu uns selbst zurückzukehren und unsere Gefühle, unser Herz – kurz: das, was uns
ausmacht – wiederzuentdecken. Beratung und therapeutische Angebote helfen dabei, unseren Körper
wieder ins Lot zu bringen und seine Selbstheilungskräfte anzuregen. Von diesen Orten kehren wir gesünder,
erfrischt, mit neuem Lebensgefühl und neuer Lebensfreude zurück. Ein Effekt, der anhalten soll, denn wir
lernen dort, wie wir auch in unserem Alltag ein gesünderes und damit glücklicheres Leben führen können.

Gesund und erfüllt zu leben, bedeutet zu verstehen, dass wir komplexe Wesen sind, in denen Geist und
Körper zusammenhängen. Es bedeutet auch zu erkennen, dass wir in einer vernetzten Welt leben, in
der wir Verantwortung für unsere Mitmenschen, die Natur, den Planeten übernehmen.

Wir danken denen, die mit ihrer Vision und Passion die hier vorgestellten Hotels und Resorts gegründet
haben und gemeinsam mit ihren Mitarbeitern einzigartige Refugien schufen. Sie schenken uns mehr
Lebensgenuss, inneres Wachstum und Frieden in uns selbst – und damit in der Welt um uns herum.

Spirit of Mother Earth
Wo die Energie von Mutter Erde spürbar ist

Gaia Retreat & Spa

This location in the Byron Bay hinterland is positively addictive. Known as the healing capital of Australia, this unique property seduces to drift into infinity with its endless beautiful vistas. You can feel the full power of this mystical region as it grounds and reconnects you to the spirit of the land. Empathetic healers and therapists skilled in intensive and deeply penetrating treatments and luxury pampering provide the guests with an opportunity to surrender and restore balance to their lives. Gaia is proudly co-owned by Olivia Newton-John and strives to deliver an authentic Australian retreat experience, tailored to the guests' individual needs. The area around Gaia is renowned for some of the finest seasonal food Mother Earth has to offer. The head chef personally chooses the freshest organic produce available from Gaia's own organic garden and the surrounding orchards and plantations for his healthy spa cuisine. After all, Gaia is the goddess known as "Mother Earth."

Dieser Ort im australischen Hinterland macht regelrecht süchtig. Die Gegend gilt als eine der heilenden Regionen Australiens und vermittelt ein Gefühl der Unendlichkeit, wenn man den Blick über die weite Landschaft schweifen lässt. Hier spürt man die Kraft dieses mystischen Kontinents, die es den Gästen leicht macht, die Verbindung zwischen sich und der Natur wiederherzustellen. Einfühlsame Heiler und Therapeuten verstehen sich auf intensive, tief gehende und verwöhnende Behandlungen, die helfen, loszulassen und die Lebensbalance wiederzufinden. Olivia Newton-John ist stolze Mitbesitzerin dieses Rückzugsortes, der ein authentisch australisches Flair vermittelt und auf die persönlichen Bedürfnisse seiner Gäste eingeht. Die Gegend um Gaia ist bekannt für das beste Gemüse und Obst, sodass der Koch für seine Gesundheitsküche persönlich in den eigenen biologischen Gärten und Obstplantagen ernten kann. Gaia ist übrigens die Göttin „Mutter Erde".

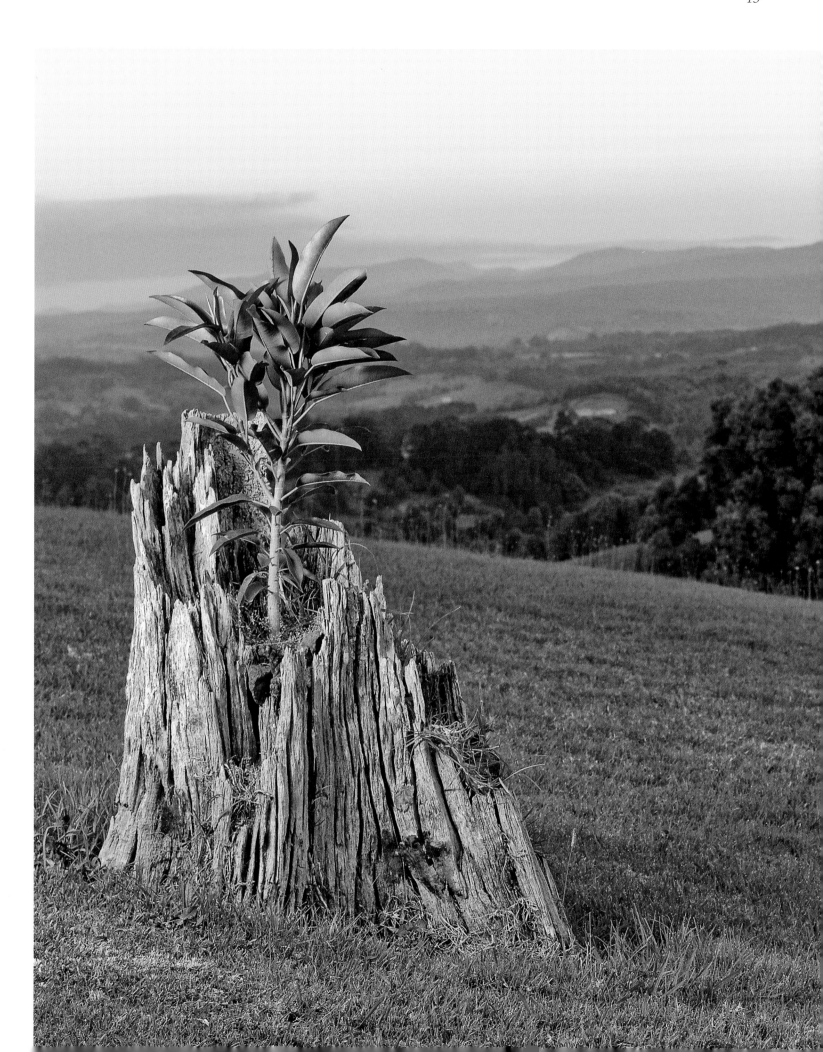

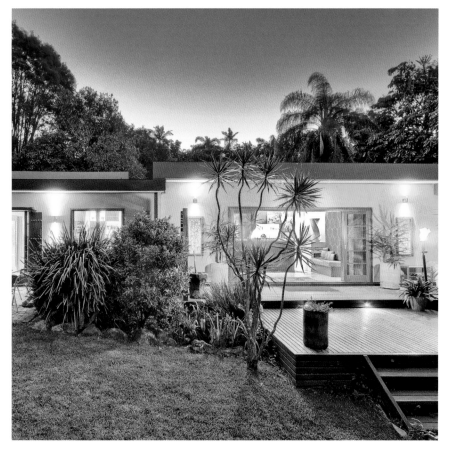

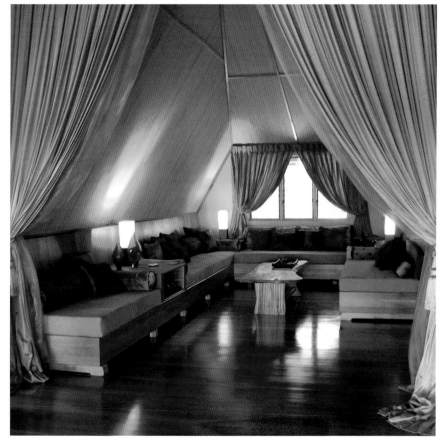

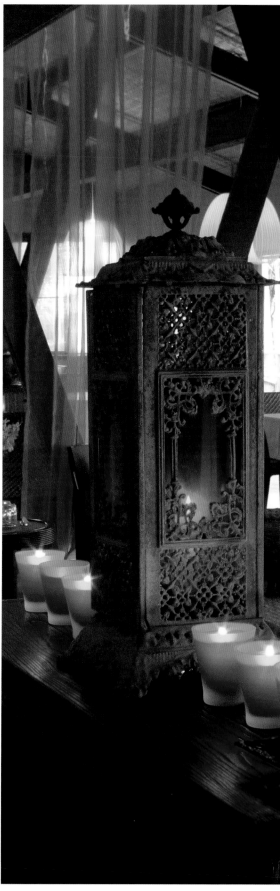

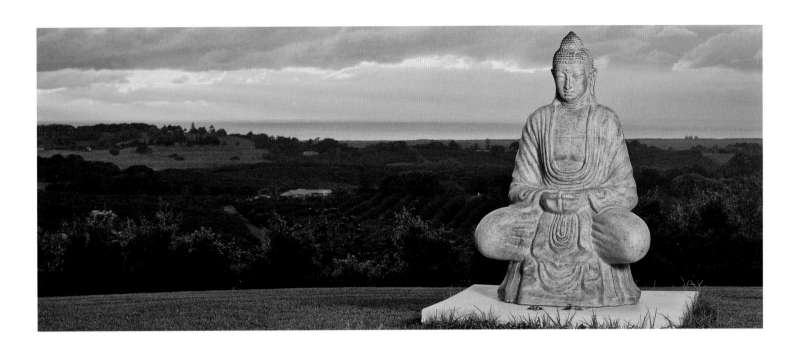

Spa, Health & Other Facilities
Gaia Day Spa including 10 spa treatment rooms, spa hot tub, swimming pool, outdoor sauna, steam room, gym. Organic spa cuisine restaurant (for in-house and Day Spa guests), yoga room, tennis court, walking tracks, conference facilities for up to 40 people, CD/DVD/book library.

Treatments & Services
Acupuncture, aqua aerobics, Ayurvedic therapies, beauty therapies, body balance, Chinese medicine, energy and spiritual healing, Hawaiian massage, hot rock massage, hypnotherapy, indigenous healing treatments, let's get physical classes, meditation, massage, naturopathic and wellness consultations, nutritional health and well-being talks, Pilates, Qigong, reflexology, Reiki, sauna/steam bath treatments, Swedish massage, sound meditation, stretch classes, Tai Chi, yoga. Private guidance and focus add-on packages also available.

Activities
Biking, boxing, clay sculpture, nature walks, organic cooking classes.

Rooms
12 Layana Rooms, 4 Sura Terraces (premium), 2 Acala Suites (private exclusive suites), 4 Platinum Villas.

Located
In the subtropical hinterland of Byron Bay. It takes about 2 hours by car to get to Brisbane.

933 Fernleigh Road
Brooklet, NSW 2479, Australia
www.gaiaretreat.com.au

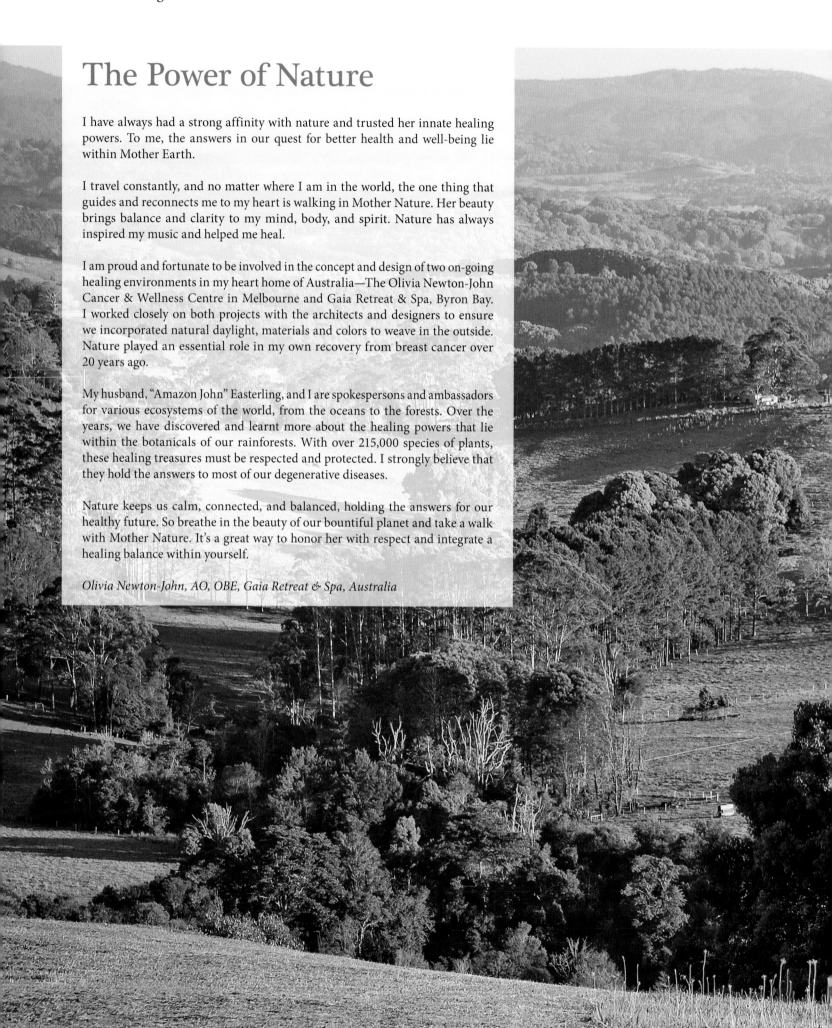

The Power of Nature

I have always had a strong affinity with nature and trusted her innate healing powers. To me, the answers in our quest for better health and well-being lie within Mother Earth.

I travel constantly, and no matter where I am in the world, the one thing that guides and reconnects me to my heart is walking in Mother Nature. Her beauty brings balance and clarity to my mind, body, and spirit. Nature has always inspired my music and helped me heal.

I am proud and fortunate to be involved in the concept and design of two on-going healing environments in my heart home of Australia—The Olivia Newton-John Cancer & Wellness Centre in Melbourne and Gaia Retreat & Spa, Byron Bay. I worked closely on both projects with the architects and designers to ensure we incorporated natural daylight, materials and colors to weave in the outside. Nature played an essential role in my own recovery from breast cancer over 20 years ago.

My husband, "Amazon John" Easterling, and I are spokespersons and ambassadors for various ecosystems of the world, from the oceans to the forests. Over the years, we have discovered and learnt more about the healing powers that lie within the botanicals of our rainforests. With over 215,000 species of plants, these healing treasures must be respected and protected. I strongly believe that they hold the answers to most of our degenerative diseases.

Nature keeps us calm, connected, and balanced, holding the answers for our healthy future. So breathe in the beauty of our bountiful planet and take a walk with Mother Nature. It's a great way to honor her with respect and integrate a healing balance within yourself.

Olivia Newton-John, AO, OBE, Gaia Retreat & Spa, Australia

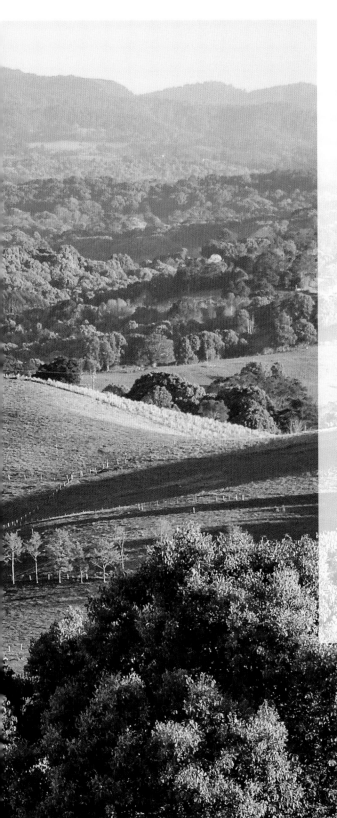

Die Kraft der Natur

Tiefe Naturverbundenheit habe ich schon immer verspürt. Seit jeher vertraue ich auf natürliche Heilkräfte und glaube, dass wir in unserem Streben nach mehr Gesundheit und Wohlbefinden auf Mutter Erde hören müssen.

Ich bin ununterbrochen auf Reisen, und überall auf der Welt finde ich durch Bewegung in der freien Natur wieder zu mir selbst. Die Schönheit der Natur verleiht meiner Seele, meinem Körper und Geist Gleichgewicht und Klarheit. Die Natur war schon immer Muse meiner Musik und hat mir zur Heilung verholfen.

Es erfüllt mich mit Stolz und Freude, in meiner geliebten Heimat Australien am Entwurf und Design des Olivia Newton-John Cancer & Wellness Centre Melbourne und des Gaia Retreat & Spa Byron Bay mitgewirkt zu haben. Beides sind wunderbare Orte für Gesundheit und Heilung. Bei den Projekten habe ich eng mit den Architekten und Designern zusammengearbeitet, um sicherzustellen, dass sowohl das natürliche Sonnenlicht als auch Materialien und Farben der natürlichen Außenwelt in das Design einfließen. Als ich vor mehr als 20 Jahren an Brustkrebs erkrankte, war die Natur ein wichtiger Bestandteil meiner eigenen Genesung.

Mein Mann, „Amazon John" Easterling, und ich sind Sprecher und Botschafter für verschiedene Ökosysteme dieser Welt, von den Ozeanen bis hin zu den Wäldern. Im Laufe der Jahre haben wir mehr über die Heilkräfte der Pflanzen unserer Regenwälder herausfinden und lernen können. Mit über 215 000 Pflanzenarten verdienen diese heilsamen Schätze unsere Achtung und unseren Schutz. Ich bin fest davon überzeugt, dass diese Pflanzen zur Heilung der meisten degenerativen Krankheiten beitragen können.

Die Natur vermittelt uns Ruhe, Verbundenheit und Gleichgewicht, und ist der Schlüssel zu einer gesunden Zukunft. Atmen Sie also die Schönheit unseres freigebigen Planeten ein und genießen Sie einen Spaziergang mit Mutter Erde. Es ist ein guter Weg, Respekt für die Natur zu zeigen und gleichzeitig inneres Gleichgewicht zu finden.

Olivia Newton-John, AO, OBE, Gaia Retreat & Spa, Australien

Blissful Creation

Glückselige Schöpfung

Saffire Freycinet

The Creator must have been in a good mood on the day this place was made. The vast land of Tasmania stretches out like an incredibly beautiful movie set. White, sandy beaches, sapphire-blue water, the pink granite of the Hazards, and the grayish green scrubland—the colors of the Freycinet Peninsula have an ideal effect on your well-being. Whales pass through Great Oyster Bay, dolphins drop by to play, and with a bit of luck, you can experience it all without even getting out of bed. Inspiration permeates the entire hotel, and materials such as wood, stone, and leather make the beauty and depth of nature a tangible experience. Guests can choose delightful, rejuvenating, and refreshing treatments from Spa Saffire's menu of services. And only the best of what Tasmania has to offer ends up on the menu of healthy, fresh culinary dishes. Incidentally, the courses offered by the chef give you insight into his skill. After all, cooking is known to be an extremely meditative activity.

An diesem Tag muss der Schöpfer besonders gute Laune gehabt haben. Unfassbar schön wie eine Filmkulisse liegt es da, das weite Land Tasmaniens. Weiße Sandstrände, saphirblaues Wasser, der pinkfarbene Granit der Hazards und das Graugrün des Buschlandes – die Farben der Halbinsel Freycinet beeinflussen das Wohlbefinden optimal. Wale ziehen durch die Great Oyster Bay, Delfine schauen zum Spielen vorbei, und mit etwas Glück kann man all das von seinem Bett aus erleben. Inspiration liegt über dem ganzen Haus, und Materialien wie Holz, Stein und Leder sorgen für eine fühlbare Erfahrung der Schönheit und Tiefe der Natur. Aus dem Spa Saffire-Menü wählen die Gäste köstliche Spa-Behandlungen zur Verjüngung und Erfrischung. Und auf dem Menü der gesunden, frischen Küche steht das Beste, was Tasmanien zu bieten hat. Der Chefkoch gewährt übrigens in Kursen Einblick in sein Können, denn Kochen ist ja bekanntlich eine äußerst meditative Beschäftigung.

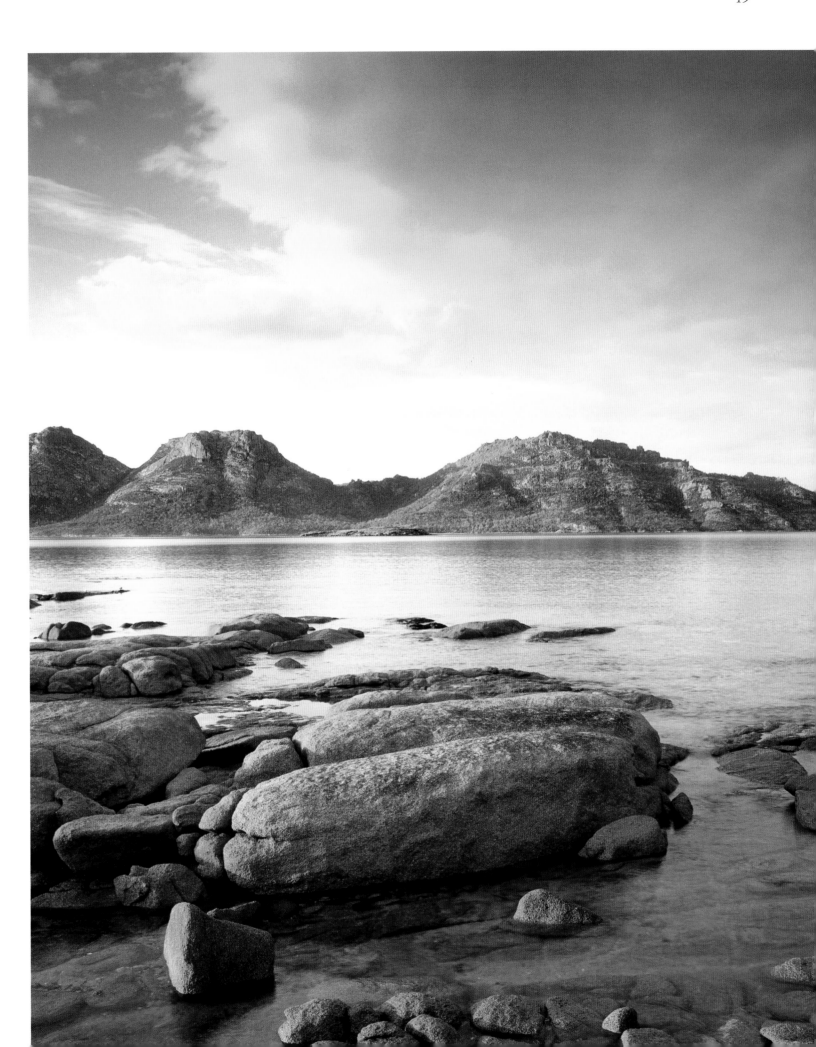

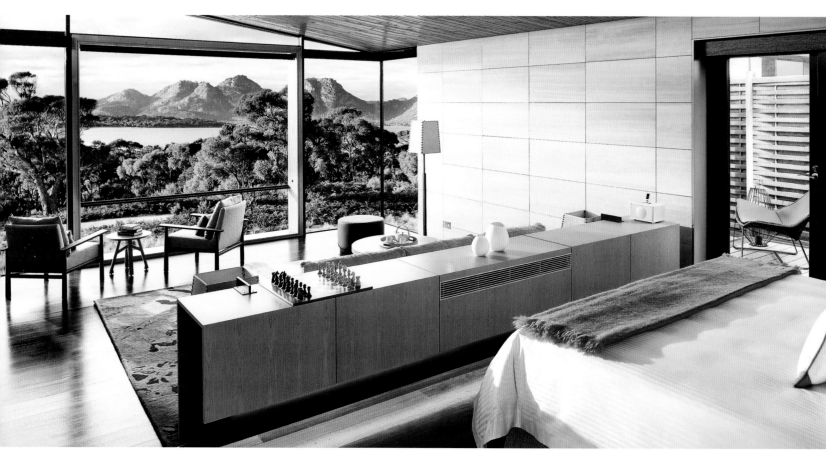

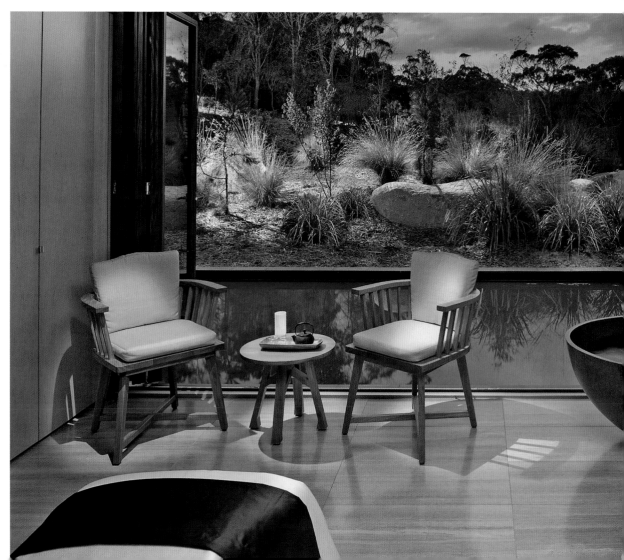

Spa, Health & Other Facilities
Spa Saffire, sauna/steam bath, gym. Palate restaurant, hammocks, business center, conference rooms.

Treatments & Services
Anti-stress, crystal massage, graceful aging, hot stone massage, individually designed programs for relaxation, restoration, and transformation, welcoming Spa Experience Menu. 24-hour front desk, concierge service, laundry service, newspapers.

Activities
Beach games, board games, cooking class with the chef, fishing, helicopter tours, jogging, kayaking, mountain biking, Pelican Bay canoeing and bird-watching, quad biking, Schouten Island Signature Experience, star gazing, visiting Freycinet Marine Oyster Farm, wine and vine adventures, Wineglass Bay Lookout walk.

Rooms
20 suites – 3 categories: deluxe, luxury, premium.

Located
2.5 hours by car from the major cities of Hobart and Launceston.
Reachable by road or air, arrangements can be made by the Saffire team.

2352 Coles Bay Road
Coles Bay, TAS 7215, Australia
www.saffire-freycinet.com.au

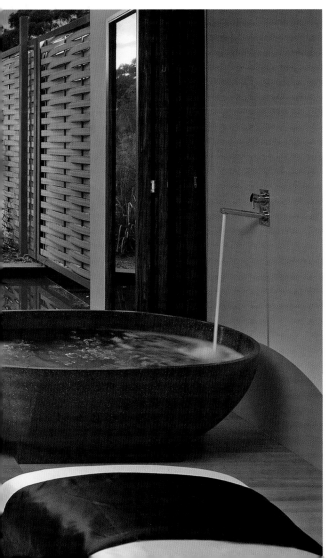

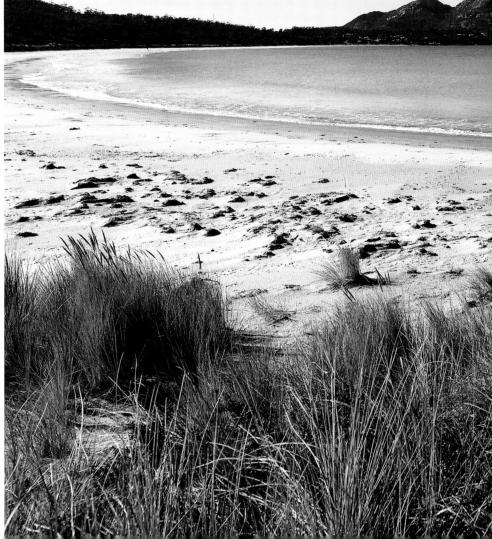

Beauty Lies in Health

Gesundheit macht schön

The Lyall Hotel and Spa

The Lyall is famous for its service, which is tailored to the personal needs of its guests. Although it is situated only a few steps from the chic Toorak Road and Chapel Street, the hotel is an oasis of tranquility. This is the reason why Olivia Newton-John stays here whenever she is in Melbourne. The Lyall Spa's holistic philosophy is that inner health results in visible beauty. Visitors to the spa will find a sense of equilibrium in relaxation treatments such as massages and body wraps, or programs aimed at lifestyle improvement. The comfortable suites are exquisitely appointed with a mini-kitchen, daily fresh fruit, and an excellent assortment of coffee and tea that makes it easier to wake up in the morning.

Berühmt ist The Lyall für einen Service, der auf die persönlichen Bedürfnisse der Gäste zugeschnitten ist. Obwohl es nur wenige Schritte von der schicken Toorak Road und Chapel Street entfernt liegt, ist das Haus eine Oase der Ruhe. Aus diesem Grund hat Olivia Newton-John dieses Hotel für ihre Besuche in Melbourne ausgewählt. Der holistische Ansatz im Lyall Spa lautet: Innere Gesundheit führt zu sichtbarer Schönheit. Die nötige Ausgeglichenheit finden Spa-Besucher bei Entspannungsbehandlungen wie Massagen oder Körperwickeln sowie bei Programmen zur Verbesserung des persönlichen Lebensstils. Die gemütlichen Suiten sind erstklassig ausgestattet mit eigener Miniküche, täglich frischem Obst und ausgezeichneten Tee- und Kaffeesorten, die das Aufwachen jeden Morgen erleichtern.

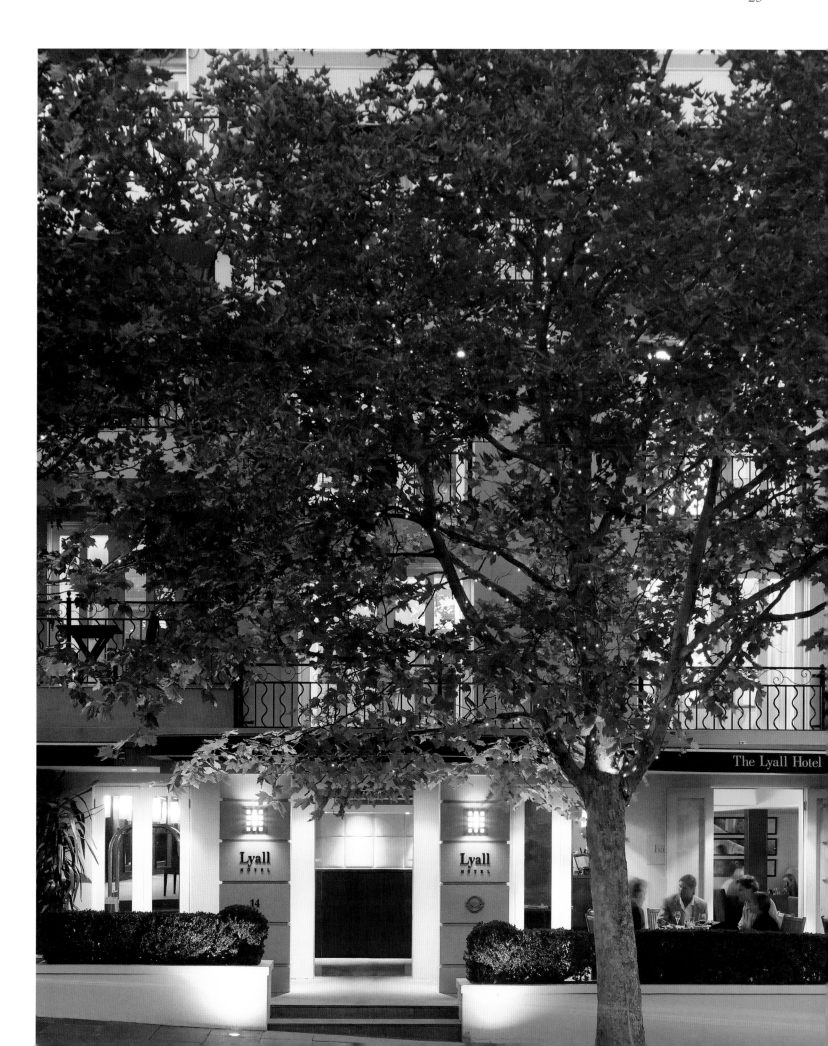

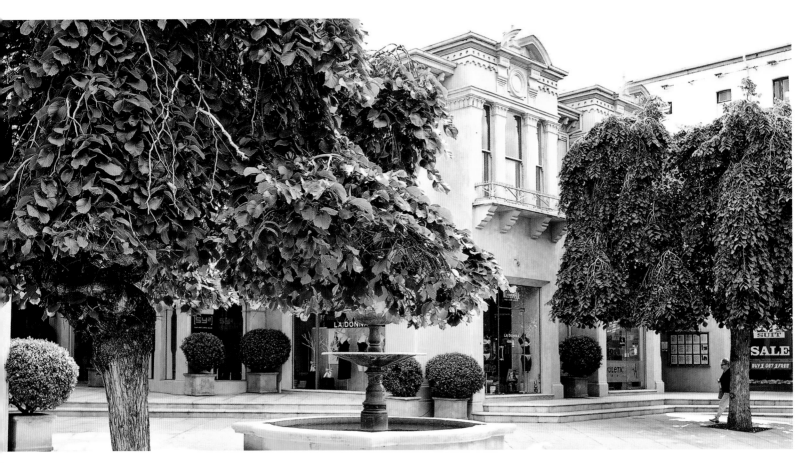

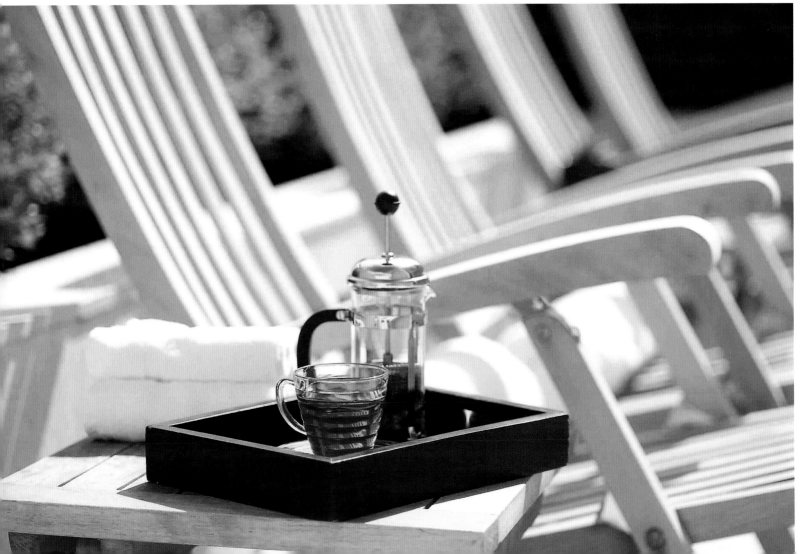

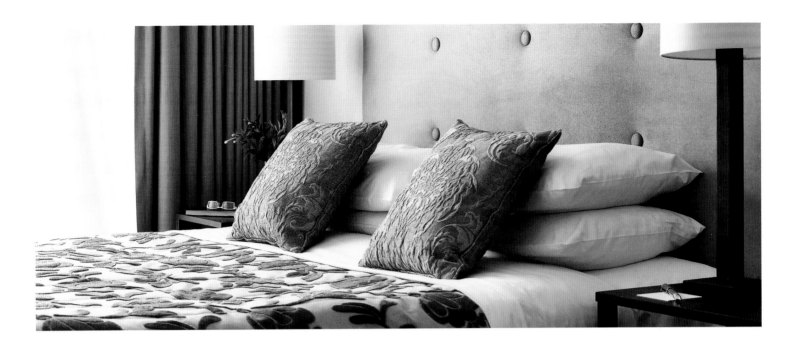

Spa, Health & Other Facilities
Spa with 8 treatment rooms including steam rooms with Swiss and drench showers, outdoor relaxation terrace, and a gymnasium featuring Life Fitness equipment. The Lyall Bistro, Champagne Bar, well-equipped business center and conference room, DVD/book/magazine library.

Treatments & Services
Hydrotherapy, naturopathy, Pilates, reflexology, remedial and relaxation massage, Sodashi and Payot products and treatments, yoga. 24-hour concierge, 24-hour room service, Exclusive Shopping Privilege Card, laundry and dry cleaning service, pillow menu.

Activities
Bicycling, bird-watching, canoeing, fitness, golf (nearby), horseback riding, hot air ballooning, jogging, swimming, Toorak Road and Chapel Street shopping and dining, tennis, windsurfing.

Rooms
40 1 and 2-bedroom suites including 3 Grand Suites and The Platinum Suite. All have a spacious separate living area and kitchen, marble bathrooms with twin head shower and separate bath.

Located
The Lyall Hotel is situated in South Yarra, Melbourne. The central business district is a 10-minute drive from the hotel and public transport is easily accessible.

16 Murphy St, South Yarra
Melbourne, VIC 3141, Australia
www.thelyall.com

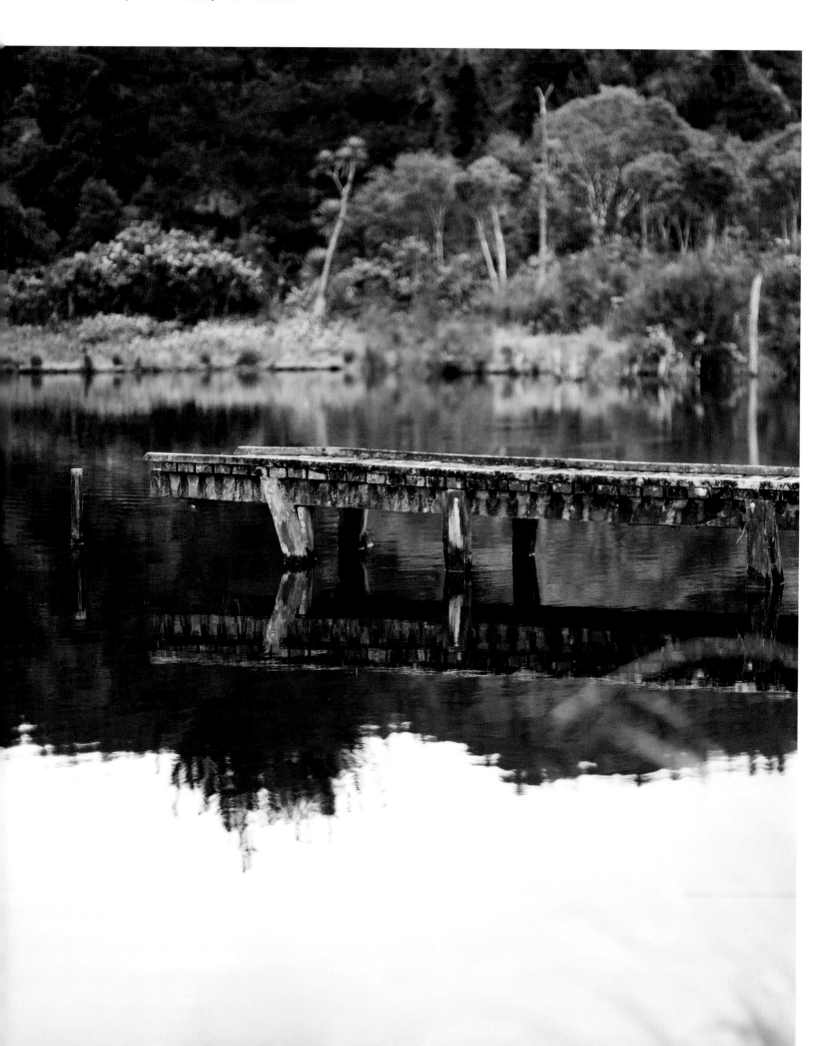

Wilderness Meets Prosperity

Wildnis trifft Wohlstand

Treetops Lodge & Estate

New Zealand has an ancient history. It is where the Maori culture is still very much alive, especially in the mystical region around Rotorua on the North Island. This place is known as the world's capital for trout fishing, and it is famous for its mineral springs. In an 800-year-old forest of rivers and lakes, John Sax built his Treetops Lodge, whose architecture blends perfectly with the landscape. The resort's motto is "nature meets luxury." A variety of programs introduces guests to the world of the Maori—such as the "Maori Indigenous Food Trail." This program is a tour of the forest, in which a local guide points out herbs and plants that are used to prepare traditional dishes, and which are said to have healing properties. In the eco-spa, holistic treatments and massages, as well as skin and beauty care rituals stimulate the body's natural healing process.

Neuseeland hat eine uralte Geschichte, und besonders in der mystischen Umgebung von Rotorua auf der Nordinsel ist die Kultur der Maori noch immer sehr lebendig. Der Ort gilt als Welthauptstadt der Forellenfischer und ist bekannt für sein Heilwasser. Hier – in einem über 800 Jahre alten Wald mit Flüssen und Seen – gründete John Sax das Treetops, das sich architektonisch perfekt in die Landschaft einfügt. „Natur trifft Luxus" lautet das Motto. Verschiedene Programme führen die Gäste in die Welt der Maori ein, zum Beispiel der „Maori Indigenous Food Trail". Dabei handelt es sich um eine Waldtour, bei der ein einheimischer Führer Kräuter und Pflanzen vorstellt, aus denen traditionelle Speisen zubereitet werden und denen eine heilende Wirkung nachgesagt wird. Im Öko-Spa regen ganzheitliche Anwendungen, Massagen sowie Haut- und Schönheitsbehandlungen den natürlichen Heilungsprozess des Körpers an.

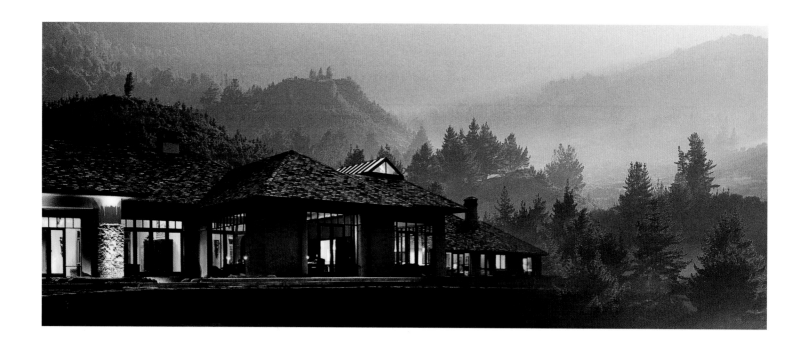

Spa, Health & Other Facilities
2 spa therapy rooms, 2 wooden outdoor Jacuzzis, healing lounge. Restaurant, vegetable garden, golf course, business center, conference rooms, library, video rental.

Treatments & Services
Maori body treatments and massages, skin and beauty rituals, wellness programs.
Childcare/babysitting, free Wi-Fi, wedding service.

Activities
Archery, fishing, golf, hiking, horse trekking, hunting, mountain biking, sightseeing, surfing.

Rooms
4 Valley Villas, 4 Forest Villas, 4 Lodge Wing Suites,
3-bedroom and 2-bathroom owners' Cottage.

Located
Located in Rotorua, approximately 2 hours by car from Auckland.
11 miles (18 kilometers) from Rotorua Regional Airport.

351 Kearoa Road
RD1 Horohoro
Rotorua, New Zealand
www.treetops.co.nz

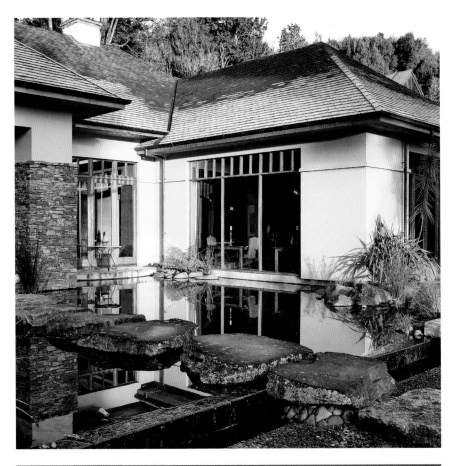

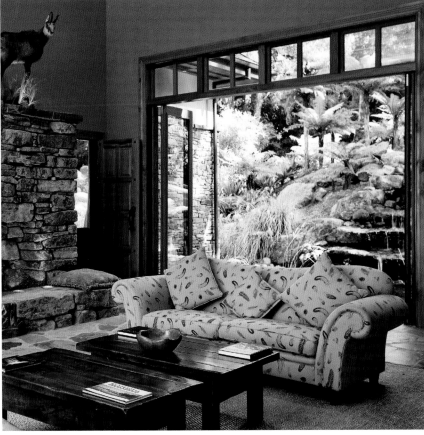

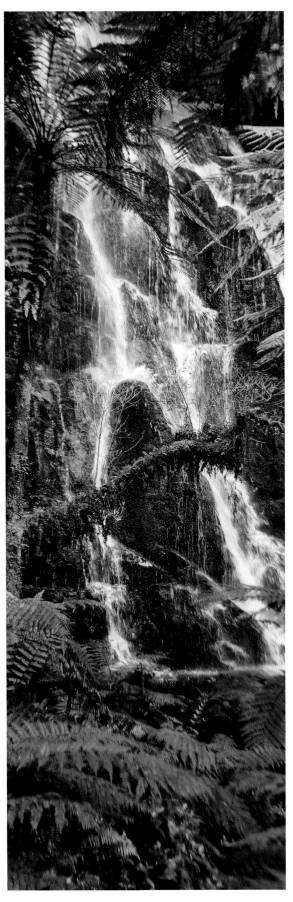

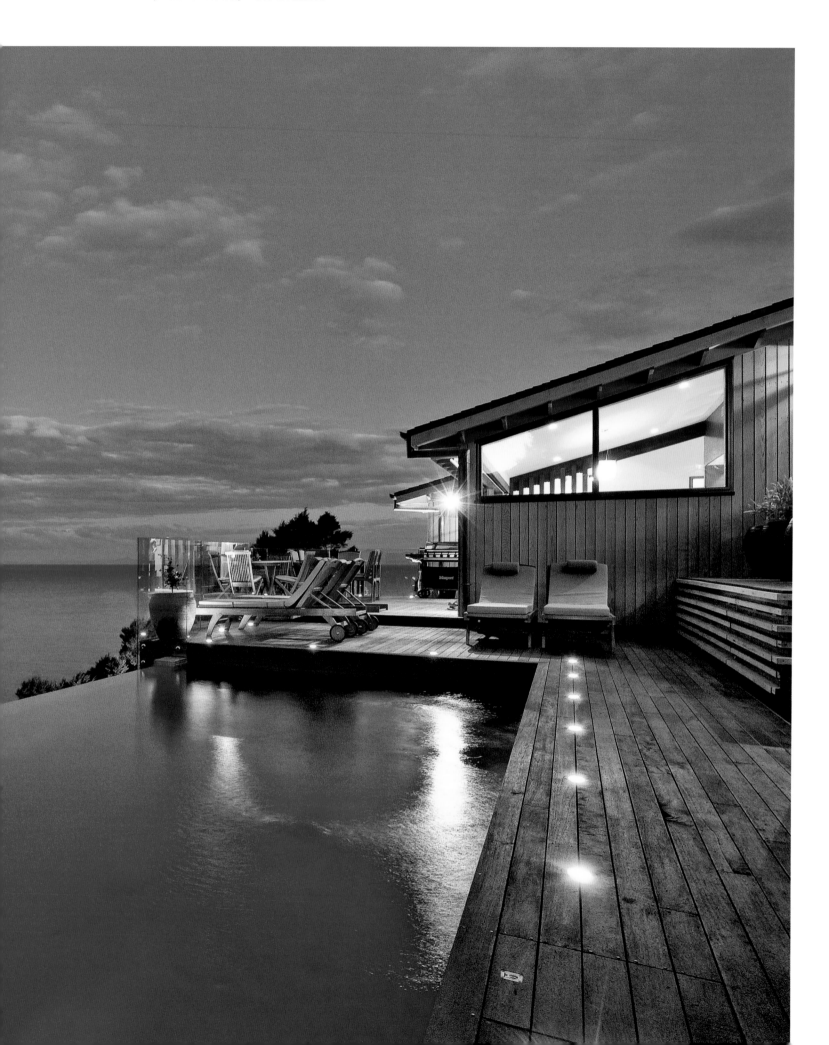

More Than Just an Apple a Day

Mehr als nur ein Apfel pro Tag

Split Apple Retreat

It is situated at the *end* of the world and can be the *beginning* of something entirely new. An international clientele comes to this exclusive retreat to find the peace and serenity they need to recuperate or to devote themselves to a particular project. Many books have been written in this place, which is treasured by authors. The earth's healing powers and the ocean's vast expanse cause us to look beyond what our minds can perceive. Named after nearby Split Apple Rock—a boulder that resembles an apple split in half—everything here revolves around food, specifically around a healthy, healing diet. Situated on a cliff high above the ocean, near the Abel Tasman National Park, the resort is dedicated to life and healing according to the principle of "you are what you eat." Founder Dr. Lee Nelson has devoted himself to this notion for many years. Guests can benefit from a wellness and nutrition consultation tailored to their individual needs. Nelson's Thai wife transforms her husband's findings into a real experience in the form of delicious meals. Along with salmon, pomegranate juice, blueberries, and avocado crepes, massages, meditation, aromatherapy, and two private beaches revitalize stressed souls.

Es liegt am *Ende* der Welt und kann der *Anfang* für etwas komplett Neues sein. Ein internationales Publikum kommt in dieses exklusive Retreat, um die Ruhe und Gelassenheit zu finden, die notwendig ist, um sich zu erholen oder einem bestimmten Projekt zu widmen. Viele Bücher wurden hier bereits verfasst, an diesem von Autoren geschätzten Ort. Die heilenden Kräfte der Erde und die unendliche Weite des Ozeans geben Raum, über das rational Erfassbare hinauszugehen. Benannt nach dem nahe gelegenen Split Apple Rock – einem Felsen, der einem in der Mitte geteilten Apfel gleicht – dreht sich hier tatsächlich alles ums Essen, genauer gesagt um gesunde, heilende Ernährung. Nahe dem Abel Tasman National Park auf einer Klippe hoch über dem Meer wird nach dem Prinzip „Du bist, was Du isst" gelebt und geheilt. Gründer Dr. Lee Nelson beschäftigt sich seit vielen Jahren mit diesem Thema. So bietet das Retreat eine individuell abgestimmte Wellness- und Ernährungs-beratung an. Nelsons thailändische Gattin setzt die Erkenntnisse ihres Mannes in Form von feinen Speisen in die Praxis um. Neben wildem Lachs, Granatapfelsaft, Blaubeeren und Avocado-Crèpes revitalisieren Massagen, Meditation, Aromatherapie und zwei private Strände die gestressten Geister.

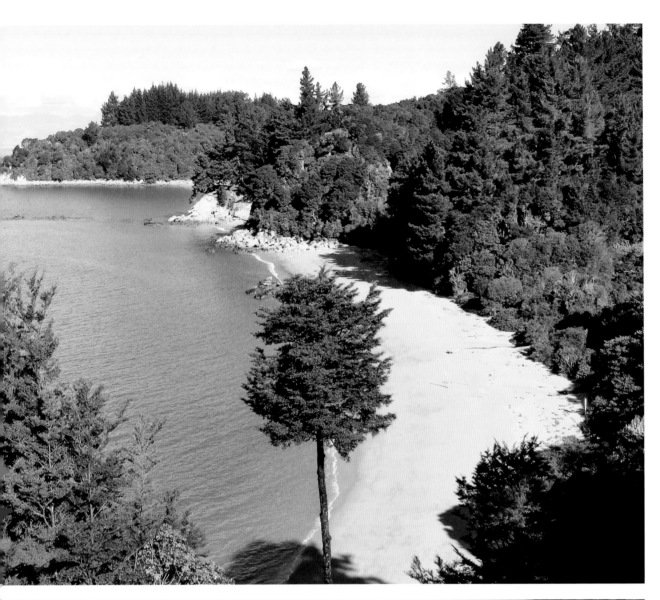

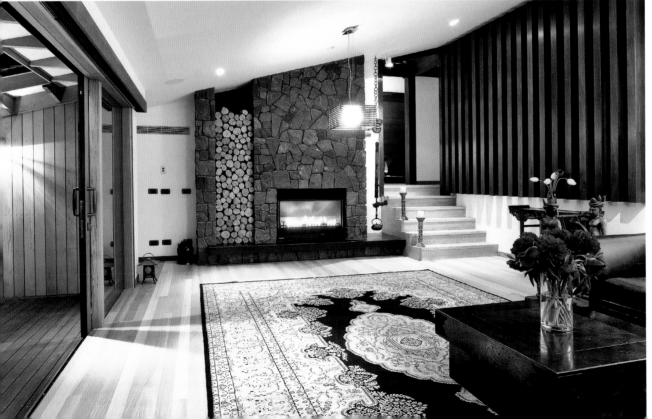

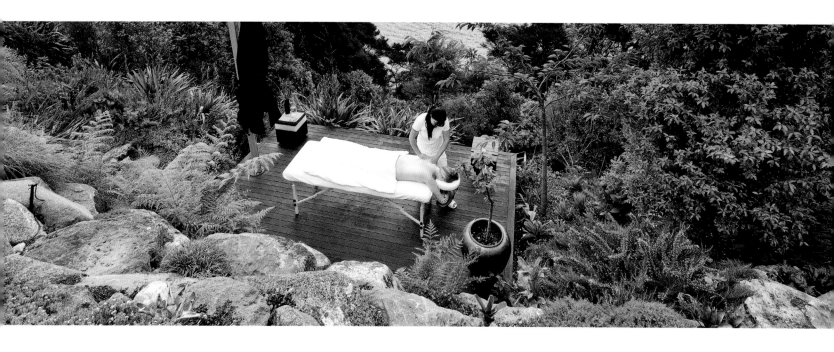

Spa, Health & Other Facilities
Outdoor spa pool, infinity swimming pool and outdoor shower, far infrared sauna, steam room, gymnasium. Gourmet restaurant, 8-seater theater.

Treatments & Services
Acupuncture; deep tissue, reflexology, and aromatherapy massages; meditation guidance and other stress reduction therapies, physical trainer, Pilates. Health programs for executive de-stressing, improved fitness, rejuvenation and pampering, relaxation, weight reduction. Free parking.

Activities
Cooking lessons, fishing, horseback riding, kayaking, sailing, sky-diving, swimming with the seals and dolphin-spotting, walking. Helicopter can be arranged to drop you at remote spots for walking or private picnics at otherwise inaccessible beaches.

Rooms
3 guest suites and 1 guest suite villa for 3 persons.

Located
A 50-minute drive or 15-minute heli flight from Nelson Airport.

195 Tokongawa Drive
RD2 Motueka
Tasman 7197, New Zealand
www.splitapple.com

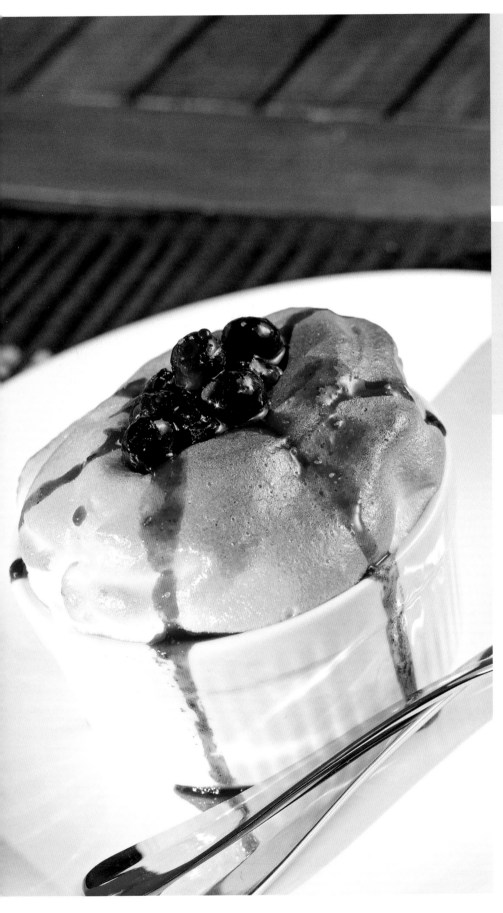

› 500 g fresh or frozen blueberries
› 1 tbsp xylitol
› 3 egg whites (room temperature)
› 1/2 tsp lemon zest
› 1 tbsp buckwheat flour
› 1/4 tsp vanilla extract
› pinch of cinnamon

Serves 4

› 500 g frische oder gefrorene Blaubeeren
› 1 EL Xylit
› 3 Eiweiß (Zimmertemperatur)
› 1/2 TL abgeriebene Zitronenschale
› 1 EL Buchweizenmehl
› 1/4 TL Vanilleextrakt
› Prise Zimt

Für 4 Personen

Blueberry Soufflé

Method
Preheat the oven to 34 °F (200 °C). Coat four 3.5 inches soufflé dishes with non-stick spray. If you are using frozen blueberries: Combine the blueberries with the xylitol and cinnamon for about 3–5 minutes in a small pot over medium heat. If you are using fresh blueberries: There is no need to heat them, combine the blueberries with the xylitol and cinnamon.

Put aside 50 g of the blueberry mixture for the topping. Divide the remaining mixture into 4 soufflé dishes. It should be about 3/4 full.

Beat the egg whites in a bowl until stiff. Add flour, lemon zest, and vanilla extract, then beat for another 1–2 minutes. Gently spoon the egg white mixture on top of the soufflé dishes and mould into the shape of a cup cake. Bake in the oven for 10–15 minutes or until it has risen and turned golden brown. Cut a cross into the top to make a space for the remaining blueberry mixture, spoon the blueberry mixture so that it sits on top. Serve immediately.

Health Benefits
Blueberries, along with pomegranates, wild salmon, and green tea are real superfoods. Blueberries and longevity go hand in hand.
Blueberries may be the ultimate brain food. Regular consumption may help preserve brain function, cognition, and coordination as we age by potentially staving off the onset of cognitive dysfunction. If combined with walnuts—another brain food—blueberries may help avoid memory loss associated with aging. Their strong anti-inflammatory effect also has multiple benefits.

Blaubeeren-Soufflé

Zubereitung
Den Ofen auf 200 °C vorheizen. Vier Souffléförmchen (8–10 cm Durchmesser) einfetten. Falls Sie gefrorene Blaubeeren verwenden, Xylit und Zimt unter die Blaubeeren mischen und für 3–5 Minuten in einem kleinen Topf bei mittlerer Hitze auftauen lassen. Falls Sie frische Blaubeeren verwenden, müssen sie nicht erhitzt, sondern können direkt mit Xylit und Zimt vermengt werden.

Stellen Sie etwa 50 g der Blaubeerenmischung für den Belag beiseite. Verteilen Sie den Rest der Mischung auf die vier Souffléförmchen, sodass sie ungefähr zu drei Vierteln gefüllt sind.

Das Eiweiß in einer Schüssel steif schlagen. Das Mehl, die abgeriebene Zitronenschale und den Vanilleextrakt hinzugeben und weitere 1–2 Minuten schlagen. Die Eiweißmischung vorsichtig mit dem Löffel auf die Souffléförmchen verteilen und zu einem Häubchen formen. Im Ofen 10–15 Minuten backen oder so lange, bis das Soufflé aufgegangen und goldbraun ist. In die Spitze ein Kreuz einschneiden und die restliche Blaubeermischung mit dem Löffel auftragen, sodass sie die oberste Schicht bildet. Sofort servieren!

Gesundheitlicher Nutzen
Blaubeeren sind neben Granatäpfeln, wildem Lachs und grünem Tee echte Supernahrungsmittel. Der Genuss von Blaubeeren verspricht ein langes Leben.
Blaubeeren gelten als optimale Nahrung für das Gehirn. Der regelmäßige Verzehr kann im Alter die Gehirnfunktion, die Wahrnehmung und das Koordinationsvermögen fördern, indem das Einsetzen kognitiver Störungen potenziell abgewehrt wird. In Kombination mit Walnüssen, auch optimal für das Gehirn, können Blaubeeren dem altersbedingten Gedächtnisverlust entgegenwirken. Außerdem ist die stark entzündungshemmende Wirkung der Blaubeere in vielerlei Hinsicht von Vorteil.

Learning to Love in Balinese

Lieben lernen auf balinesisch

Fivelements

"Learn how to love" is the motto of Fivelements. Small wonder, since Bali is where the resort's founders first met and fell in love. They decided to build a resort in this beautiful location based on the philosophies and traditions of Bali, including the rituals, healing practices, and sacred arts that have existed and evolved for centuries. Designed in accordance with eco-conscious principles, ancient Balinese architectonic guidelines, and sacred geometry, Fivelements embraces an authentic approach to healing and wellness. The resort is inspired by the Balinese way of life, "Tri Hita Karana," which encourages us to nurture harmony with spirit, the environment, and one another. Their holistic integrative approach combines Balinese healing rituals for purification, balancing, and regeneration, raw vegan, "living foods" cuisine for revitalizing, and sacred arts for inner strength, alignment, and dedication. The overall aim is to inspire healthy living through a highly personalized "healing journey" and the guests' will to transform through love.

„Learn how to love" ist das Motto von Fivelements. Kein Wunder, denn die Gründer des Resorts lernten sich einst hier auf Bali kennen und lieben. Sie beschlossen, auf diesem wunderschönen Fleckchen Erde ein Resort zu gründen, welches die Philosophien und Traditionen Balis vermittelt, seine Rituale, Heilverfahren und heiligen Künste, die sich über die Jahrhunderte entwickelt haben. Nach ökologischen Prinzipien und alten balinesischen Geometrie- und Architekturgesetzen gebaut, setzt das Fivelements auf die Authentizität seiner Heil- und Wellnessangebote. Alles hier ist von der balinesischen Lebenskunst „Tri Hita Karana" inspiriert: In Harmonie mit Menschen, Göttern und Natur zu leben, ist eine Grundvoraussetzung für nachhaltiges körperliches und seelisches Wohlbefinden. Der holistische integrative Ansatz verbindet balinesische Heilrituale für Reinigung, Ausgleich und Regeneration mit einer veganen Rohkostküche zur Revitalisierung, den „living foods", sowie den „sacred arts" für Stärke und Zielgerichtetheit. So will Fivelements die Gäste durch eine persönliche Heilreise zu einem gesunden Leben inspirieren und zur Bereitschaft zu einer Transformation durch Liebe.

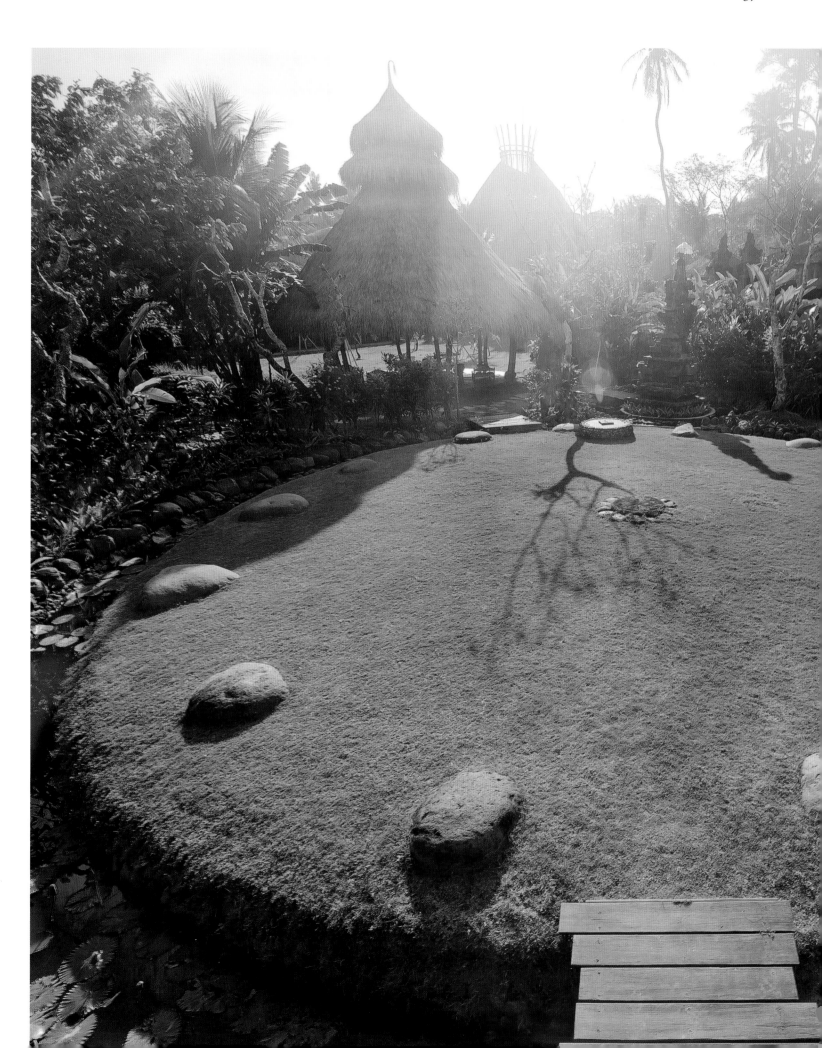

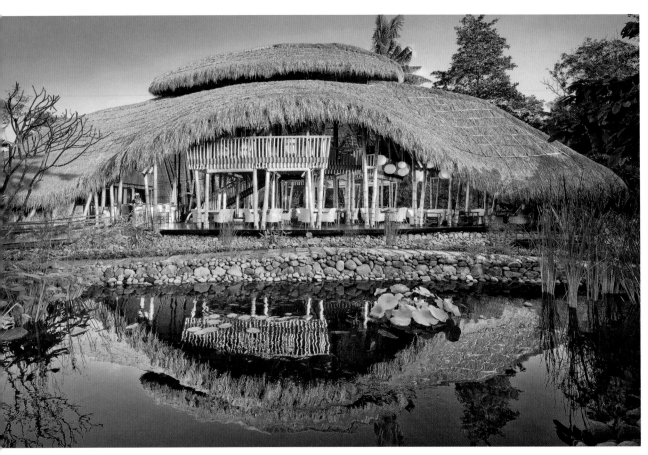

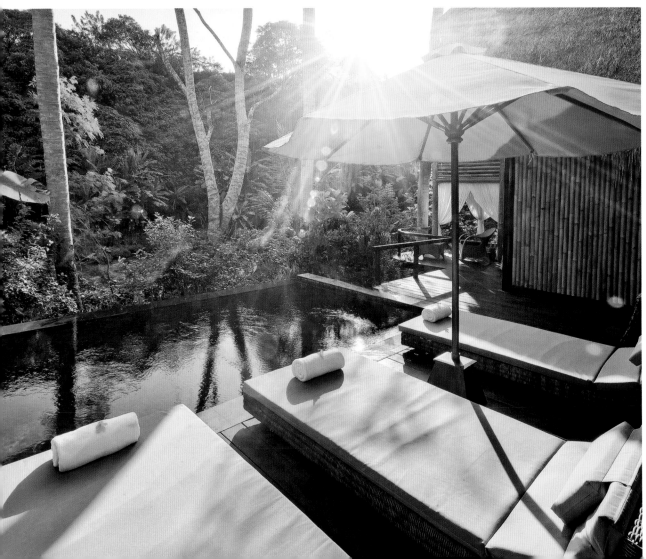

Spa, Health & Other Facilities
Beauty sanctuary with pool and relaxation lounge, water healing pools with riverside terrace, Sakti dining room, 3 multifunction mandala meeting rooms, sacred space meditation areas, healing reception, laboratory, boutique with signature Fivelements products, property-wide music sound system.

Treatments & Services
Aikido, aromatherapy; body, face, and nail care rituals; deep energy healing and massage, expressive arts, holistic healing, meditation, nutrition consultations and trainings, raw vegan living foods cuisine, sacred sound healing, soma, soul dance, water healing, wellness consultations, yoga. 24-hour room service, babysitting/childcare, transfer service from the airport, valet parking.

Activities
Art, biking, ceremonies and sacred sites, culture, Fivelements Eco-Cultural Healing Journey excursions, rafting and trekking, shopping.

Rooms
7 exclusive sleeping suites.

Located
Nestled alongside the sacred Ayung River in the highlands of Bali nearby Ubud;
45 minutes from Seminyak or Sanur; 75 minutes from Bali's International Airport by car.

Banjar Baturning, Mambal
80352 Bali, Indonesia
www.fivelements.org

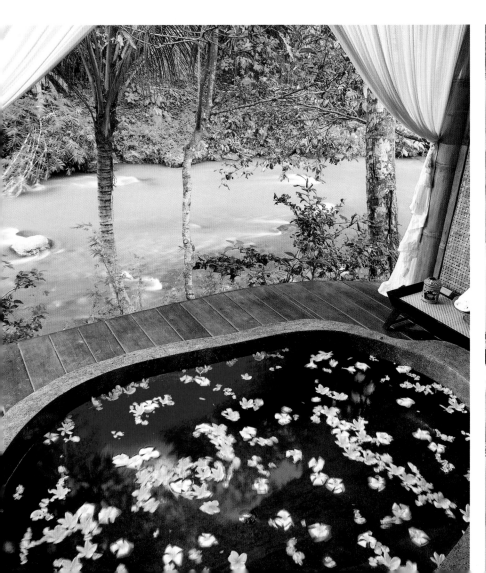

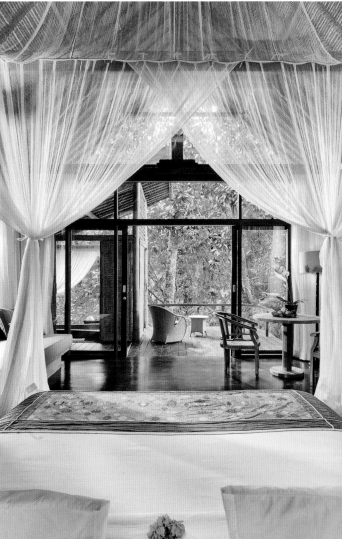

A Feelgood Place on a Coffee Plantation

Wohlfühlort auf der Kaffeeplantage

MesaStila

Anyone who travels a lot has seen plenty of train stations. But this one is something special. Dating back to Dutch Colonial times, this station is over 150 years old and built on a 55-acre coffee plantation, surrounded by eight mountains, in the Javanese jungle. It is the reception for MesaStila, a luxury retreat property which consists of various historical buildings located in the cool highlands of Central Java. The island of Java is known for its traditional healing methods and its natural beauty. Here, the resort offers a peaceful escape from everyday stress. Since illness is a waste of lifetime, the spa provides treatments to ensure stable health and more energy—such as hammam and unique services like Javanese lulur body scrubs (Javanese for "skin protection")—as well as local healers who have mastered the traditional Indonesian folk medicine called "jamu."

Wer viel reist, hat schon viele Bahnhöfe gesehen. Doch dieses Exemplar ist etwas Besonderes: Die Station aus der niederländischen Kolonialzeit ist über 150 Jahre alt und liegt auf einer 200 000 Quadratmeter großen Kaffeeplantage im javanesischen Dschungel, die von acht majestätischen Bergen umgeben ist. Dies ist die Rezeption des MesaStila, ein Luxus-Retreat im kühlen Hochland von Zentral-Java, das aus verschiedenen historischen Gebäuden besteht. Die Insel Java ist für ihre heilenden Kräfte und die Schönheit ihrer Natur bekannt. In dieser Umgebung bietet das Resort einen friedlichen Rückzugsort vom Alltagsstress. Da Krankheit eine Verschwendung von Lebenszeit ist, ermöglicht das Spa Behandlungen, die für eine stabile Gesundheit und mehr Energie sorgen – darunter Hamam-Massagen und außergewöhnliche Behandlungen wie javanesische Lulur-Körperpeelings (javanesisch für „Hautschutz"). Außerdem gibt es einheimische Heiler, die die traditionelle indonesische Volksmedizin „Jamu" beherrschen.

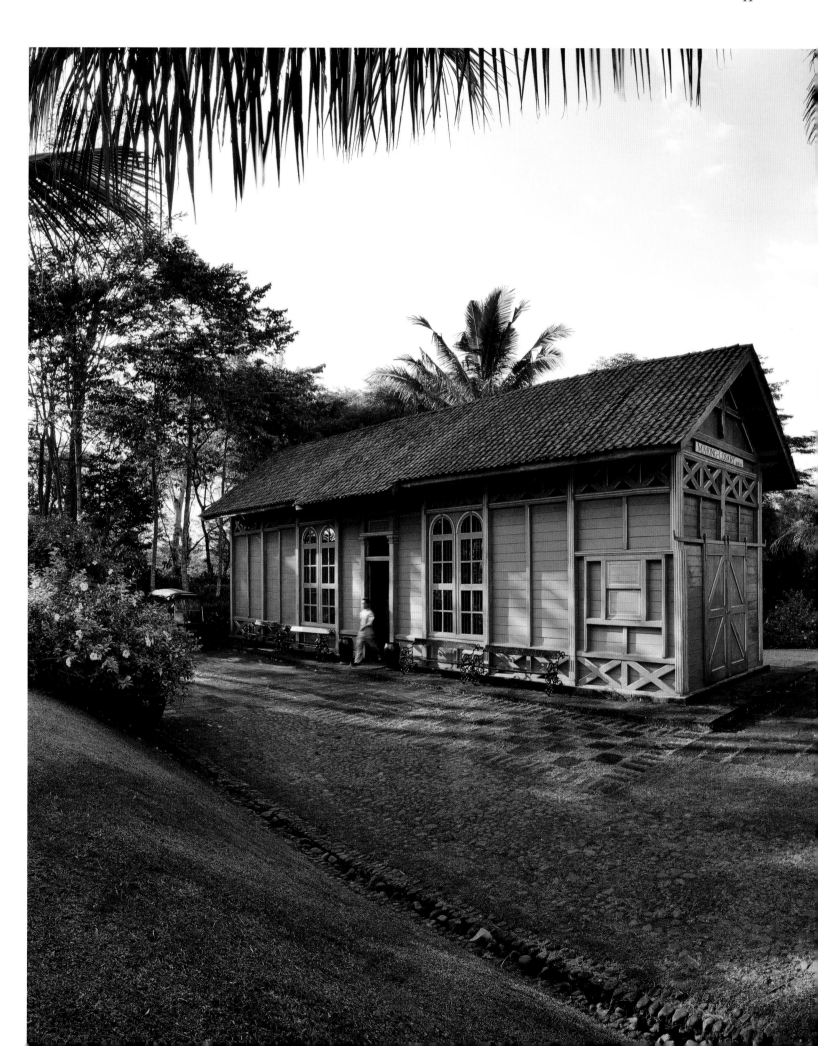

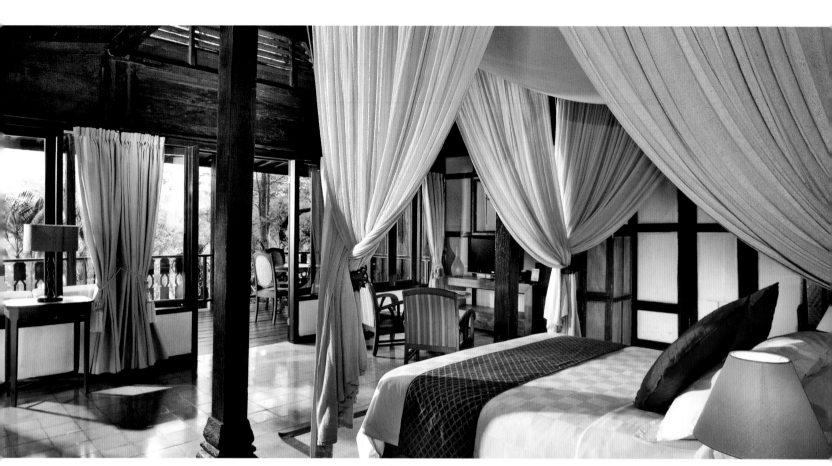

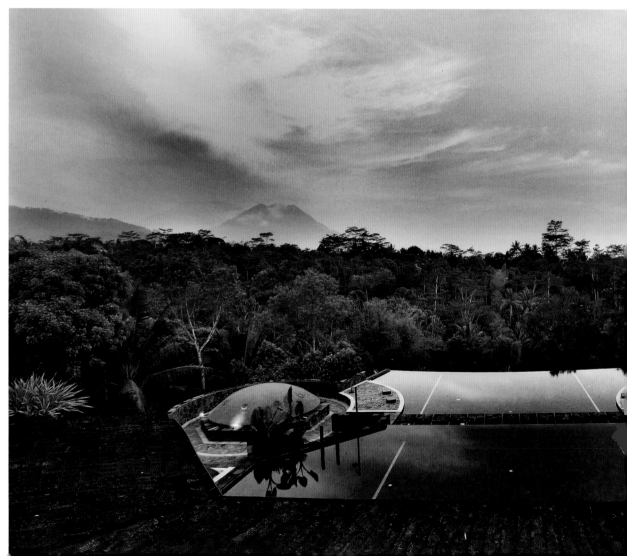

Spa, Health & Other Facilities
Hammam spa, swimming pool, fitness center, jungle gym, labyrinth, yoga pavilion. Expansive coffee plantation.

Treatments & Services
Aromatherapy, cleansing programs, deep tissue massage, hammam steam spa scrubs and massages, heart-healing retreats, jade facials, lifestyle coaching, lymphatic drainage, Pencak Silat classes, personal training, reflexology, sleep retreat, sound therapy, traditional Javanese healing treatments including Jamu and Javanese massage, TRX and jungle gym bootcamp programs, tuina massage, yoga. Endurance training workshops for competitive age-grouper, nutritional counseling, weight management.

Activities
Cultural activities, golf, hiking and trekking, horseback riding, jogging, mountain biking, road cycling, tennis, white water rafting.

Rooms
22 luxury villas with large living areas, outdoor verandas offering views of the jungle, coffee plantation or nearby mountains.

Located
Between Semarang, Jogjakarta, and Solo Airport, all 1.5 to 2 hours away. It takes 45 minutes by plane from Jakarta to Semarang Airport, 1 hour from Jakarta to Yogyakarta or Solo Airport, and 1 hour from Bali to Yogyakarta or Solo Airport.

PO Box 108
56100 Magelang, Indonesia
www.mesahotelsandresorts.com/mesastila

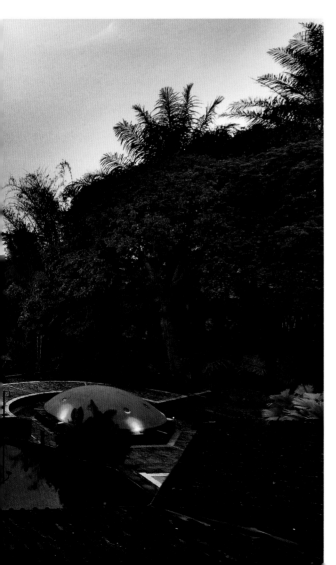
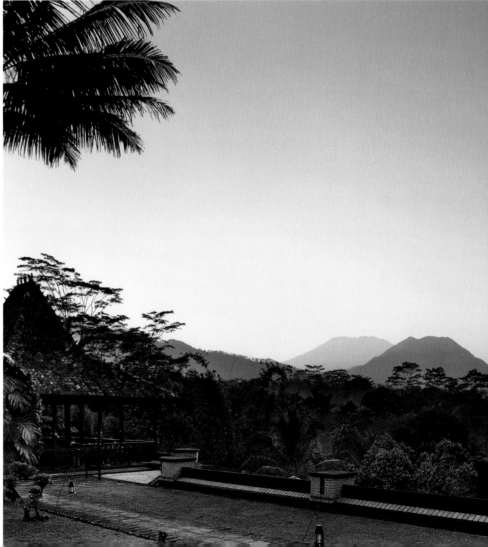

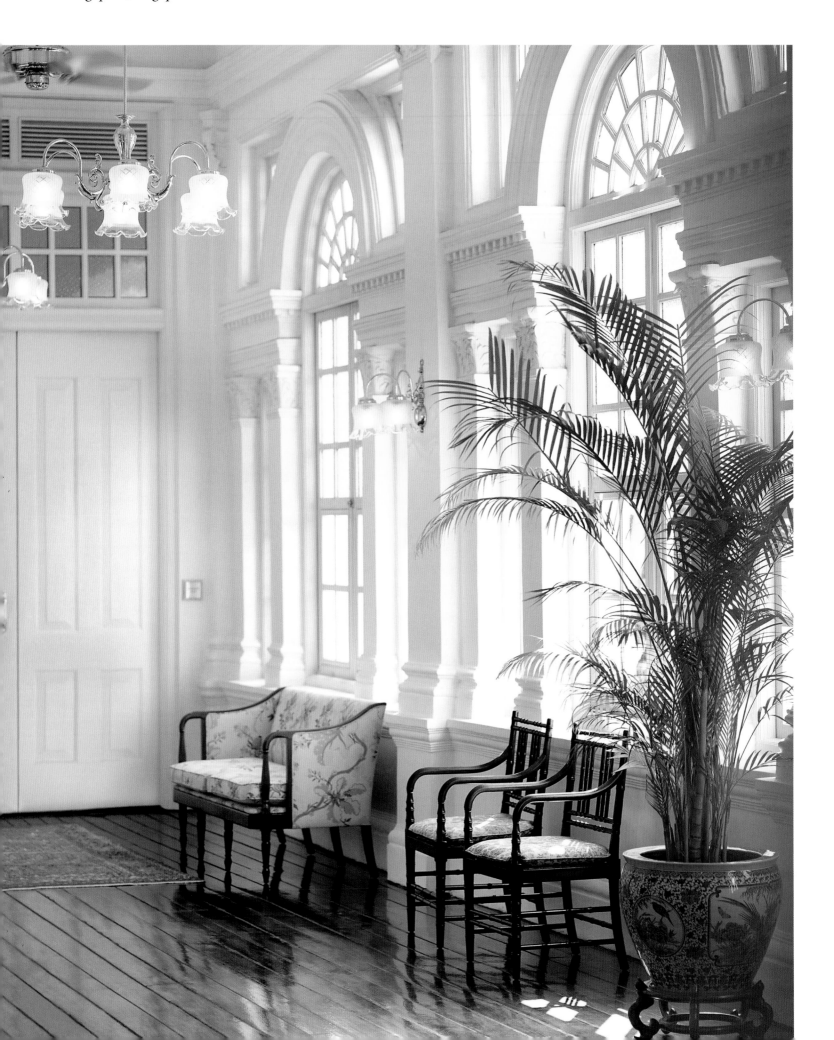

Eternal Beauty

Unsterbliche Schönheit

Raffles Hotel Singapore

Anyone who still remembers the charm of the old Raffles—when bird cages hung in the lush gardens and frangipani perfumed the air—is certain to recapture many of these memories in the new Raffles. Guests of the world-renowned grand hotel situated in the heart of Singapore include celebrities, royals, writers, and ordinary mortals. The birthplace of the legendary Singapore Sling is now a destination where travelers can unwind and recover. And the best place to do this is the Raffles Spa, a true paradise of tranquility, away from the bustle of the metropolis. The hotel's extensive range of spa and health treatments and the steam baths promise a relaxing effect. The VIP suite or "couple room" is for guests who want to share a unique experience of recreation and togetherness.

Diejenigen, die sich noch an den Charme des alten Raffles erinnern können – als in den üppigen Gärten noch Vogelkäfige hingen und der Geruch von Frangipani in der Luft war – werden sicher viel davon im neuen Raffles wiederentdecken. Zu den Gästen des weltberühmten Grand Hotels mitten in Singapur zählen Prominente, Royals, Schriftsteller und Normalsterbliche. Die Geburtsstätte des legendären Singapore Sling ist heute ein Ort, an dem sich Reisende ausruhen und erholen können. Und das geht am besten im hoteleigenen Spa, einem wahren Traumland der Stille, abseits der Hektik der Metropole. Das Angebot an Spa- und Gesundheitsanwendungen sowie Dampfbädern verspricht Erholung und Frische für Körper, Geist und Seele. Die VIP-Suite ist geeignet, um Spa-Therapien zu zweit zu genießen – ungestörte Zweisamkeit und absolute Entspannung sind garantiert.

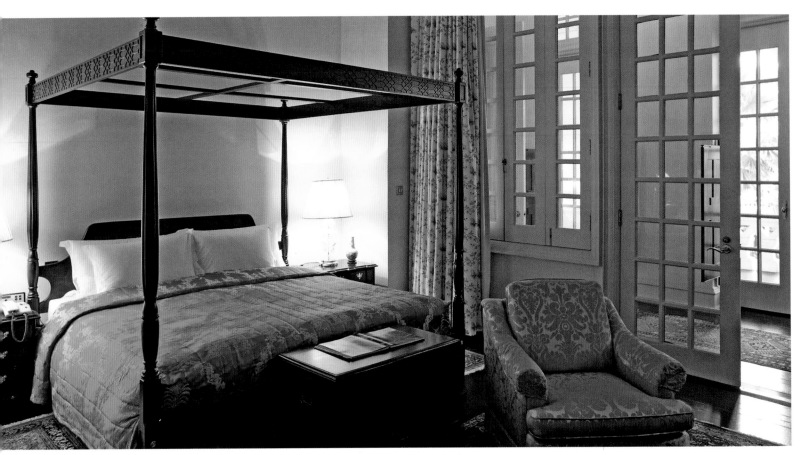

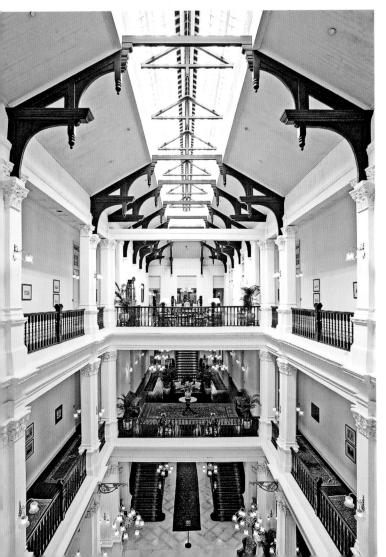

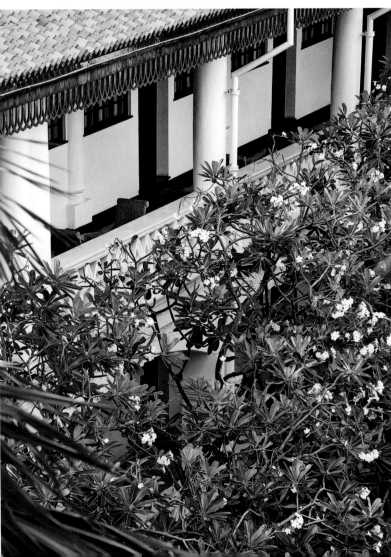

Spa, Health & Other Facilities
6 private treatment rooms including 2 VIP suites and 4 individual multifunctional therapy rooms; outdoor swimming pool, fitness center. Pool bar, meeting and function rooms.

Treatments & Services
Back massage, body scrubs, body wraps, facial treatments, foot massage, full body massage (aromatherapy massage, Swedish massage, deep tissue massage, lavender dreams massage), hair care, manicure, pedicure, spa body therapies, spa ritual packages. 24-hour front desk, babysitting/childcare.

Activities
Jogging, squash, swimming, tennis.

Rooms
103 individually designed suites: 84 Courtyard and Palm Court Suites, 12 Personality Suites, 5 Grand Hotel Suites and 2 Presidential Suites, many with private verandas.

Located
In the heart of Singapore's business and civic district, just 20 minutes from Changi International Airport and a 5-minute train ride from Singapore's bustling shopping district Orchard Road.

1 Beach Road
189673 Singapore
www.raffles.com/singapore

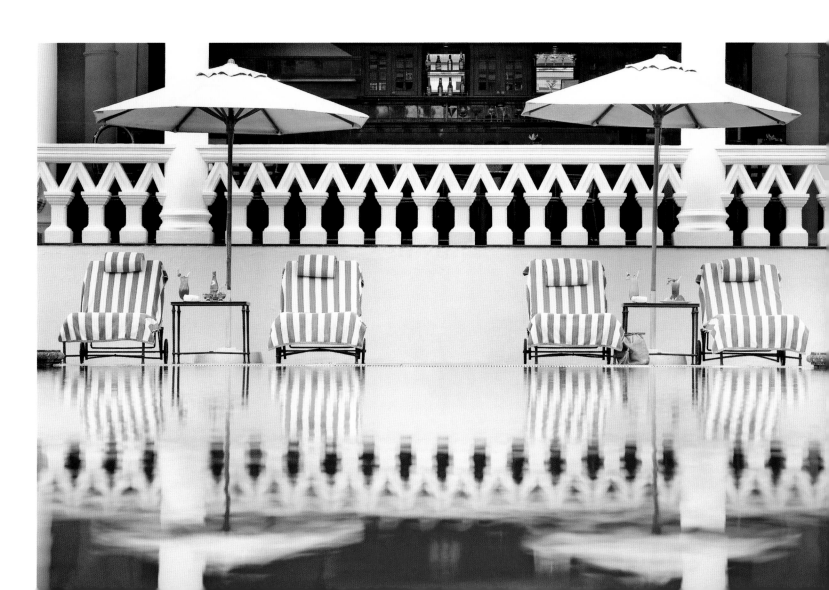

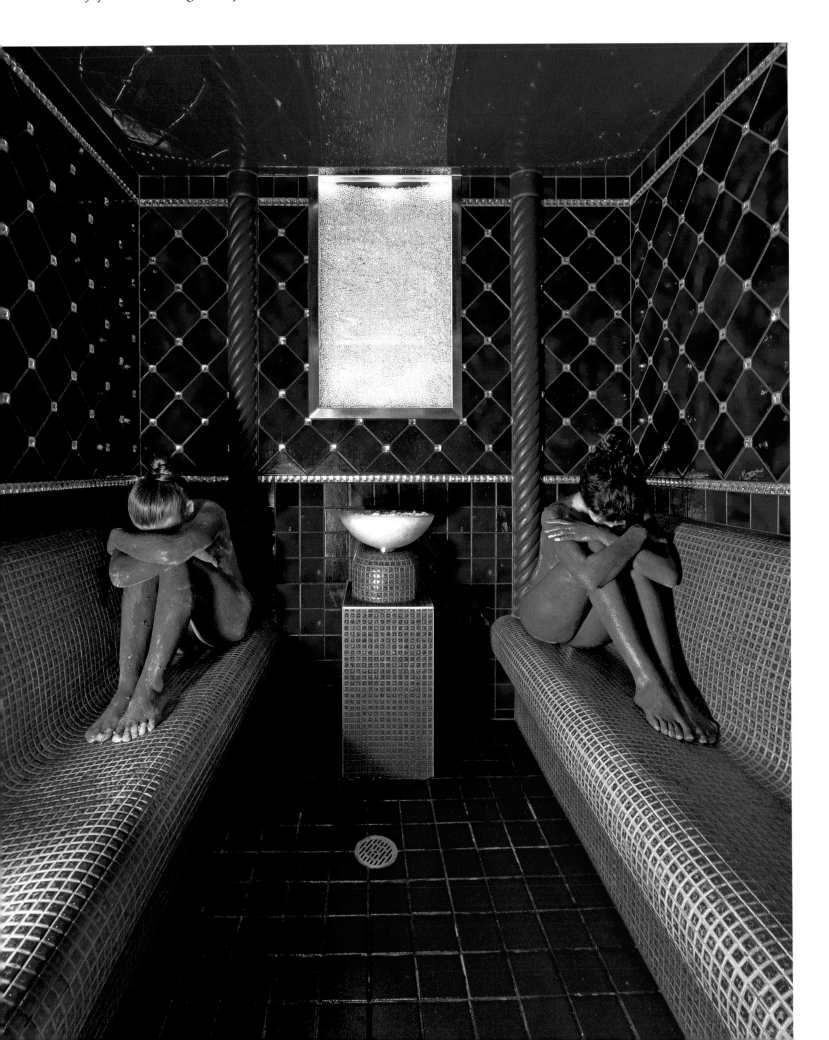

A Journey Towards Wellness
Eine Reise zum Wohlbefinden

The Chateau Spa & Organic Wellness Resort

It's not exactly the first thing that comes to mind: a medieval castle in the heart of the Malaysian rain forest. The castle is a reproduction of Haut-Kœnigsbourg in Alsace, France, and yet combined with its Malaysian setting, it never ceases to surprise. This merging of cultures continues inside the organic spa and wellness resort, where European treatment methods meet Asian hospitality in the La Santé spa. There is something to welcome every guest, depending on his or her individual needs: an herbal sauna and salt grotto, a massage table with automatic exfoliator or an aroma hydropool, therapies for body pampering or weight loss, and special programs aimed at men or pregnant women. People come here from all over the world to benefit from the exclusive, doctor-supervised health programs for holistic well-being. For an alternative experience, you can stroll around The Chateau's organic farm, participate in a tea ceremony in the Japanese Village, admire tiger orchids in the Botanical Gardens, or explore the jungle on horseback.

Auf diese Idee muss man erst einmal kommen: Ein mittelalterliches Schloss im Dickicht des malaysischen Regenwaldes. Zwar ist das Schloss eine Kopie von Haut-Kœnigsbourg im Elsass, doch die Kombination bleibt überraschend. Die Verschmelzung der Kulturen setzt sich im Innern des biologischen Spa- und Wellness-Resorts fort: Im La Santé Spa treffen europäische Behandlungsmethoden auf asiatische Gastfreundschaft. Ob Kräutersauna oder Salzgrotte, Massageliege mit Peeling-Automatik oder Aroma-Hydropool, ob zum Verwöhnen des Körpers oder Gewichtsabnahme, ob spezielle Angebote für Männer oder für Schwangere: Jeder Gast ist mit seinen individuellen Bedürfnissen willkommen. Menschen aus aller Welt kommen hierher, um die exklusiven, ärztlich betreuten Gesundheitsprogramme zum ganzheitlichen Wohlbefinden zu erfahren. Alternativ kann man im Chateau über einen Bio-Bauernhof schlendern, eine Teezeremonie im japanischen Dorf erleben, im botanischen Garten Tigerorchideen bewundern oder den Dschungel mit dem Pferd erkunden.

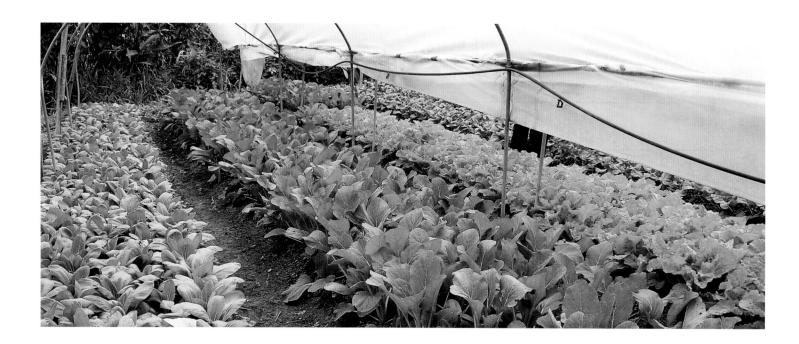

Spa, Health & Other Facilities
Treatment rooms, aroma hydropool, herbal bath, salt grotto, mud chamber, relaxation whirlpool, changing rooms with integrated sauna and steam areas, deluxe treatment room with whirlpool, outdoor relaxation pavilions, gymnasium, consultation rooms, manicure and pedicure cabin, Mind & Body Studio. Spa cafe, spa boutique, hair salon.

Treatments & Services
Spa packages for body, mind, and beauty: Aquaveda bed/Soap Brush treatment, beauty, body cleansing, couple retreat, detox and weight loss programs, Fit for Life program, packages especially for men, pre- and postnatal therapy, stress relief, wellness. Airport transfers, concierge service, free high-speed Internet, free parking, heli/limo service, laundry.

Activities
18-hole award-winning golf course, adventure park Flying Fox, animal park, horse trails, Japanese village, Papillon Terrace, salt pool, sport complex, The Pavilion.

Rooms
128 rooms and suites.

Located
45 minutes from the Kuala Lumpur city center and 90 minutes from Kuala Lumpur International Airport.

Berjaya Hills, Km 48 Persimpangan Bertingkat Lebuhraya Karak
28750 Bukit Tinggi, Pahang, Malaysia
www.thechateau.com.my

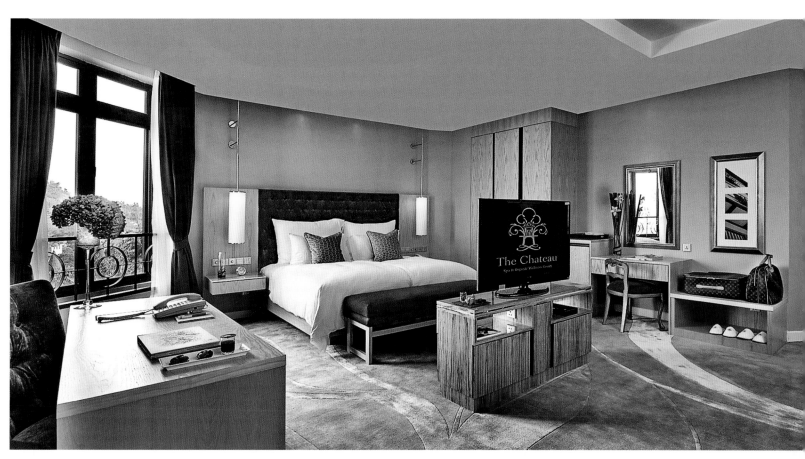

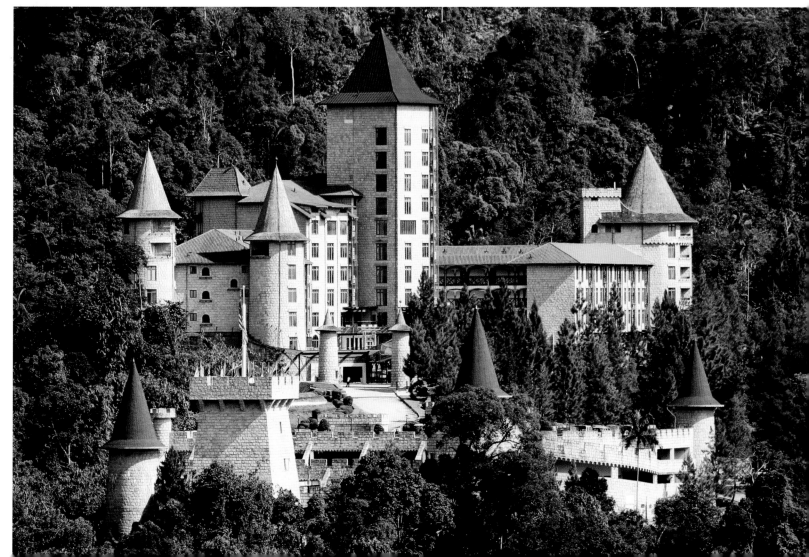

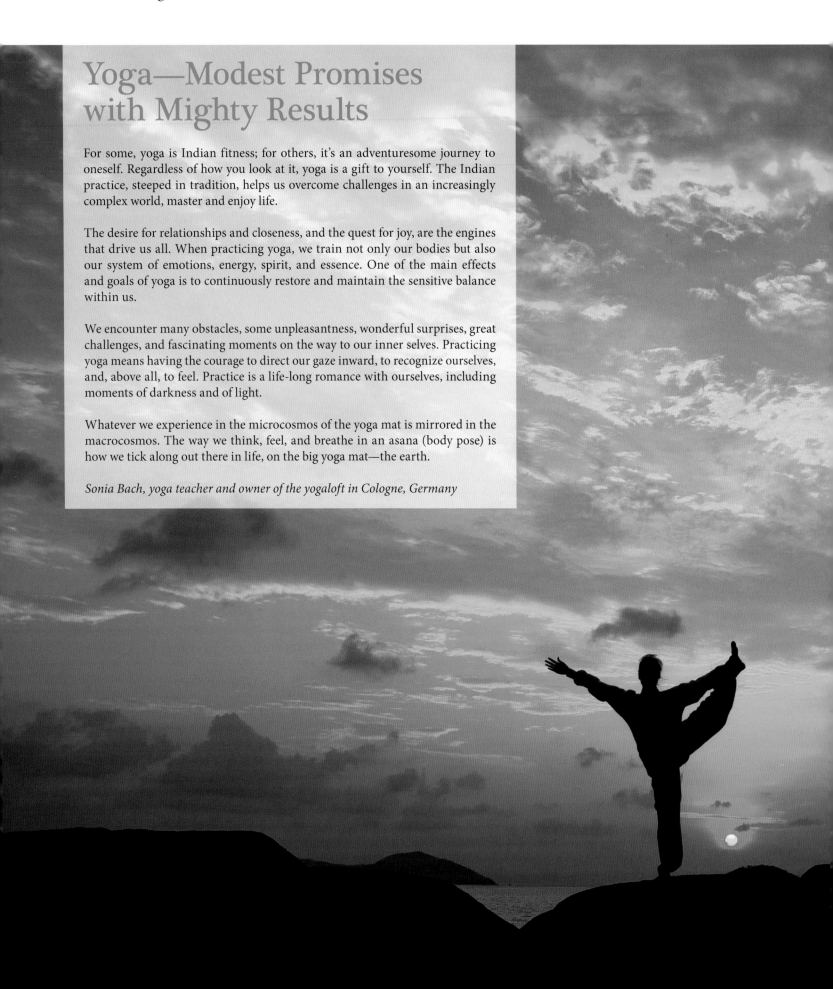

Yoga—Modest Promises with Mighty Results

For some, yoga is Indian fitness; for others, it's an adventuresome journey to oneself. Regardless of how you look at it, yoga is a gift to yourself. The Indian practice, steeped in tradition, helps us overcome challenges in an increasingly complex world, master and enjoy life.

The desire for relationships and closeness, and the quest for joy, are the engines that drive us all. When practicing yoga, we train not only our bodies but also our system of emotions, energy, spirit, and essence. One of the main effects and goals of yoga is to continuously restore and maintain the sensitive balance within us.

We encounter many obstacles, some unpleasantness, wonderful surprises, great challenges, and fascinating moments on the way to our inner selves. Practicing yoga means having the courage to direct our gaze inward, to recognize ourselves, and, above all, to feel. Practice is a life-long romance with ourselves, including moments of darkness and of light.

Whatever we experience in the microcosmos of the yoga mat is mirrored in the macrocosmos. The way we think, feel, and breathe in an asana (body pose) is how we tick along out there in life, on the big yoga mat—the earth.

Sonia Bach, yoga teacher and owner of the yogaloft in Cologne, Germany

Yoga verspricht nicht viel, hält aber einiges

Für die einen ist es indische Fitness, für die anderen eine abenteuerliche Reise zu sich selbst. Wie auch immer, Yoga zu praktizieren ist ein Geschenk an sich selbst. Die indische, traditionsreiche Praxis hilft dabei, in einer immer komplexer werdenden Welt voller Herausforderungen zu bestehen und das Leben zu meistern beziehungsweise zu genießen.

Der Wunsch nach Verbindung und Verbundenheit, das Streben nach Glück sind der Motor, der alle Menschen antreibt. In der Yogapraxis trainieren wir nicht nur unseren Körper, sondern das gesamte System von Emotionen, Energie und Seele. Das darin verborgene empfindliche Gleichgewicht immer wieder herzustellen und zu bewahren, gehört zu den wichtigsten Effekten und Zielen von Yoga.

Auf dem Weg zum eigenen Selbst gibt es viele Hindernisse, einige Unannehmlichkeiten, tolle Überraschungen, große Herausforderungen und faszinierende Augenblicke. Yoga zu praktizieren bedeutet mutig zu sein, den Blick nach innen zu richten, sich selbst zu erkennen und vor allem sich zu fühlen. Die Praxis ist eine lebenslange Romanze mit sich selbst, inklusive aller Schatten- und Lichtmomente.

Alles, was auf der Yogamatte im Mikrokosmos erlebt wird, spiegelt sich im Makrokosmos wider. Wie wir in einer Asana (Körperübung) denken, fühlen, atmen, so „ticken" wir auch draußen im Leben, auf der großen Yogamatte – der Erde.

Sonia Bach, Yogalehrerin, Inhaberin von the yogaloft, Köln, Deutschland

All-inclusive Natural Living

Natürlich leben all-inclusive

Fusion Maia Resort

Simple, modest, down to earth—perfect. This resort has everything to offer: It includes such things as the only spa-inclusive concept in Asia, one that offers guests a full range of holistic treatments at no additional charge. Experience its healing massages, body therapies, beauty treatments as well as yoga and meditation—to your heart's content. The Natural Living Program also includes sports activities, gourmet cuisine with a 24-hour breakfast service, and private villas with a sleek, modern design—each of which comes with its own pool and garden. And best of all: There is a private beach. Together with General Manager Michelle Ford, the Fusionistas design programs tailored to individual needs and provide their guests with an unforgettable experience at My Khe Beach.

Simpel, schlicht, bodenständig – perfekt. Dieses Resort bietet alles, nur keinen Schnickschnack. Dazu zählt zum Beispiel das asienweit einzigartige Spa-inclusive-Konzept, mit dem jedem Gast die gesamte Palette an ganzheitlichen Behandlungen ohne zusätzliche Kosten zur Verfügung steht. Heilende Massagen, Körpertherapien und Schönheitsbehandlungen sowie Yogakurse oder Meditation soviel das Herz begehrt. Zum Natural Living Programm gehören außerdem sportliche Aktivitäten, eine Gourmetküche mit einem Frühstücksservice rund um die Uhr sowie private Villen in geradlinigem, modernem Design – jede davon mit eigenem Pool und Garten. Und das Highlight: Es gibt einen privaten Strand. Abgestimmt auf die individuellen Bedürfnisse gestalten die Fusionistas rund um Geschäftsführerin Michelle Ford ihren Gästen einen unvergesslichen Aufenthalt am Strand von My Khe Beach.

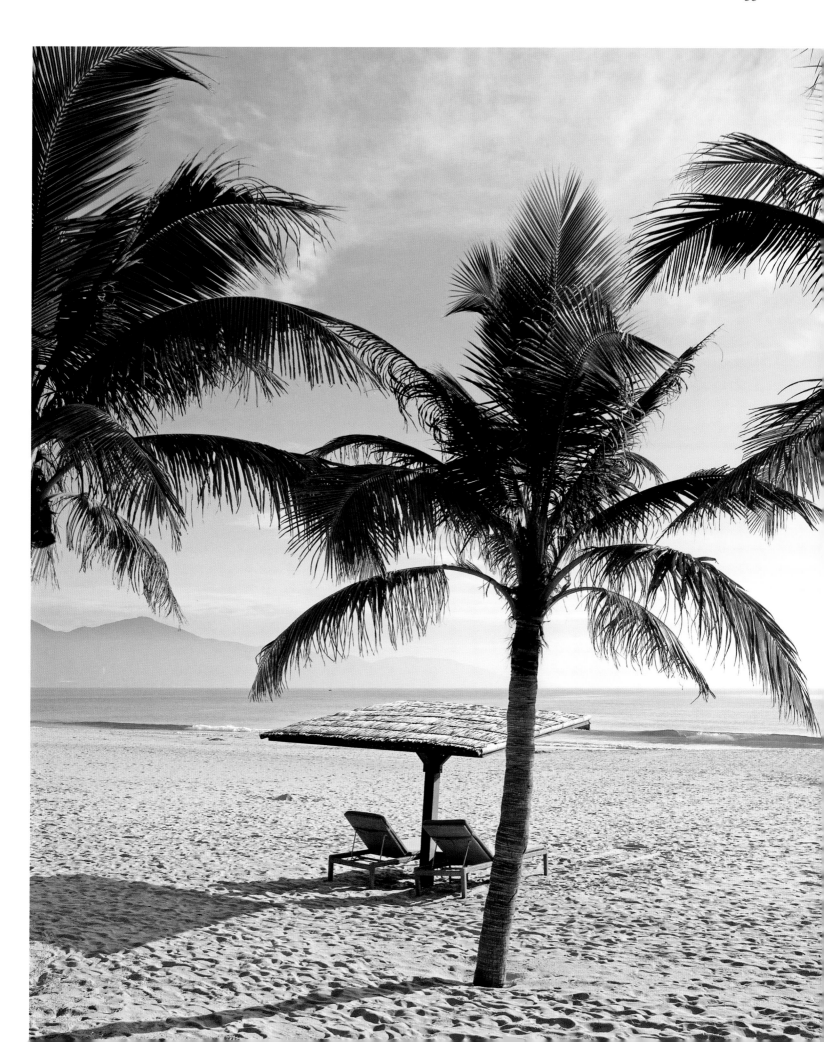

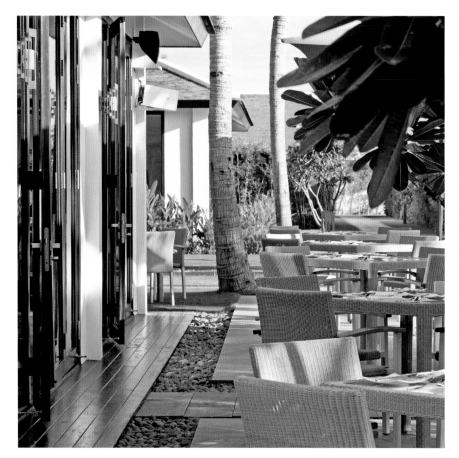

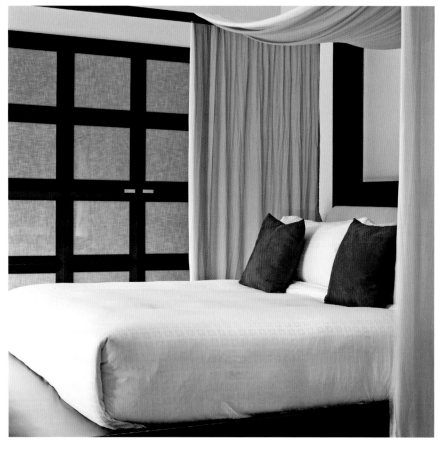

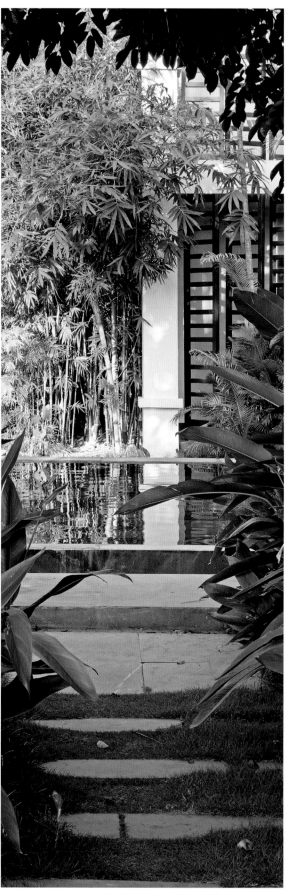

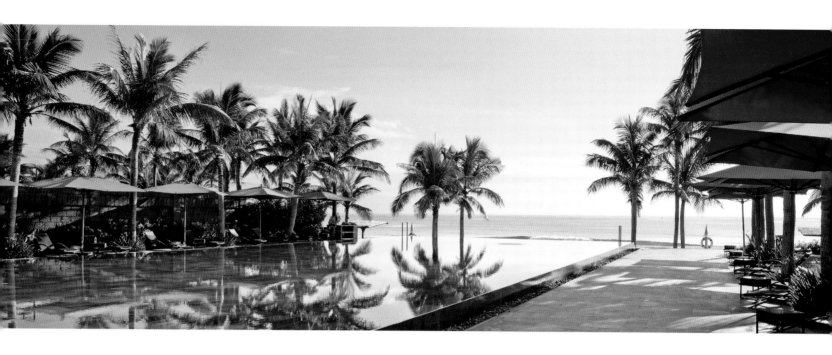

Spa, Health & Other Facilities
Spa pool with waterfall, private Jacuzzis, steam room, sauna, yoga room, tropical spa garden.
4 restaurants, Fusion Lounge Restaurant in Hoi An, conference rooms, library.

Treatments & Services
Balancing foot massage, be active thai fusion massage, body scrubs and envelope, calming back, facials, in-tense therapy, manicure, mindful energy therapy, natural living massage, neck and shoulder massage, nourishing hand relaxation therapy, open your mind holistic head therapy, pedicure, the fusion feeling, uplifting warm pressure massage. 24-hour front desk, airport transfer, babysitting/childcare, free parking, laundry service.

Activities
Fusion Lounge in Hoi An with complimentary bicycles, golf, scuba diving. 3 world heritage sites.

Rooms
87 villas including 80 pool villas, 4 spa villas, and 3 beach villas.

Located
Located on the My Khe Beach, the resort is only 10 minutes from Da Nang center, 20 minutes from the world's heritage town Hoi An, and 15 minutes from the airport.

Truong Sa Street, Khue My Ward, Ngu Hanh Son District
Da Nang City, Vietnam
www.fusionmaiadanang.com

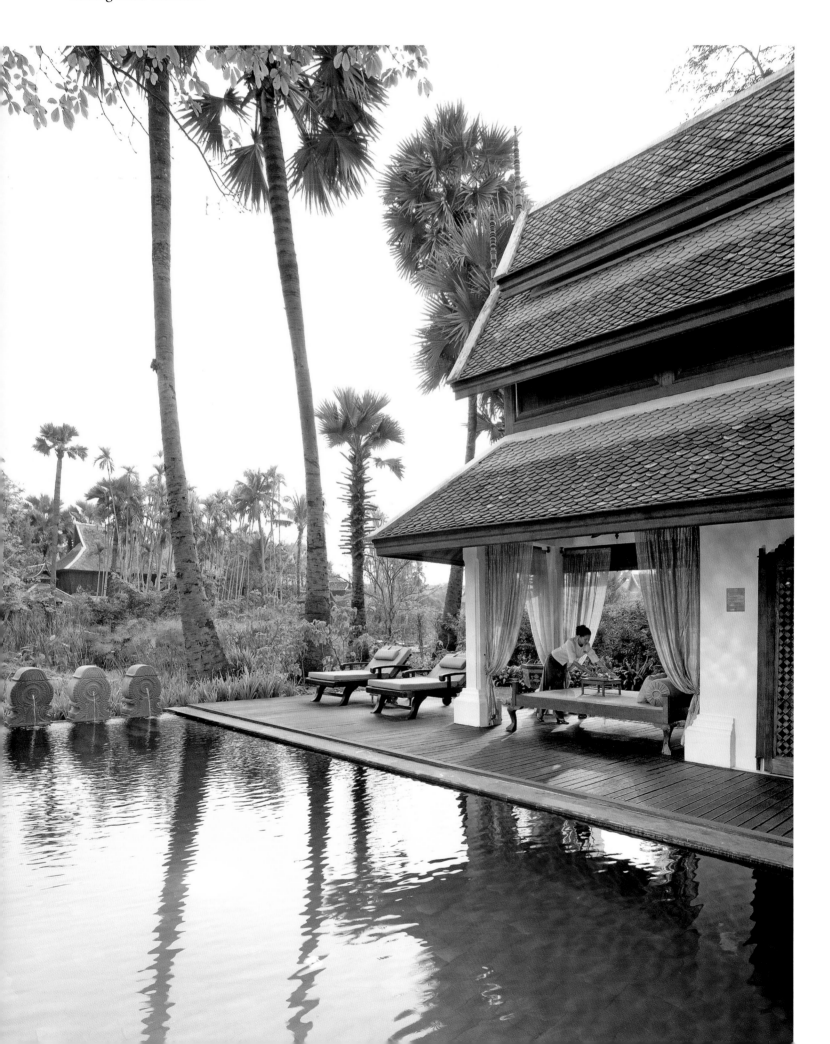

Royal Awakening in Seven Stages

Königliches Erwachen in sieben Stufen

Mandarin Oriental Dhara Dhevi

On 59 acres of land at the foot of the mountains in northern Thailand, surrounded by rice paddies, lies an unusual city. All of its buildings reflect the region's architectural history. Life in this city pulses under a seven-tiered roof, designed in the style of an ancient palace. It is where the Dheva Spa delivers its promise: Take the seven steps to Nirvana. The journey to this state of being beyond human frailty, which Buddhists can achieve only after many years of meditation, takes guests to a world-famous Ayurvedic center, where Dheva Spa products, hydrotherapy, and advanced yoga are used in healing treatments. The guides along this journey are therapists who were trained in a special academy. The final destination is a return to physical and spiritual perfection. Incidentally, dheva is a Sanskrit word that describes supernatural beings who benevolently guide us on the way to enlightenment.

Über 24 Hektar Land am Fuße der Berge Nordthailands und umgeben von Reisfeldern erstreckt sich eine besondere Stadt. All ihre Gebäude spiegeln die Architekturgeschichte der Region wider. Ihr Herz schlägt unter einem siebenfach abgestuften Dach im Stil eines antiken Palastes, unter dem das Versprechen des Dheva Spa eingelöst werden soll: In sieben Stufen zum Nirwana. Die Reise in diesen Daseinszustand jenseits menschlicher Schwächen, für den ein Buddhist lange meditieren muss, führt die Gäste in ein weltbekanntes ayurvedisches Zentrum und dort durch heilende Anwendungen mit Dheva-Spa-Produkten, Hydrotherapie und Yoga auf Meisterebene. Die Reiseleitung übernehmen Therapeuten, die an einer eigenen Akademie ausgebildet wurden. Am Ende der Reise steht das Wiedererlangen von geistiger und körperlicher Perfektion. Dheva ist übrigens ein Wort aus dem Sanskrit: Es bezeichnet überirdische Wesen, die uns auf dem Weg zur Erleuchtung wohlwollend begleiten.

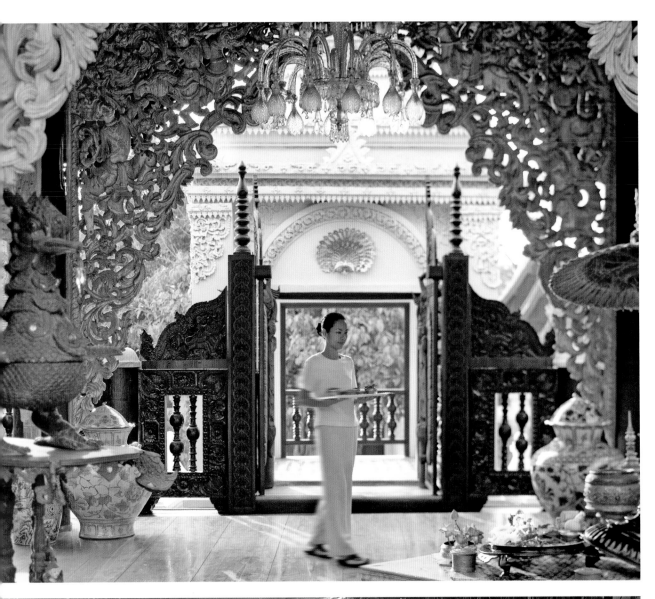

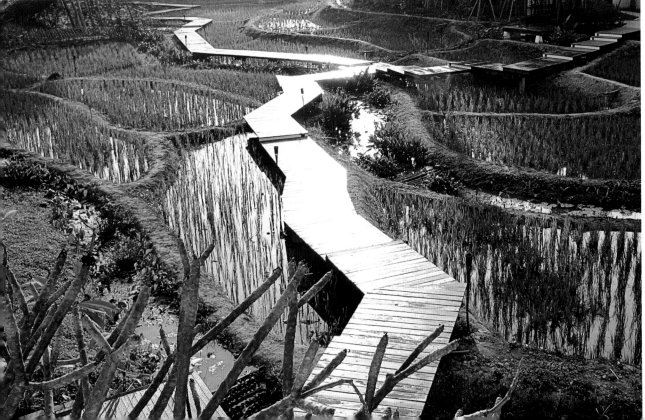

Spa, Health & Other Facilities
18 treatment rooms, 2 large swimming pools, spa residences, yoga and Tai Chi areas, outdoor exercise areas, herbal gardens for treatments and meals, Ayurvedic center. 6 restaurants, shopping village with Thai products, grand ballroom for 500 guests, handicrafts, world-class library, 2 tennis courts, amphitheater for cultural events.

Treatments & Services
A large variety of treatments including anti-stress, hydrotherapy, Lanna massage, lymphatic drainage, Mandalay Experience, reflexology, Royal Thai Ceremony, Swedish massage, Thai massage, weight loss, yoga. Ayurveda, consultations, tailor-made wellness programs, Traditional Chinese Medicine. Ayurvedic meals.

Activities
Cooking school, swimming, tennis.

Rooms
123 luxurious teak wood villas including colonial suites and signature residences with 6 bedrooms.

Located
15 minutes from Chiang Mai International Airport and 10 minutes from the city center.

51/4 Sankampaeng Road Moo 1 T. Tasala A. Muang
Chiang Mai 50000, Thailand
www.mandarinoriental.com/chiangmai

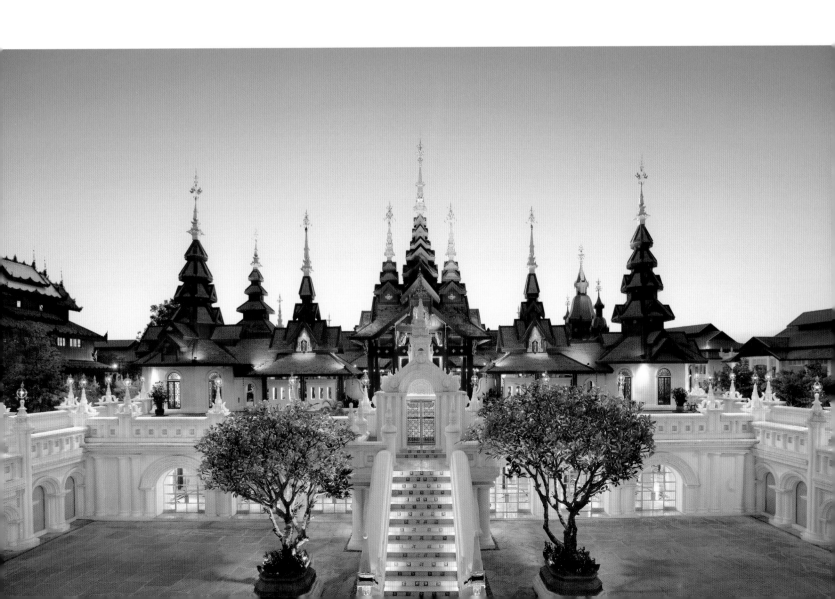

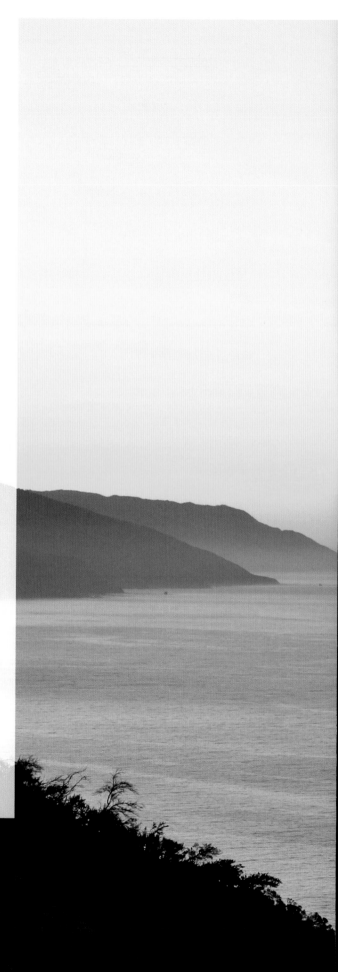

Energy—The Source of Health and Healing

"In every culture and in every medical tradition
before ours, healing was accomplished by
moving energy." – Albert Szent-Györgyi

All ancient healing traditions were familiar with the importance of subtle energies for our health and healing. The close relationships of these energies with our psychological-spiritual and mental-emotional dimensions were common knowledge as well. Concepts of subtle, invisible bodies of energy are found in most cultures on the five continents. What the earlier traditions called "breath of life," "ether," "Odem" (Germany), "qi" (China), or "prana" (India) is what modern health sciences term "vital energy" or "bioenergy."

"Feeling energy flows" is nothing extraordinary for those of us who work with energy therapies such as acupuncture and active cupping therapy. And yet for centuries, concepts of this "healing energy" were considered virtually incompatible with the conventional medical paradigm. As a result of new discoveries, initially in physics, energy concepts are slowly gaining acceptance in the medical sciences. The ability to measure "bioenergies" in and around the human body led to a new and extremely promising field of academic study—energy medicine, today one of the fastest growing fields in the health sciences.

The goal of preventive medicine—where many doctors and therapists see the greatest potential for energy medicine—is to help people avoid a long life of suffering caused by chronic degenerative disease. Instead, the idea is to guide them back to radiant health and vitality. Hence, the essence of preventive medicine lies in early intervention, when functional disorders develop on the borderline between health and illness. It is precisely this borderline that can be diagnosed and treated with energy medicine.

This is where the true potential of energy medicine unfolds, providing us with the opportunity to remove energy blockages and release disruptive energies from the body's energy field, to activate the body's own vibrations and harmonize the energy flow, thereby recharging the body's energy reserves.

With energy medicine, a new way of thinking is beginning to take shape, one that is changing the way modern scientific medicine views health and disease. Energy medicine points the way to an exciting new era, opening our hearts and minds to a new paradigm where ancient healing traditions blend with advanced medical research and health sciences to facilitate the adaptation processes needed for self-healing.

Dr. Roland G. Heber, M.D., Indeo Healing and Teaching Institute
for Integrative Medicine in Lans, Austria

Energie – Quelle von Gesundheit und Heilung

> „In jeder Kultur und in jeder medizinischen Tradition vor uns erzielte man Heilung, indem man die Energie in Bewegung brachte." – Albert Szent-Györgyi

Alle alten Heiltraditionen wussten um die Bedeutung feinstofflicher Energien für die Gesundheit und Heilung sowie deren enge Beziehungen zu seelisch-geistigen und mental-emotionalen Dimensionen. Konzepte feinstofflicher, unsichtbarer Energie-Körper gibt es in den meisten Kulturen der fünf Kontinente. Was die frühen Traditionen „Atem des Lebens", „Äther", „Odem", „Qi" (China) oder „Prana" (Indien) nannten, ist die „Vitale Energie" oder „Bio-Energie" der modernen Gesundheitswissenschaften.

„Energieflüsse zu fühlen" ist nichts Außergewöhnliches für uns, die wir mit energetischen Therapien wie Akupunktur und aktiver Schröpftherapie arbeiten. Jahrhundertelang jedoch galten Konzepte dieser „Heilenergie" als so gut wie unvereinbar mit dem konventionellen medizinischen Paradigma. Mit den neuen, zunächst in der Physik gewonnenen Erkenntnissen finden energetische Konzepte langsam Akzeptanz in den medizinischen Wissenschaften. Mit der Messbarkeit von Bio-Energien im und um den menschlichen Körper entstand ein mit Spannung zu verfolgender, neuer akademischer Zweig: Energiemedizin. Inzwischen ist sie einer der am schnellsten wachsenden Zweige der Gesundheitswissenschaften.

Es ist Zielsetzung der Präventivmedizin – in der viele Ärzte und Therapeuten das größte Potenzial der Energiemedizin sehen – zu verhindern, dass Menschen einen langen Leidensweg durch chronisch-degenerative Erkrankung gehen. Stattdessen sollen sie zu strahlender Gesundheit und Vitalität zurückbegleitet werden. Konsequenterweise besteht die Essenz der Präventivmedizin in frühzeitiger Intervention, wenn Funktionsstörungen sich im Grenzbereich zwischen Gesundheit und Krankheit abspielen. Und genau dieser Grenzbereich lässt sich mit der Energiemedizin diagnostizieren und therapieren.

Von hier aus entfaltet sich das wahre Potenzial der Energiemedizin und eröffnet uns die Möglichkeit, Energieblockaden zu öffnen und störende Energien aus dem Energiefeld des Körpers freizusetzen, körpereigene Schwingungen zu aktivieren, den Energiefluss zu harmonisieren und so die Energiereserven des Körpers wieder aufzuladen.

Mit der Energiemedizin nimmt ein Umdenken Form an, das die Sichtweise der modernen wissenschaftlichen Medizin auf Gesundheit und Krankheit verändert. Energiemedizin deutet auf den Beginn einer aufregenden neuen Ära hin, die unser Herz und unseren Verstand für ein neues Paradigma öffnet, wo alte Heiltraditionen mit fortschrittlicher medizinischer Forschung und Gesundheitswissenschaft verschmelzen, um die nötigen Adaptationsprozesse für die Selbstheilung zu ermöglichen.

Dr. med. Roland G. Heber, Indeo Heil- und Lehrinstitut für Integrative Medizin in Lans, Österreich

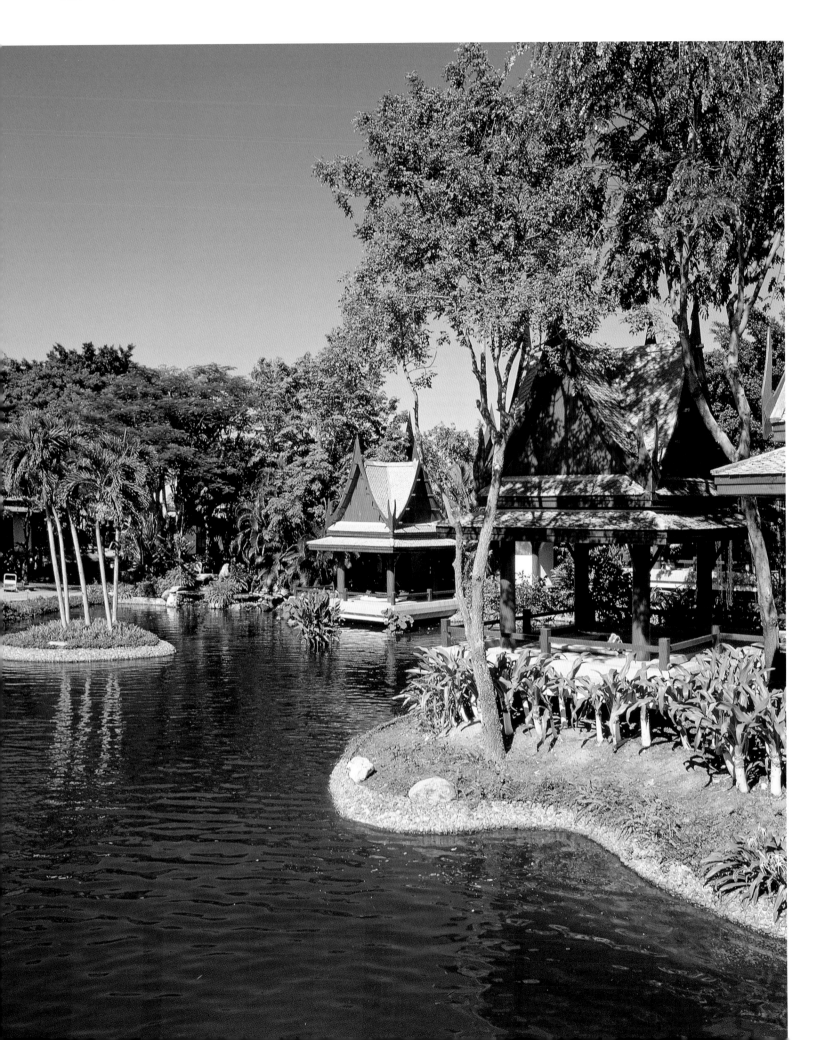

Therapeutic Combinations for Personal Fulfillment

Therapie-Kombinationen für persönliche Erfüllung

Chiva-Som

No matter who you are or what you can do—once the detoxifying juice has passed through our bodies and flushed toxins out of the liver, kidneys, and digestive tract, everyone is the same. The fact that Chiva-Som upholds guest privacy also enhances the sense of feeling good and comfortable. The name of this prize-winning health resort situated in beautiful, lush tropical gardens means nothing short of "haven of life." Happy to arrive in this haven, guests can indulge in expert treatments. The first step in this regard is to identify a person's individual mental, physical, and spiritual needs. Asian therapies such as Traditional Chinese Medicine and Indian Ayurveda, combined with Western naturopathy and wellness, gradually lead to a healthier, happier life. According to the resort's philosophy, we achieve personal fulfillment through health in body, mind, and spirit.

Egal, wer man ist und was man kann – wenn der Detox-Saft unsere Körper durchspült und Leber, Nieren und Verdauungstrakt von kleinen Sünden reinwäscht, dann sind wir alle gleich. Zu einem gesteigerten Wohlbefinden führt auch der Umstand, dass das Chiva-Som die Privatsphäre der Gäste hochhält. Der Name des vielfach ausgezeichneten Health Resorts in üppigen tropischen Gärten bedeutet nichts Geringeres als „Hafen des Lebens". Glücklich in diesem Hafen angekommen, können sich die Gäste den Behandlungen durch Experten hingeben. Diese beginnen mit einer Feststellung der individuellen mentalen, körperlichen und spirituellen Bedürfnisse. Asiatische Therapien wie Traditionelle Chinesische Medizin und indisches Ayurveda kombiniert mit westlicher Naturheilkunde und Wellness führen dann Schritt für Schritt zu einem gesünderen und glücklicheren Leben. Persönliche Erfüllung erreicht man durch die Gesundheit von Körper, Geist und Seele, lehrt die Philosophie des Hauses.

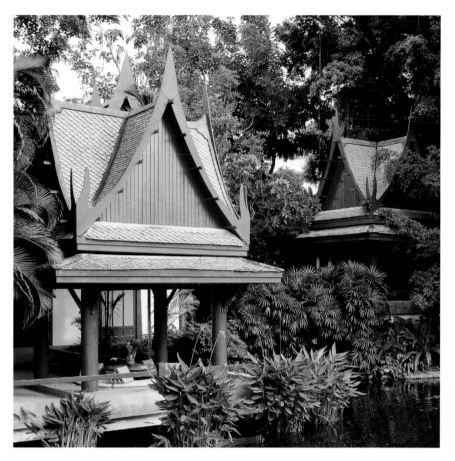

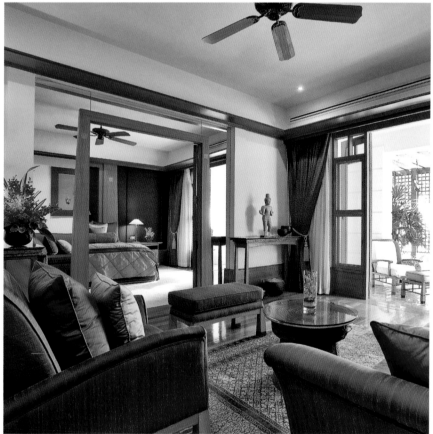

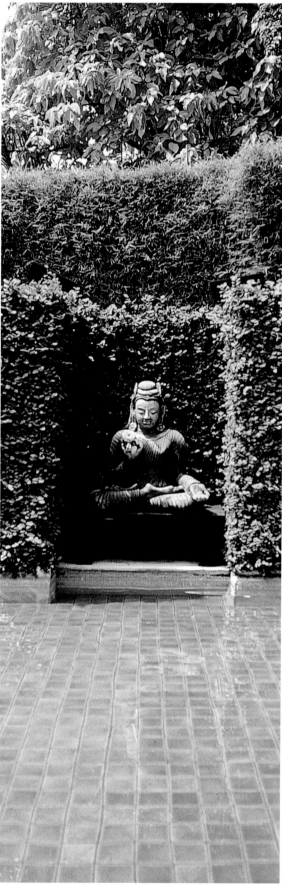

Spa, Health & Other Facilities
77 treatment rooms, large outdoor swimming pool, indoor swimming pool, Watsu pool, plunge pool, waterfalls, flotation pool, large hydro Jacuzzi, huge unisex multilevel steam room, Kneipp therapy foot bath, relaxation room, fully equipped gymnasium. Dance studio, Pilates studio, yoga pavilion, yoga sala, kinesis studio, Tai Chi pavilion, bathing pavilion. 2 restaurants.

Treatments & Services
Body wraps, Chi Nei Tsang, cleansing, firming and relaxing facials and oriental foot rituals, fitness, holistic health treatments, mind training, personal training classes, physiotherapy, Pilates, Qigong, Reiki, shiatsu, Tai Chi, Thai massage, Watsu. 24-hour room service, buggy service, laundry service, VIP airport welcome.

Activities
Biking, golf, guided tours, outdoor training, sailing, sea kayaking, sightseeing, swimming, tennis, windsurfing.

Rooms
58 rooms including 33 ocean-view rooms, 17 Thai pavilion rooms, and 8 suites.

Located
Located in Hua Hin, about 3 hours from Bangkok International Airport.

73/4 Petchkasem Road, Hua Hin
Prachuab Khirikhan 77110, Thailand
www.chivasom.com

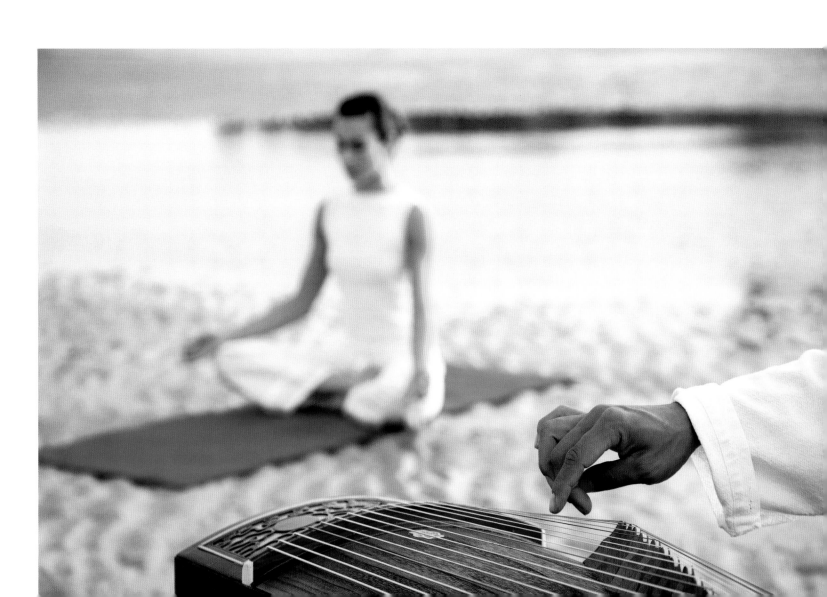

"Yam Hua Plee" Banana Blossom Salad

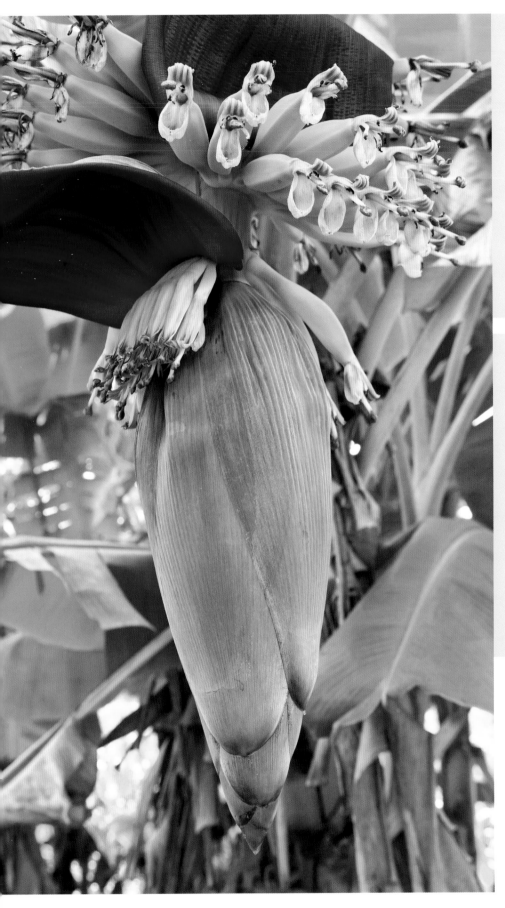

- › 2 ½ tbsp lime juice
- › 2 tbsp soy sauce
- › 1 ½ tbsp honey
- › 2 bird's eye chillies, finely chopped
- › 130 g banana blossom, peeled, diagonally sliced & socked in lime juice water
- › 3 tbsp roasted almonds, coarsely chopped
- › 2 tbsp sliced shallot
- › 2 tbsp chopped scallions
- › 1 tbsp finely diagonally sliced lemongrass
- › 3 tbsp roasted coconut flakes, tip of coriander to garnish
- › prawns, ad lib

Serves 4

- › 2,5 EL Limettensaft
- › 2 EL Sojasauce
- › 1,5 EL Honig
- › 2 Thai-Chilis, fein gehackt
- › 130 g Bananenblüte, geschält, diagonal geschnitten und in Limettensaft eingelegt
- › 3 EL geröstete Mandeln, grob gehackt
- › 2 EL geschnittene Schalotten
- › 2 EL gehackte Frühlingszwiebeln
- › 1 EL fein und diagonal geschnittenes Zitronengras
- › 3 EL geröstete Kokosraspeln, Messerspitze Koriander zum Garnieren
- › Garnelen, nach Belieben

Für 4 Personen

Chiva-Som, Thailand

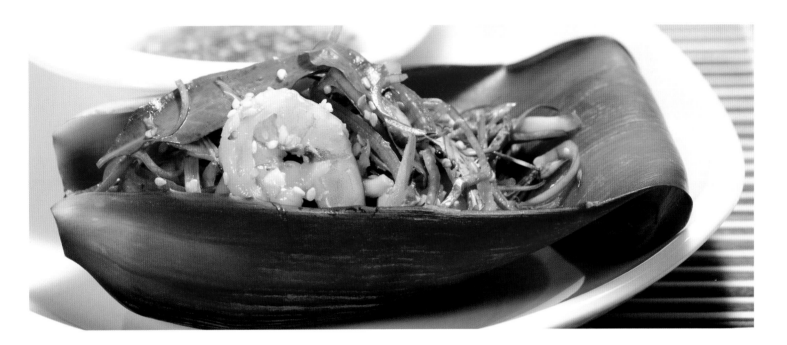

"Yam Hua Plee"
Banana Blossom Salad

Method
To prepare dressing, whisk lime juice, soy sauce, honey, and chillies in a large bowl. Set aside. To prepare salad, gently toss all remaining ingredients with all of dressing in a mixing bowl until evenly mixed. Sprinkle over coconut flakes and coriander and serve.

Health Benefits
Banana blossom is known to help increase the concentration of progesterone hormone, which reduces bleeding during menstruation. Thus, for people suffering from painful menstruation and excess bleeding, cooked banana blossom with curd or buttermilk has a soothing effect. Banana blossom is also considered to be a good source of vitamin A and C, and it is traditionally believed to be beneficial as a lactating agent.

„Yam Hua Plee"
Bananenblüten-Salat

Zubereitung
Für das Dressing den Limettensaft, die Sojasauce, den Honig und die Chilis in einer großen Schüssel mit dem Schneebesen schlagen. Dressing beiseite stellen. Für den Salat alle übrigen Zutaten mit dem Dressing in einer Rührschüssel mischen, bis alles gleichmäßig vermengt ist. Kokosnussraspeln und Koriander darüber streuen und servieren.

Gesundheitlicher Nutzen
Die Bananenblüte ist dafür bekannt, die Konzentration des Hormons Progesteron zu steigern, was zu schwächeren Menstruationsblutungen beiträgt. Gekocht mit Quark oder Buttermilch, schafft sie Linderung für Frauen mit Menstruationsbeschwerden und starken Blutungen. Die Bananenblüte ist eine reichhaltige Quelle an Vitamin A und C. Ihr wird traditionell eine positive Wirkung während der Stillzeit zugesprochen.

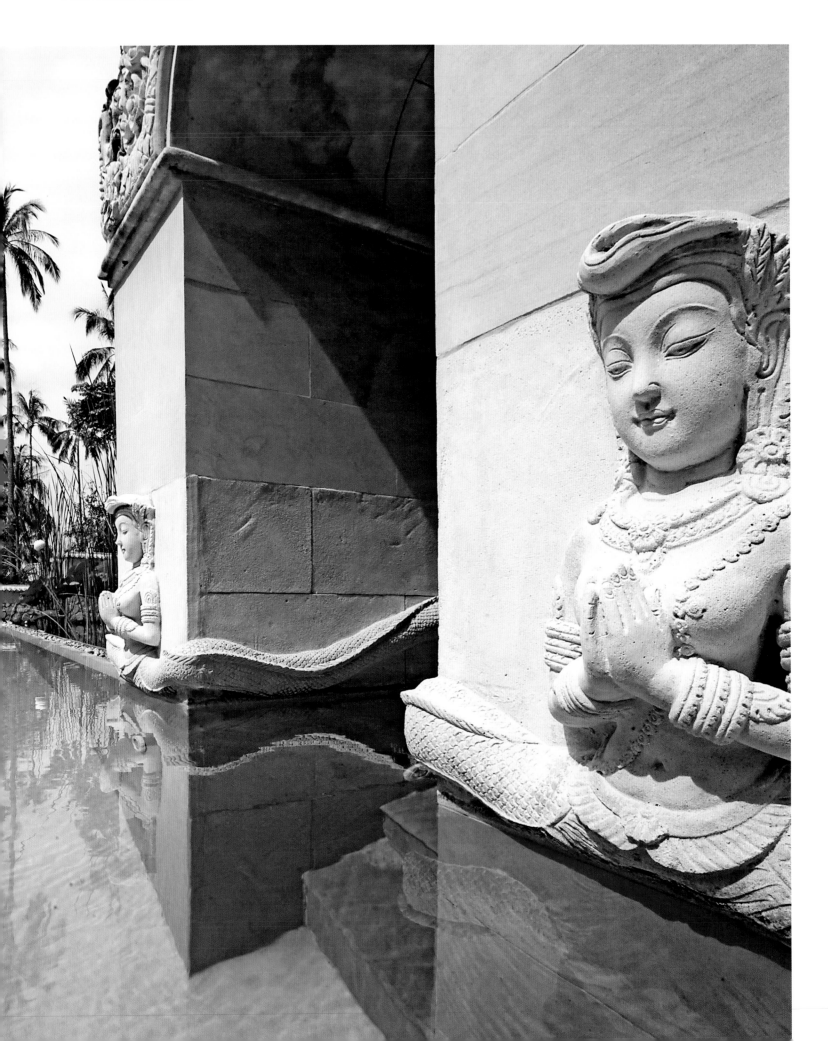

Growth, Reconnection, and Unfolding of the Human Spirit

Wachsen, entfalten und zu sich finden

Kamalaya Wellness Sanctuary & Holistic Spa

The history of the Kamalaya Wellness Sanctuary & Holistic Spa began when Karina and John Stewart met in the Himalayas in 1982. They shared a common spiritual lifestyle, knowledge of the healing power of nature, and the conviction that true happiness is to be found in giving. These principles laid the foundation for the concept behind Kamalaya, which opened on Koh Samui in 2005. Situated on a tropical hillside with a view of the island's pristine coast, the resort is laid out like a village, whose essence is revealed by its name: "Lotus (Kamal) Realm (Alaya)," an ancient symbol for the growth and unfolding of the human spirit. Holistic medicine, Eastern and Western therapies, spa treatments, and alternative fitness techniques bring body and spirit into a harmonious equilibrium. Holistic wellness programs and the strong presence of nature let the guests find their balance of soul. The heart of Kamalaya is a cave that served as a retreat for Buddhist monks hundreds of years ago. The place is permeated by a deep bond with the forces of the universe. Today, the cave is open to guests as a place of spiritual reflection.

Die Geschichte vom Kamalaya Wellness Sanctuary & Holistic Spa begann, als sich Karina und John Stewart 1982 im Himalaya begegneten. Beide verband eine gemeinsame spirituelle Lebensweise, das Wissen um die Heilkraft der Natur und die Überzeugung, dass das wahre Glück im Geben liegt. Auf dieser Grundlage entstand das Konzept für das 2005 eröffnete Kamalaya auf Koh Samui. Direkt an einem tropischen Hang mit Blick über die ursprüngliche Bucht wurde es wie ein Dorf angelegt, dessen Wesen schon der Name verrät: „Lotus (Kamal) Reich (Alaya)", ein altes Symbol für das Wachstum und die Entfaltung des menschlichen Geistes. Ganzheitliche Medizin, östliche und westliche Therapien, Spa-Behandlungen und alternative Fitness bringen Körper und Geist in Einklang. Holistische Wellness-Programme und die starke Präsenz der Natur sorgen für seelisches Gleichgewicht. Das Herz von Kamalaya ist eine alte Felsenhöhle, in die sich jahrhunderte-lang buddhistische Mönche zur Meditation zurückzogen. Sie spürten hier eine tiefe Verbundenheit mit den Kräften des Universums. Heute steht den Gästen die Höhle als ein Ort der spirituellen Besinnung offen.

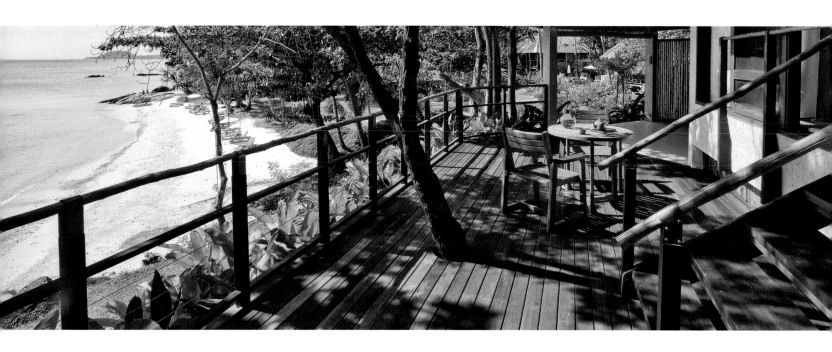

Spa, Health & Other Facilities
Plunge pools, herbal steam cavern, far infrared sauna, yoga pavilion, yoga sala, shakti fitness center.
2 restaurants, conference room.

Treatments & Services
Life enhancement programs and retreats such as Detoxification, Healthy Lifestyle, Stress & Burnout, Yoga Synergy. Consultations and healing therapies from Eastern and Western traditions including Ayurveda, homeopathy, mind-body-balance meditations, naturopathy, nutritional guidance, Traditional Chinese Medicine. Optional diagnostic procedures such as fitness, iridology, and nutritional evaluations as well as other medical testing and analysis.

Activities
Holistic fitness classes in Pilates, Qigong, Tai Chi, yoga; beach meditations, morning power walks, kayaking.

Rooms
59 rooms – 5 categories: hillside rooms, suites, villas, beach front villas, pool villas.

Located
Kamalaya is located on the southern coast of the tropical island of Koh Samui
and about 16 miles (25 kilometers) from Koh Samui Airport.

102/9 Moo 3, Laem Set Road, Na-Muang
Suratthani 84140, Thailand
www.kamalaya.com

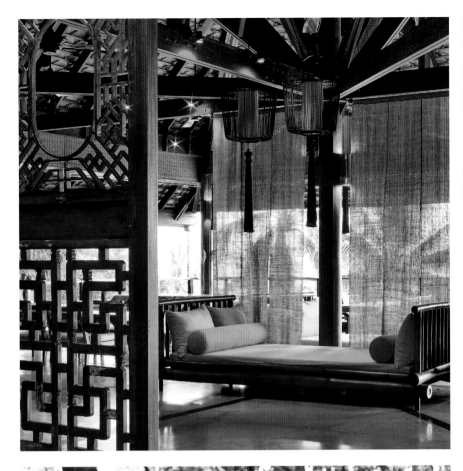

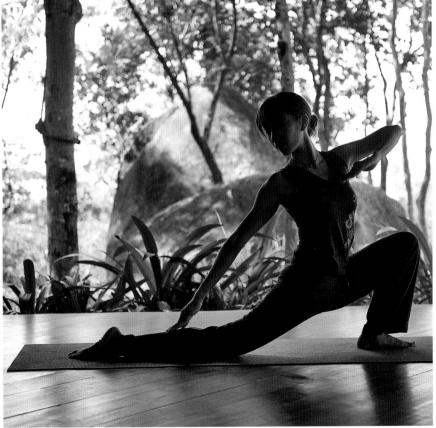

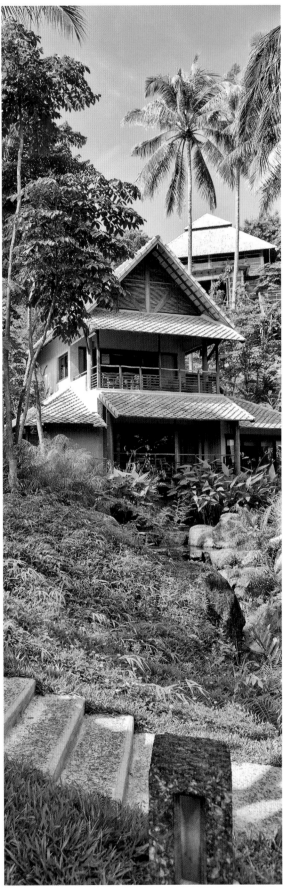

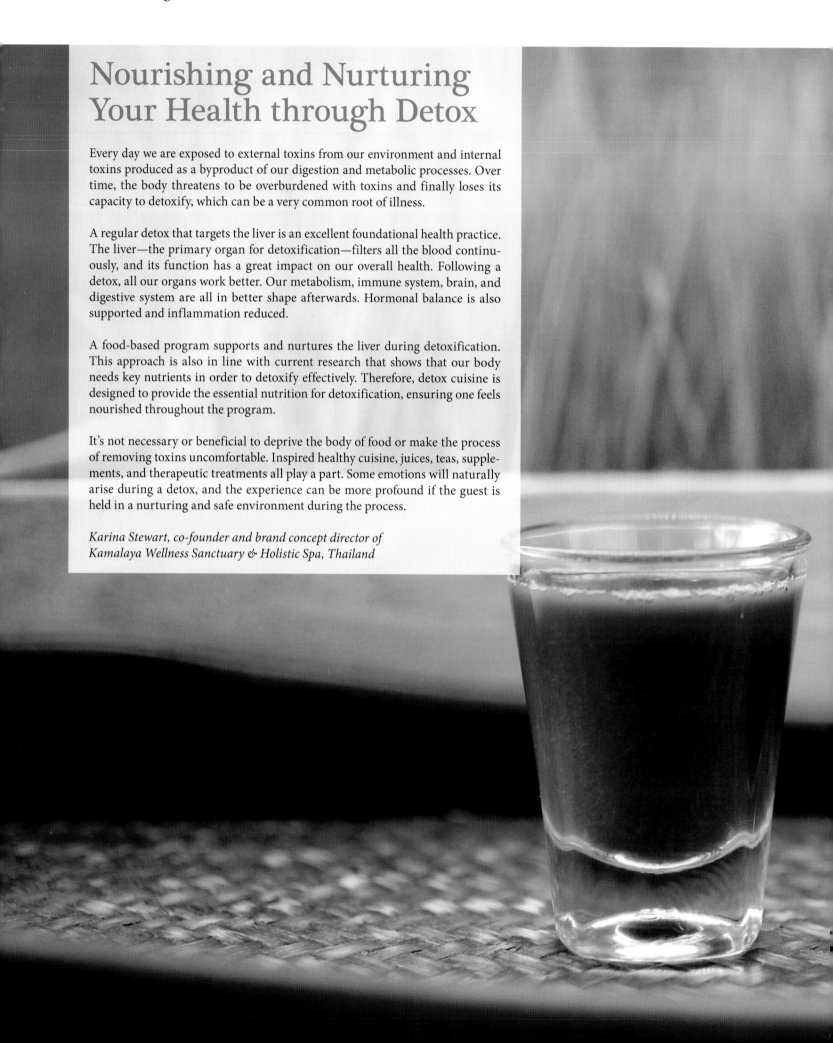

Nourishing and Nurturing Your Health through Detox

Every day we are exposed to external toxins from our environment and internal toxins produced as a byproduct of our digestion and metabolic processes. Over time, the body threatens to be overburdened with toxins and finally loses its capacity to detoxify, which can be a very common root of illness.

A regular detox that targets the liver is an excellent foundational health practice. The liver—the primary organ for detoxification—filters all the blood continuously, and its function has a great impact on our overall health. Following a detox, all our organs work better. Our metabolism, immune system, brain, and digestive system are all in better shape afterwards. Hormonal balance is also supported and inflammation reduced.

A food-based program supports and nurtures the liver during detoxification. This approach is also in line with current research that shows that our body needs key nutrients in order to detoxify effectively. Therefore, detox cuisine is designed to provide the essential nutrition for detoxification, ensuring one feels nourished throughout the program.

It's not necessary or beneficial to deprive the body of food or make the process of removing toxins uncomfortable. Inspired healthy cuisine, juices, teas, supplements, and therapeutic treatments all play a part. Some emotions will naturally arise during a detox, and the experience can be more profound if the guest is held in a nurturing and safe environment during the process.

Karina Stewart, co-founder and brand concept director of
Kamalaya Wellness Sanctuary & Holistic Spa, Thailand

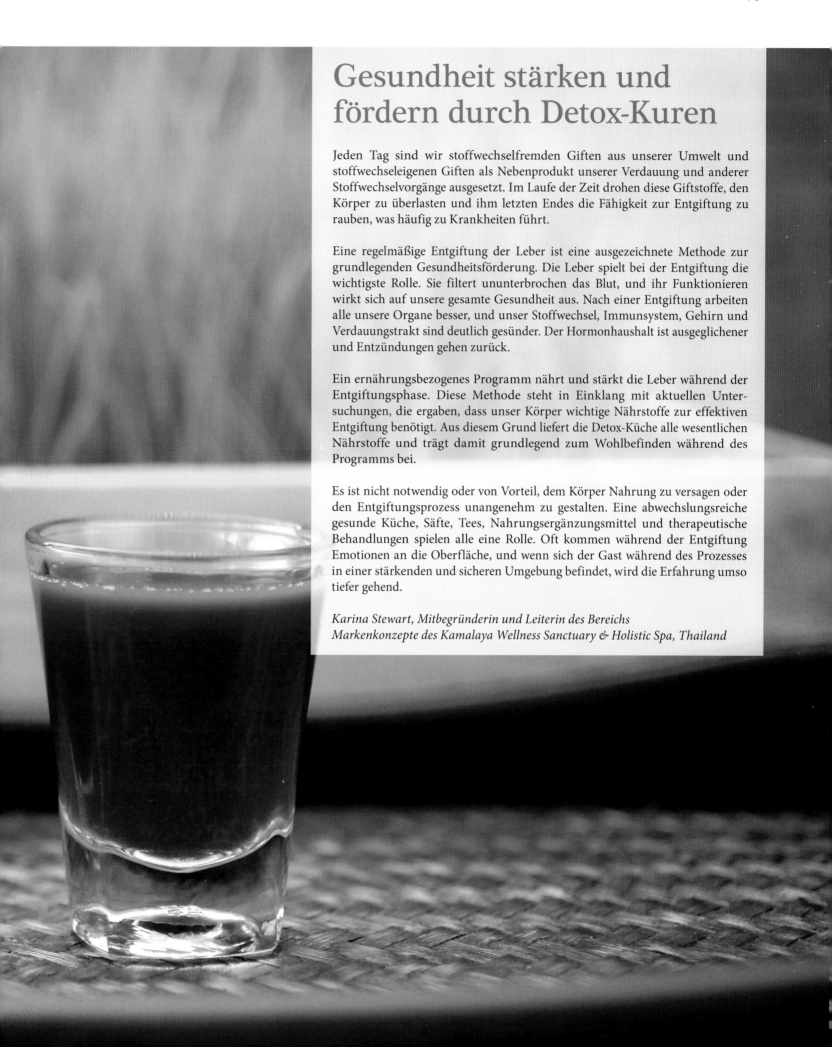

Gesundheit stärken und fördern durch Detox-Kuren

Jeden Tag sind wir stoffwechselfremden Giften aus unserer Umwelt und stoffwechseleigenen Giften als Nebenprodukt unserer Verdauung und anderer Stoffwechselvorgänge ausgesetzt. Im Laufe der Zeit drohen diese Giftstoffe, den Körper zu überlasten und ihm letzten Endes die Fähigkeit zur Entgiftung zu rauben, was häufig zu Krankheiten führt.

Eine regelmäßige Entgiftung der Leber ist eine ausgezeichnete Methode zur grundlegenden Gesundheitsförderung. Die Leber spielt bei der Entgiftung die wichtigste Rolle. Sie filtert ununterbrochen das Blut, und ihr Funktionieren wirkt sich auf unsere gesamte Gesundheit aus. Nach einer Entgiftung arbeiten alle unsere Organe besser, und unser Stoffwechsel, Immunsystem, Gehirn und Verdauungstrakt sind deutlich gesünder. Der Hormonhaushalt ist ausgeglichener und Entzündungen gehen zurück.

Ein ernährungsbezogenes Programm nährt und stärkt die Leber während der Entgiftungsphase. Diese Methode steht in Einklang mit aktuellen Untersuchungen, die ergaben, dass unser Körper wichtige Nährstoffe zur effektiven Entgiftung benötigt. Aus diesem Grund liefert die Detox-Küche alle wesentlichen Nährstoffe und trägt damit grundlegend zum Wohlbefinden während des Programms bei.

Es ist nicht notwendig oder von Vorteil, dem Körper Nahrung zu versagen oder den Entgiftungsprozess unangenehm zu gestalten. Eine abwechslungsreiche gesunde Küche, Säfte, Tees, Nahrungsergänzungsmittel und therapeutische Behandlungen spielen alle eine Rolle. Oft kommen während der Entgiftung Emotionen an die Oberfläche, und wenn sich der Gast während des Prozesses in einer stärkenden und sicheren Umgebung befindet, wird die Erfahrung umso tiefer gehend.

Karina Stewart, Mitbegründerin und Leiterin des Bereichs Markenkonzepte des Kamalaya Wellness Sanctuary & Holistic Spa, Thailand

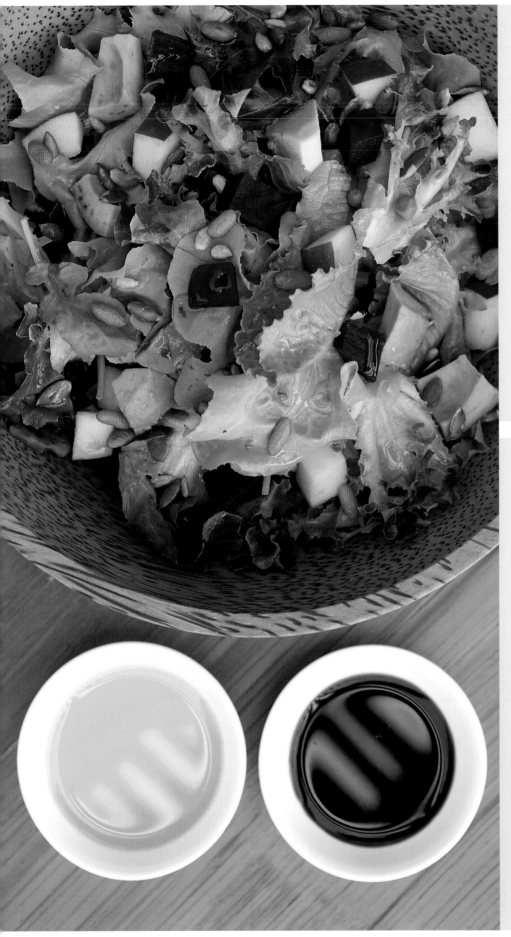

Salad
› 40 g baby cos lettuce, picked & washed
› 40 g green oak lettuce, picked & washed
› 40 g red oak lettuce, picked & washed
› 20 g rocket salad, picked & washed
› 60 g rose apple, peeled and cubed
› 60 g avocado flesh, cubed
› 100 g beetroot, cooked, peeled & cubed
› 10 g pumpkin seeds
› 10 g sunflower seeds
› 5 g flax seed, ground
› 10 g wolfberries (goji berries)

Wasabi Dressing
› 120 ml coconut water
› 80 ml apple cider vinegar
› 100 ml virgin olive oil
› to taste wasabi powder
› to taste lime juice

Serves 2

Salat
› 40 g Mini-Romana, gepflückt & gewaschen
› 40 g grüner Eichblattsalat, gepflückt & gewaschen
› 40 g roter Eichblattsalat, gepflückt & gewaschen
› 20 g Rucola, gepflückt & gewaschen
› 60 g Rosenapfel, geschält & gewürfelt
› 60 g Avocado, gewürfelt
› 100 g Rote Bete, gekocht, geschält & gewürfelt
› 10 g Kürbiskerne
› 10 g Sonnenblumenkerne
› 5 g Leinsamen, gemahlen
› 10 g Wolfsbeeren (Goji-Beeren)

Wasabi-Sauce
› 120 ml Kokoswasser
› 80 ml Apfelessig
› 100 ml natives Olivenöl
› nach Geschmack Wasabi-Pulver
› nach Geschmack Limettensaft

Für 2 Personen

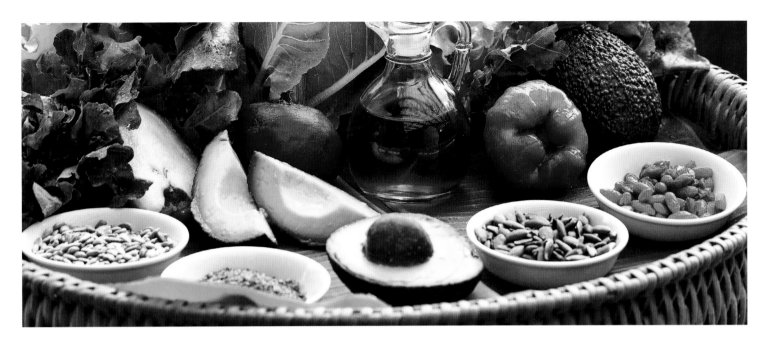

Detox Garden Salad with Wasabi Dressing

Method

To prepare dressing, place all ingredients, except olive oil, into a blender. Blend on medium setting for about 30 seconds. Switch to the lowest setting, and very slowly pour the olive oil into the blender. Add the oil slowly, otherwise the dressing will separate. Prepare the salad. Tear the baby cos, green oak, and red oak leaves into bite-size pieces. Leave the rocket leaves whole. Place all the salad leaves in a large salad bowl and toss lightly.

Sprinkle the salad leaf mix with the rose apple, avocado, beetroot, seeds, and wolfberries. Lightly lift the salad with your fingers to distribute the ingredients.

Drizzle with salad dressing just before serving.

Health Benefits

Wolfberry, also known as goji berry, is traditionally regarded as one of the most nutrient dense and important medicinal herbs in China. Recent scientific research has resulted in its often being touted as a "super food." As an excellent source of micronutrients it has many medicinal benefits including among others strengthened immune system function and protection of liver cells. Due to its high antioxidant activity goji berries are believed to slow down the aging process.

Detox-Gartensalat mit Wasabi-Sauce

Zubereitung

Für die Sauce alle Zutaten mit Ausnahme des Olivenöls in einen Küchenmixer geben. Bei mittlerer Stärke circa 30 Sekunden lang mixen. Auf niedrigster Stufe ganz langsam das Olivenöl dazugeben. Gießen Sie das Öl langsam hinzu, da es sich sonst nicht mit der Sauce vermischt. Für den Salat den Mini-Romana und den grünen und roten Eichblattsalat in mundgerechte Stücke zupfen. Den Rucola ganz lassen. Die Salatblätter in eine große Salatschüssel geben und vorsichtig mischen.

Darüber die Rosenäpfel, Avocado, Rote Bete, Kerne und Wolfsbeeren streuen. Vermengen Sie die Zutaten, indem Sie den Salat leicht mit den Fingern anheben.

Kurz vorm Servieren mit Salatsauce beträufeln.

Gesundheitlicher Nutzen

Die Wolfsbeere, auch bekannt als Goji-Beere, gilt traditionell als eines der nährstoffreichsten und wichtigsten Heilkräuter in China. Sie wird angesichts aktueller wissenschaftlicher Ergebnisse häufig als „Superfood" angepriesen. Goji-Beeren sind außerordentlich reich an wichtigen Nähr- und Vitalstoffen und haben daher vielerlei medizinischen Nutzen. So stärken sie unter anderem das Immunsystem und schützen die Leberzellen. Aufgrund ihrer anti-entzündlichen Wirkung wird zudem angenommen, dass sie den Alterungsprozess verlangsamen.

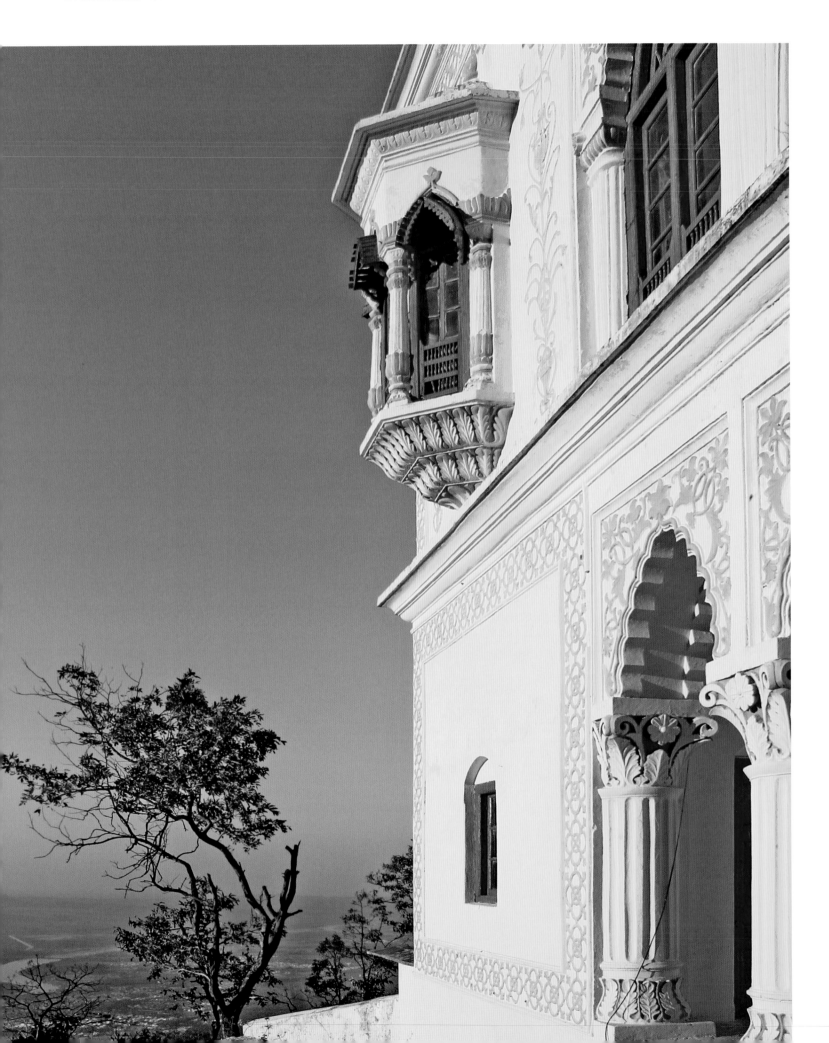

Achieving Bliss through Yoga and Ayurveda

Durch Yoga und Ayurveda zur Glückseligkeit

Ananda In The Himalayas

Ananda means bliss. It fills travelers who see the breathtaking view of the sacred Ganges and the Himalaya mountains from the Ayurvedic spa. Once the residence of a maharaja, the resort lies in the foothills of the mysterious mountain range, surrounded by the timeless traditions of Indian mysticism. With a focus on the Indian sciences of yoga and Ayurveda, the spa blends thousand-year-old therapies with modern spa technology. For years, it has topped the list of the world's best spas and features renowned yoga instructors. The guest's personal needs and health goals form the basis of tailor-made therapies and activities. From stress relief, detoxification, and deep relaxation to healthier eating and exercise habits—everyone finds a new path to well-being up here on the roof of the world. Incidentally, the yoga hall lies next to a small room, where the Indian saint, Anandamayi Ma, once spent her summers. It is truly a magical place for meditation!

Ananda bedeutet Seligkeit. Damit ist der Reisende erfüllt beim atemberaubenden Blick vom Ayurveda-Spa auf den heiligen Ganges und die Berge des Himalaya. Die einstige Residenz eines Maharadschas liegt auf den ersten Anhöhen des geheimnisvollen Gebirges, umgeben von den zeitlosen Traditionen indischer Mystik. Mit Fokus auf die indischen Wissenschaften Yoga und Ayurveda erschafft das Spa eine Synthese von jahrtausendealten Therapien und moderner Spa-Technologie. Seit Jahren führt es die Ranglisten der weltweit besten Spas an und zeichnet sich durch angesehene Yoga-Lehrer aus. Die persönlichen Bedürfnisse und Gesundheitsziele des Gastes bilden die Grundlage für maßgeschneiderte Therapien und Aktivitäten. Destress, Detox, tiefe Entspannung oder gesündere Ess- und Bewegungsgewohnheiten – hier oben auf dem Dach der Welt findet jeder Suchende neue Wege zum Wohlbefinden. Neben der Yogahalle liegt übrigens ein kleines Zimmer, in dem sich einst die indische Heilige Anandamayi Ma im Sommer aufhielt. Ein wahrhaft magischer Platz für Meditationen!

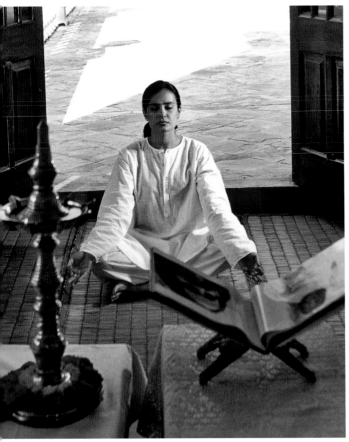

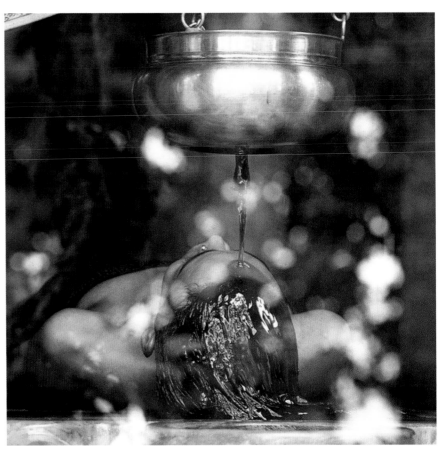

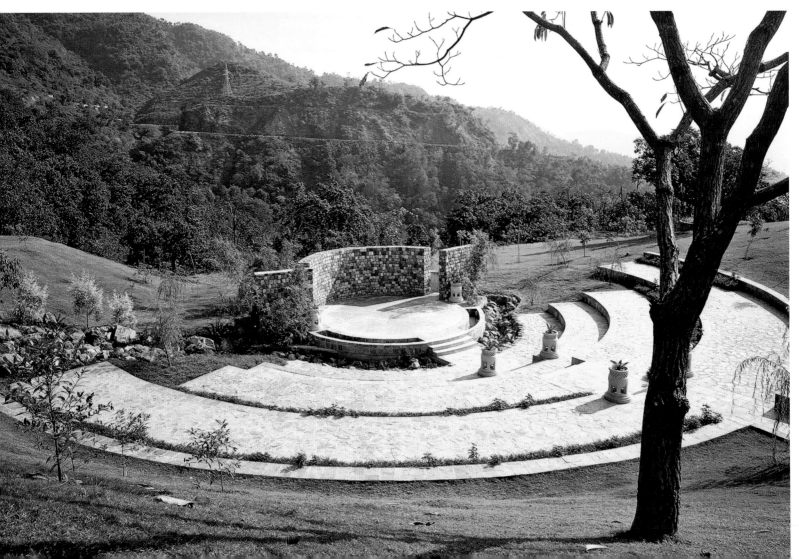

Spa, Health & Other Facilities
24,000 square feet (2,200 square meters) spa facility with 24 treatments rooms, saunas, steam bath, hydrotherapy center, yoga pavilion, gym. Restaurant, beauty salon, boutique, conference rooms, library, amphitheater.

Treatments & Services
79 body and beauty treatments, aromatherapy, Ayurveda, crystal therapy, hot stone massage, hydrotherapy, reflexology, Swedish massage, Thai massage, yoga and meditation. 24-hour front desk, tourist information.

Activities
Art and culture programs, billiards, cooking classes, golf, off-site activities including rafting, trekking, Wildlife Safari.

Rooms
70 deluxe rooms, 5 suites, with view of the Ganges valley or the palace.

Located
162 miles (260 kilometers) north of New Delhi, 3,280 feet (1,000 meters) above Rishikesh. 45 minutes of flight from Delhi to Dehradun plus transfer, 4 hours by train from Delhi to Haridwar plus transfer, 6–8 hours by car from New Delhi to Ananda In The Himalayas.

Narendra Nagar, Tehri – Garhwal
249175 Uttaranchal, India
www.anandaspa.com

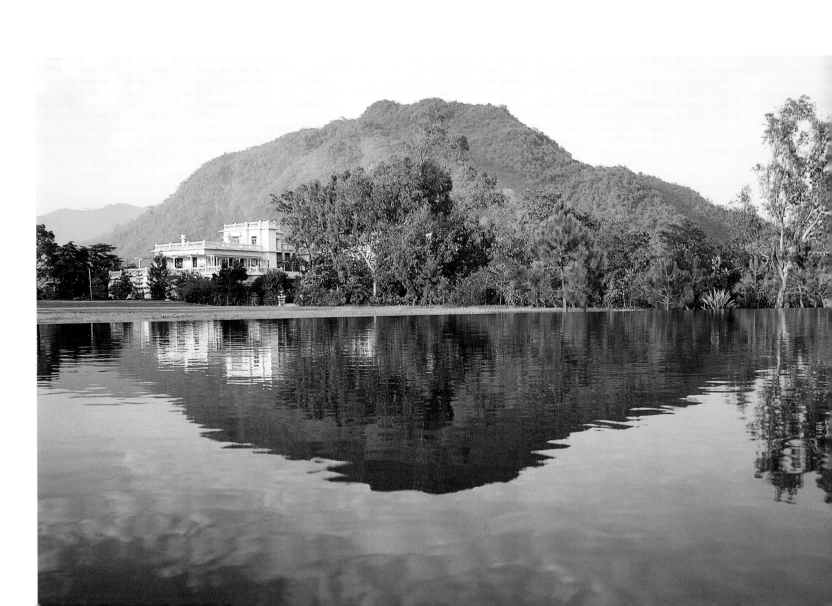

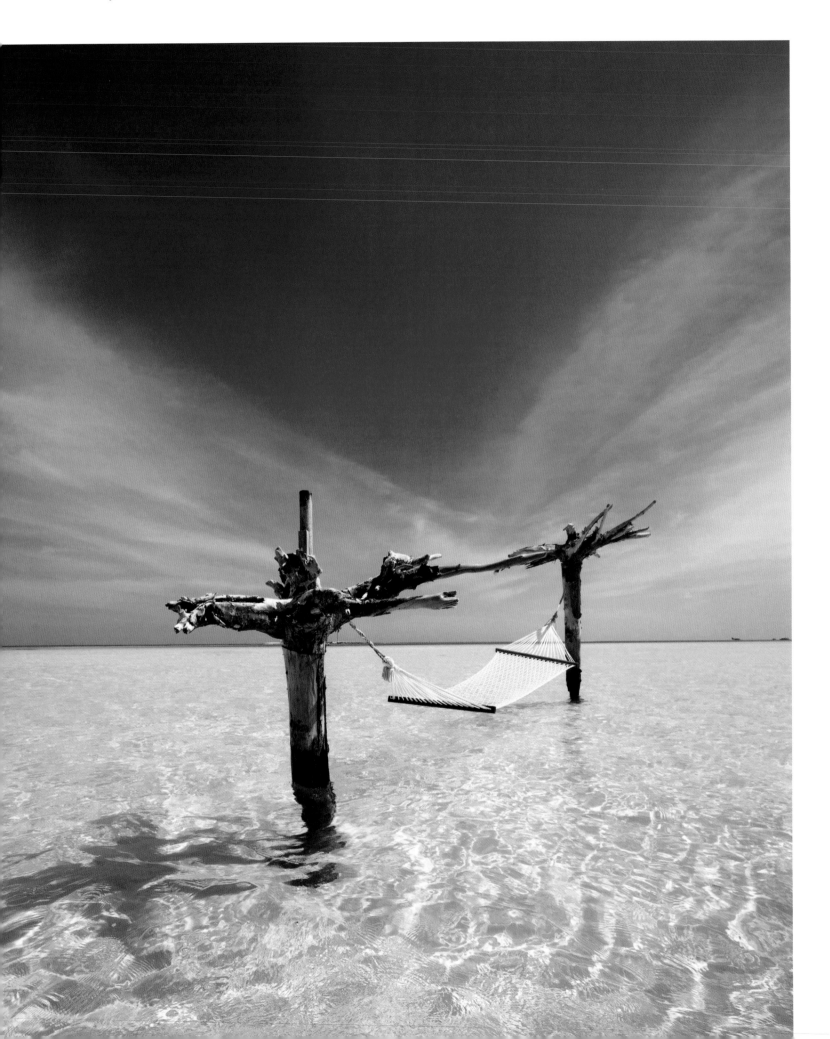

Lankanfushi Island, North Malé Atoll, Maldives

Harmony of Body and Mind in the Indian Ocean

Einklang von Körper und Geist im Indischen Ozean

Gili Lankanfushi

The island of Lankanfushi is situated six nautical miles from Malé, in the middle of a turquoise lagoon. Guests who come to this Robinson Crusoe paradise seeking holistic relaxation will find assistance from their own personal "Man Friday." Taking the name of Robinson's companion, Friday makes the vacation even more pleasant and helps organize excursions, pack your bags, and even assists with childcare. This leaves you time to get in touch with your inner self out on the Indian Ocean—for the wooden villas are not situated *on* the waterfront but on pilings *in* the ocean. You reach your accommodations from the island via jetties, and some are accessible only by boat (thus promising absolute privacy). Each villa offers decks with daybeds, a water garden, and an outdoor shower. On the island, the Meera Spa's staff help guests bring their body and spirit into balance. The services include massages with bamboo rods and warm aromatic oils as well as detoxifying body treatments utilizing hand-harvested seaweed. While your body enjoys this attention, your gaze drifts down through the glass paned floor right into the underwater realm.

Sechs Seemeilen von Malé entfernt, inmitten einer türkisfarbenen Lagune, liegt die Insel Lankanfushi. Wer in diese Robinson-Crusoe-Idylle kommt, um ganzheitlich zu entspannen, wird von seinem persönlichen „Herrn Freitag" dabei unterstützt. Benannt nach Robinsons Freund, macht er den Urlaub noch angenehmer und hilft beim Organisieren von Ausflügen oder beim Kofferpacken und übernimmt sogar die Kinderbetreuung. So bleibt mehr Zeit, mitten auf dem Indischen Ozean zu sich zu finden – denn die hölzernen Villen stehen nicht *am* Wasser, sondern auf Pfählen *im* Meer. Von der Insel aus erreicht man sie über Stege, manche (und das verspricht absolute Privatsphäre) auch nur per Boot. Jede der Unterkünfte bietet Terrassen mit Tagesbetten, Wassergarten und Außendusche. Auf der Insel bringen die Mitarbeiter des Meera Spa Körper und Geist der Gäste in Einklang. Massagen mit Bambusstangen und warmen Aromaölen sowie entgiftende Körperanwendungen mit handgesammeltem Seegras stehen auf dem Programm. Während der Körper genießt, taucht der Blick durch den verglasten Fußboden direkt in die Unterwasserwelt ab.

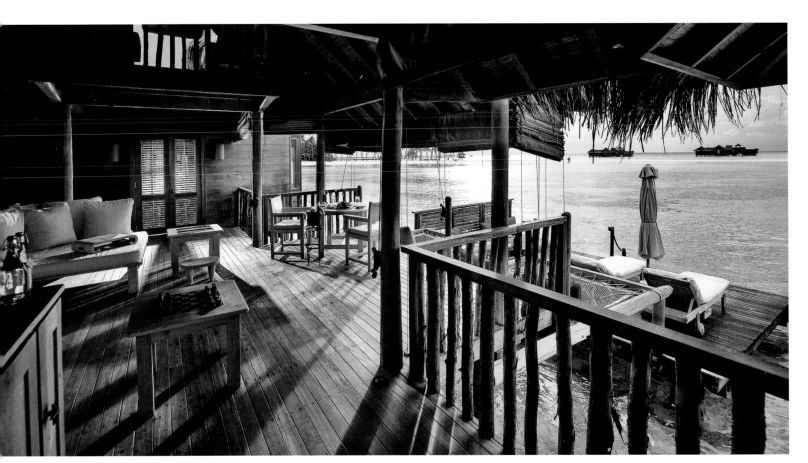

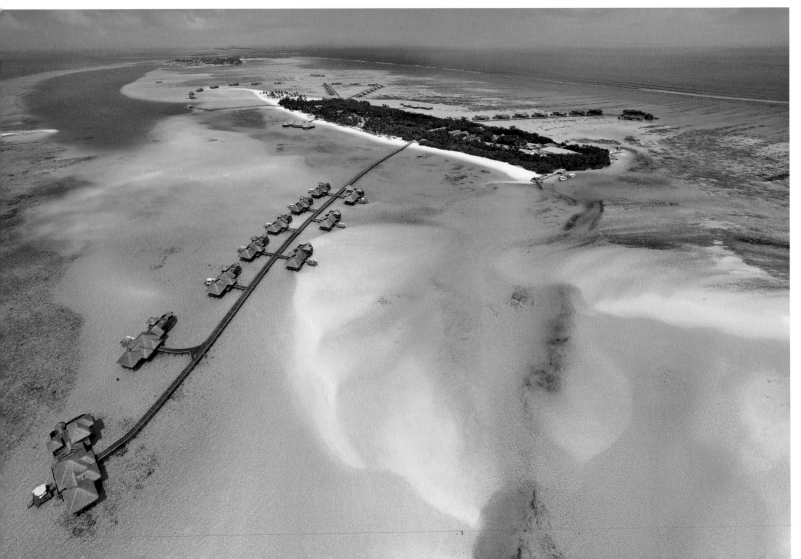

Spa, Health & Other Facilities
Meera spa comprising 7 treatment rooms, outdoor Ayurvedic treatment room, swimming pool with lounges around the beach, gym with latest equipment, yoga pavilion. Over Water Grill, Japanese Fusion restaurant, underground wine cellar.

Treatments & Services
Bamboo massage, Meera facial therapy, Sodashi facial, Tibetan singing bowl massage, Voya Organics.
24-hour front desk, airport transfer, babysitting/childcare, butler.

Activities
Badminton, canoeing, catamaran sailing, scuba diving, dolphin cruises around the atoll, kayaking, morning yoga, sailing, table tennis, tennis, traditional dhoni, volleyball, wakeboard, water-skiing, windsurfing.

Rooms
45 luxurious overwater villas.

Located
On the private island of Lankanfushi in the North Malé Atoll.
20 minutes by speedboat from Malé International Airport.

Lankanfushi Island
North Malé Atoll, Maldives
www.gili-lankanfushi.com

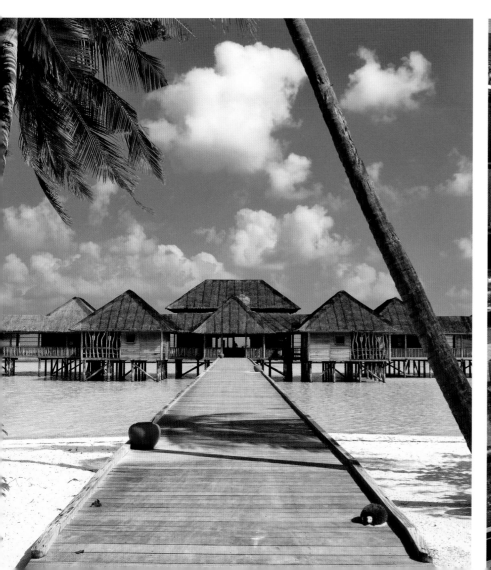

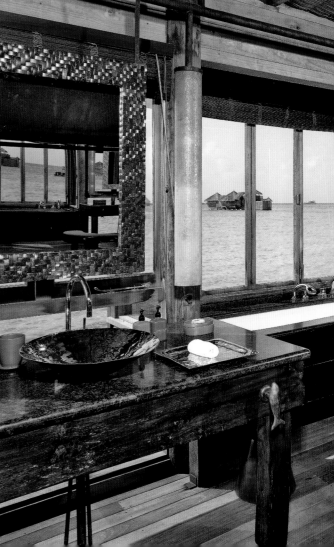

A Timeless Experience under the Sign of the White Antelope

Zeitlosigkeit im Zeichen der weißen Antilope

Al Maha Desert Resort & Spa

Where but in the desert can one find absolute peace and quiet? In an enchanting landscape of sand dunes under a cloudless sky, time loses all meaning. So it's natural that guests also find the right treatments in the Timeless Spa. Rejuvenating rhassoul ceremonies remove the outer signs of time, while detoxifying algae baths make you feel young on the inside. A jet lag recovery treatment gives you back the hours lost while getting here. Therapists with ancient knowledge and healing hands offer treatments that use local products and thereby bring body, mind, and spirit into balance. From the terrace, guests can watch a magnificent sunrise over the desert's red dunes and lose themselves in the immense power of nature. Incidentally, the Al Maha Resort takes its name from the Arabian oryx, a rare species of white antelope that can be seen in the wild.

Wo, wenn nicht in der Wüste, findet man absolute Ruhe und Frieden? In einer märchenhaften Landschaft aus Sanddünen unter wolkenlosem Himmel löst sich die Bedeutung von Zeit in nichts auf. So finden die Gäste denn auch im Timeless Spa die passenden Anwendungen: Verjüngende Rasul-Zeremonien entfernen die äußeren Zeichen der Zeit, entgiftende Algenbäder die inneren. Und die „Jet Lag Recovery" (Jet-Lag-Erholungsbehandlung) holt die Stunden zurück, die die Anreise gekostet hat. Therapeuten mit uraltem Wissen und heilenden Händen benutzen für die Anwendungen einheimische Produkte und bringen auf diese Weise Körper, Geist und Seele ins Gleichgewicht. Von der Terrasse können die Gäste den wundervollen Sonnenaufgang über den roten Wüstendünen beobachten und sich dabei von der immensen Kraft der Natur überwältigen lassen. Namensgeberin für das Al Maha Resort ist übrigens die Arabische Oryx, eine seltene weiße Antilope, die sich in freier Natur beobachten lässt.

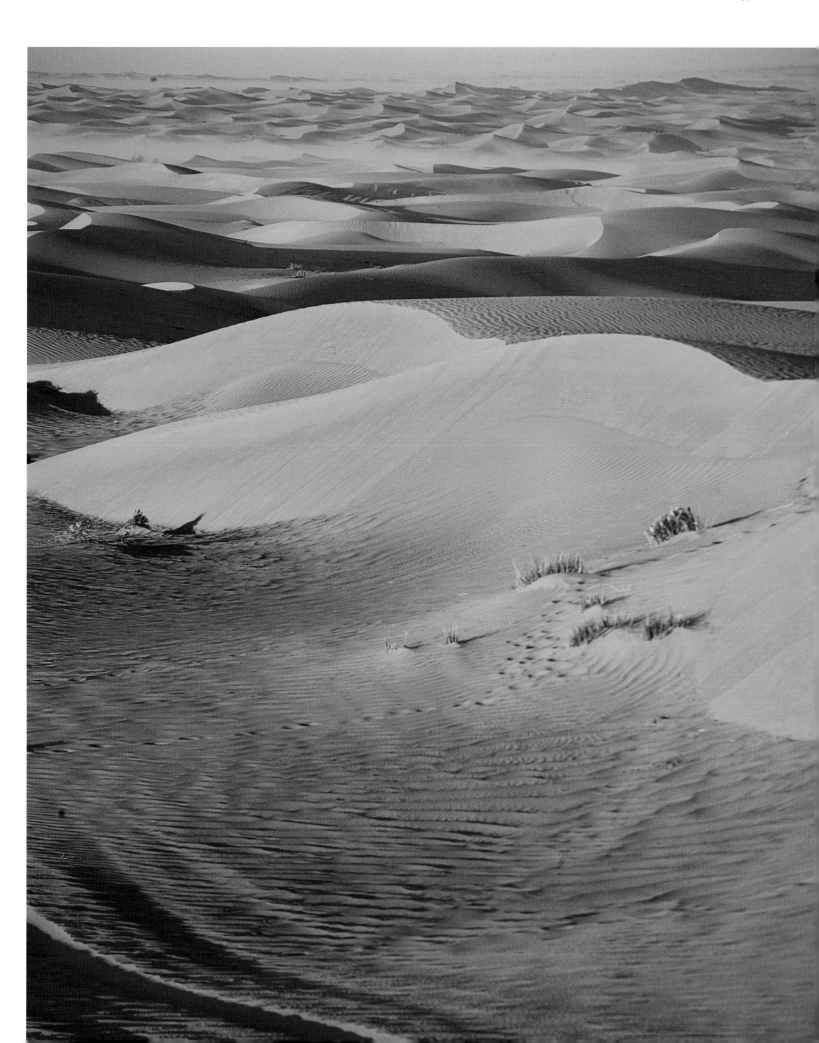

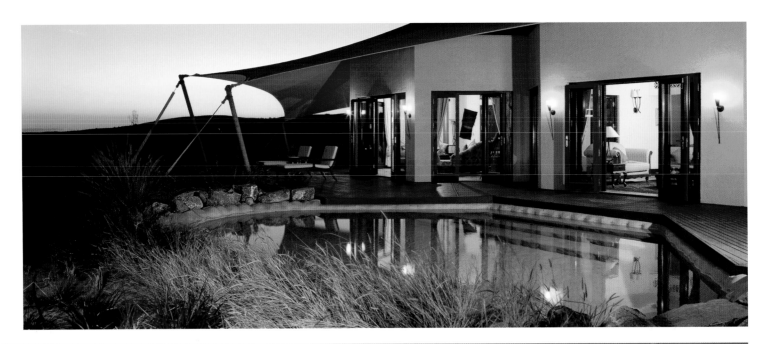

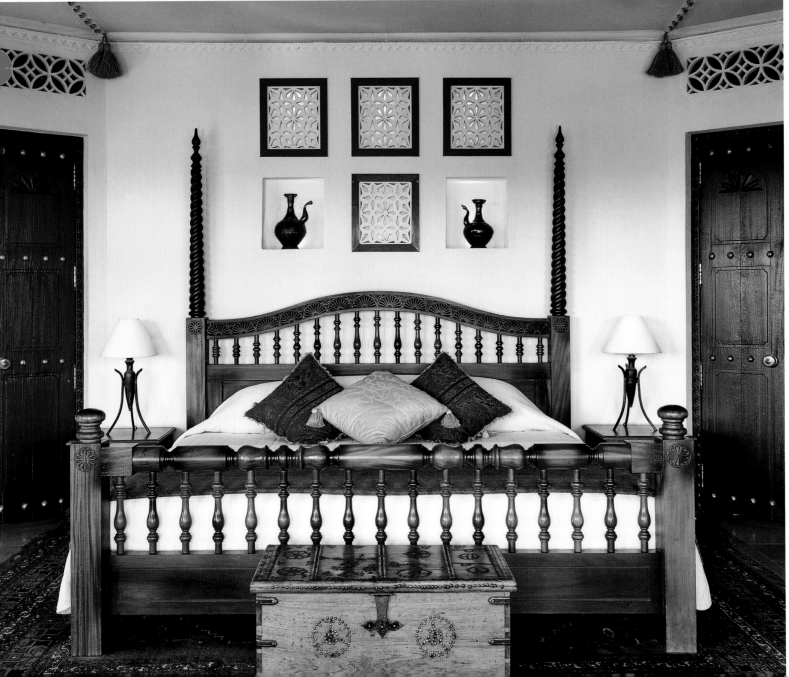

Spa, Health & Other Facilities
Private swimming pools, Jacuzzi, sauna. Bar, lounge, garden surrounded by cascading water features, patio, private decks, event facilities measuring 2,900 square feet (280 square meters), library.

Treatments & Services
Aromatherapy, hammam, Hawaiian massage, hot stone massage, hydrotherapy, reflexology, Reiki, shiatsu, sound therapy, Swedish massage, Thai massage. 24-hour front desk, free parking, free Wi-Fi, laundry service, multilingual staff.

Activities
Archery, bird-watching, camel trekking, desert safaris, falconry, hiking, horseback riding, nature walks, wildlife drives.

Rooms
42 suites with balcony and desert views.

Located
In the Dubai Desert Conservation Reserve. 31 miles (50 kilometers) away from Dubai Airport, Dubai City.

Dubai Desert Conservation Reserve, Dubai – Al Ain Road
11887 Dubai, United Arab Emirates
www.al-maha.com

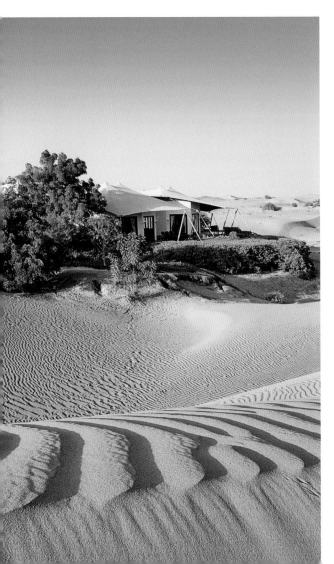

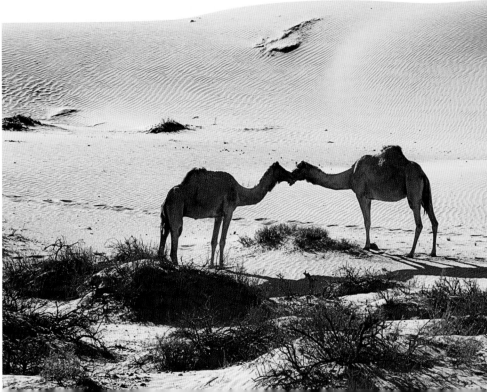

Oasis of Tranquility and Style

Stil(l)ikone

Park Hyatt Dubai

Higher, faster, wider. Dubai is one of the fastest growing cities on earth. Everything has to be bigger, crazier, more golden. In this concrete desert of excess, the Park Hyatt Dubai is a true oasis of tranquility and style. You can feel the desert's stillness here. The resort is situated right on Dubai Creek, far enough from the tremendous city hype that plays out on the other side of the river. Small boats dock at a narrow jetty right in front of the hotel, where you can go for a beautiful walk along the river. The square pool is probably the smallest and simplest anywhere in Dubai, no more than 270 square feet in size. Surrounded by tropical plants and the sound of birds chirping, it radiates an elegance rarely experienced in Dubai. This very principle permeates the entire hotel. To quote Coco Chanel, "simplicity is the keynote of all true elegance." Even the spa is a genuine style icon, one where local and international therapists work the desert stillness into their treatments, and where they use the healing power of real diamonds, rubies, and sapphires. Those who like to meditate will find the tranquility and energy they need at the Park Hyatt Hotel.

Höher, schneller, weiter. Dubai ist eine der am schnellsten wachsenden Städte der Erde. Alles muss noch mehr Gold, noch größer und noch verrückter sein. In dieser Betonwüste der Übertreibungen ist das Park Hyatt Dubai eine regelrechte Oase der Ruhe und des Stils. Die Stille der Wüste ist hier spürbar. Das Resort liegt direkt am Dubai Creek, weit genug entfernt vom gigantischen City-Hype, der sich auf der anderen Flussseite abspielt. An einem schmalen Steg direkt vor dem Hotel halten kleine Boote an. Man kann dort wunderschön am Fluss spazieren gehen. Der quadratische Pool ist wahrscheinlich der kleinste und einfachste in ganz Dubai. Er misst gerade einmal 25 Quadratmeter. Inmitten tropischer Pflanzen und umgeben von Vogelgezwitscher strahlt er eine Klasse aus, wie sie in Dubai selten ist. Und genau dieses Prinzip zieht sich durch das gesamte Haus. Um es mit den Worten Coco Chanels zu sagen: „Simplicity is the keynote of all true elegance." Auch das Spa, in dem einheimische und internationale Therapeuten die Stille der Wüste in ihre Behandlungen einfließen lassen und die Heilkraft echter Diamanten, Rubine und Saphire zum Einsatz kommt, ist eine wahre Stilikone. Wer gerne meditiert, findet im Park Hyatt die nötige Ruhe und Energie dazu.

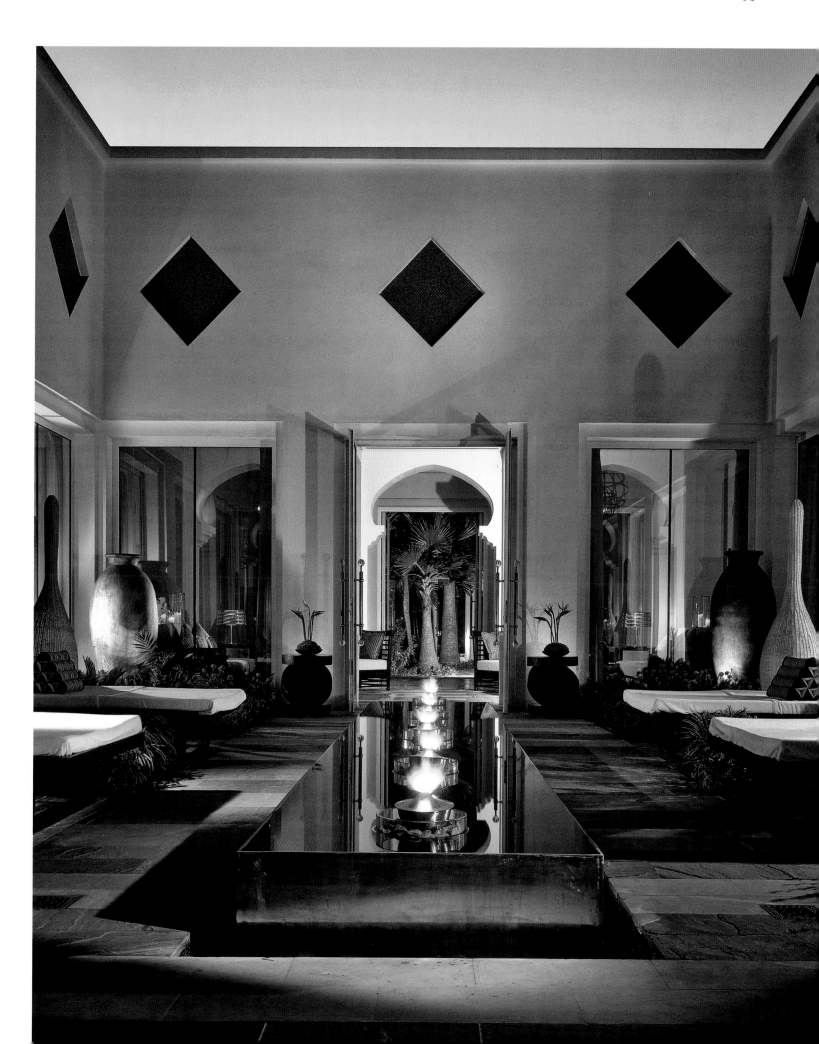

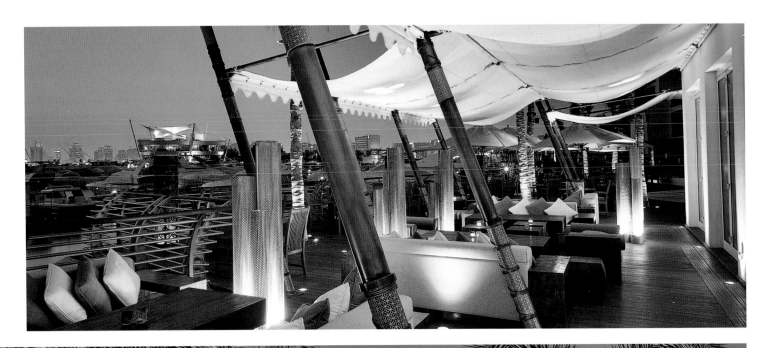

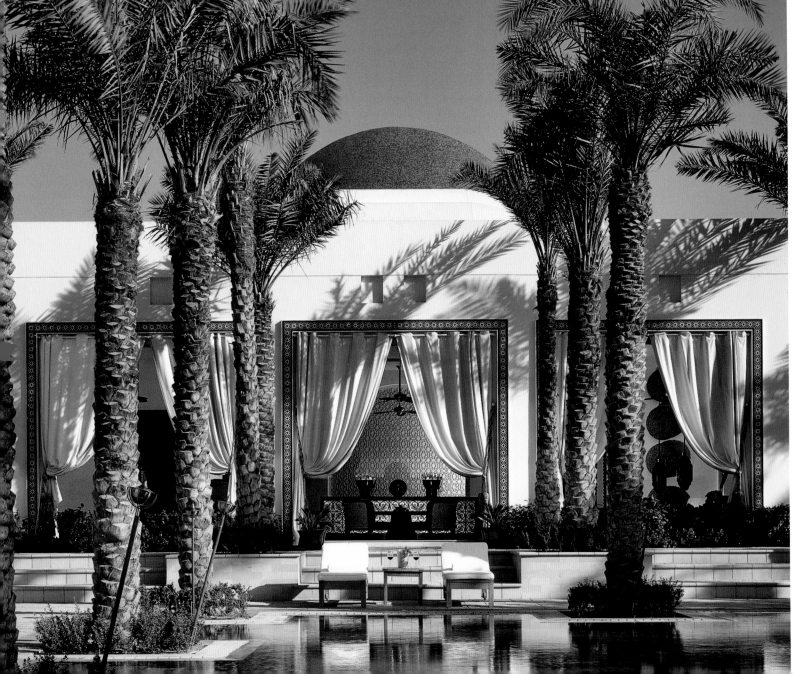

Spa, Health & Other Facilities
8 treatment rooms with private courtyards, 25 meter swimming pool with relaxation area, 4 Jacuzzis, gym with latest equipment, tranquility garden. 7 restaurants, bars, and lounges, full service business center, golf club nearby.

Treatments & Services
Aromatherapy, exclusive rituals, hammam, hot stone massage, luxury massages, reflexology, rejuvenating facials, Swedish massage, Thai massage. 24-hour concierge service, 24-hour in-room dining, housekeeping service (twice daily), laundry and dry cleaning service, valet car parking.

Activities
Bird-watching, boating, golf on the 18-hole championship Dubai Creek Golf Course, jogging, swimming.

Rooms
225 rooms and 35 suites with views of the Dubai Creek and marina, 10 categories.

Located
In Dubai, adjacent to the Dubai Creek Golf and Yacht Club. Just a few minutes from the city center. 2.5 miles (4 kilometers) from Dubai International Airport.

PO Box 2822
Dubai, United Arab Emirates
www.dubai.park.hyatt.com

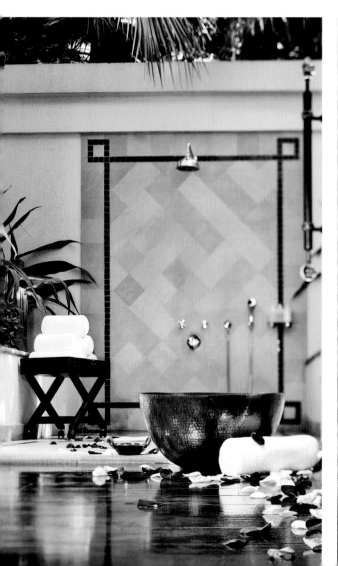

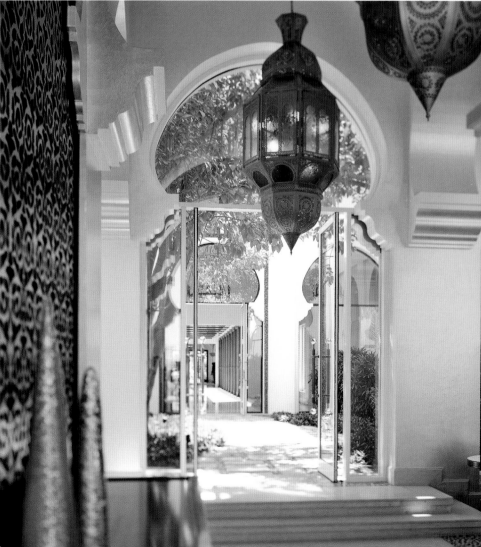

Embracing Freedom

Mut zur Freiheit

Six Senses Zighy Bay

Whether they arrive by paraglider, speed boat, or luxury 4x4, a trip of less than two hours from Dubai, guests of Six Senses Zighy Bay will certainly not want to leave this blissful place quite as fast. Rugged coves, rocky mountains up to 4,500 feet high, beaches, and the sea have lent this area its name, "Norway of the Middle East" —and for good reason. Six Senses, a company known for its spas and environmental friendliness, runs the resort in the style of a traditional Omani village. The villas provide an unforgettable stay, situated so that you can watch a sunrise from the beach—without leaving your villa. The experience appeals to your senses on all levels. Guests can *view* the dramatic mountain landscape or the colorful underwater realm. They will *hear* the early morning song of the myna birds as they work out on the Jungle Gym. *Smell* the fresh fragrance in the Spice Market restaurant. *Taste* delicious Arab specialties prepared by Bedouins in the traditional Shua Shack. *Feel* the sand between their toes. For the sixth sense, visit the spa, which will tempt you with an extrasensory adventure, such as the four-hand Sensory Spa Journey or the Wonders of Oman Journey. In addition, the resort offers five different programs, ranging from a detox package to de-stress and local experiences through adventure and fitness. These individually tailored programs can be taken over three, five, and seven days.

Es ist egal, ob man mit dem Segelflugzeug, Schnellboot oder komfortablem Jeep in weniger als zwei Stunden von Dubai anreist. Sicher ist, dass Gäste des Six Senses Zighy Bay diesen seligen Ort so schnell nicht mehr verlassen wollen. Schroffe Buchten, Felsberge von bis zu 1 400 Metern Höhe, Strand und Meer gaben diesem Ort zu Recht den Namen „Norwegen des Nahen Ostens". Betrieben wird das Resort im Stil eines traditionellen omanischen Dorfes von dem für seine Spas und seine Umweltfreundlichkeit bekannten Unternehmen Six Senses. Für ein unvergessliches Erlebnis sorgen die Villen, deren Lage es ermöglicht, den Sonnenaufgang vom Strand aus zu erleben – ohne die Villa zu verlassen. Die Sinne werden hier auf allen Ebenen angesprochen: Man kann die dramatische Berglandschaft oder die bunte Unterwasserwelt *sehen*. Die Gäste *hören* die Rufe der aufgeweckten Beos bei ihrem Workout im Jungle Gym. *Riechen* frische Gewürze im Restaurant Spice Market. *Schmecken* leckere, arabische Spezialitäten der Beduinen beim traditionellen Shua Shack. *Fühlen* den Sand zwischen ihren Zehen. Für den sechsten Sinn gibt es den Spa-Bereich, der auf eine Reise ins Übersinnliche entführt, zum Beispiel bei der vierhändigen „Sensory Spa Journey" oder der „Wonders of Oman Journey". Zusätzlich bietet das Resort fünf maßgeschneiderte Programme, von Entgiftung und Entspannung bis zu Abenteuer und Fitness, die der Gast für drei, fünf oder sieben Tage buchen kann.

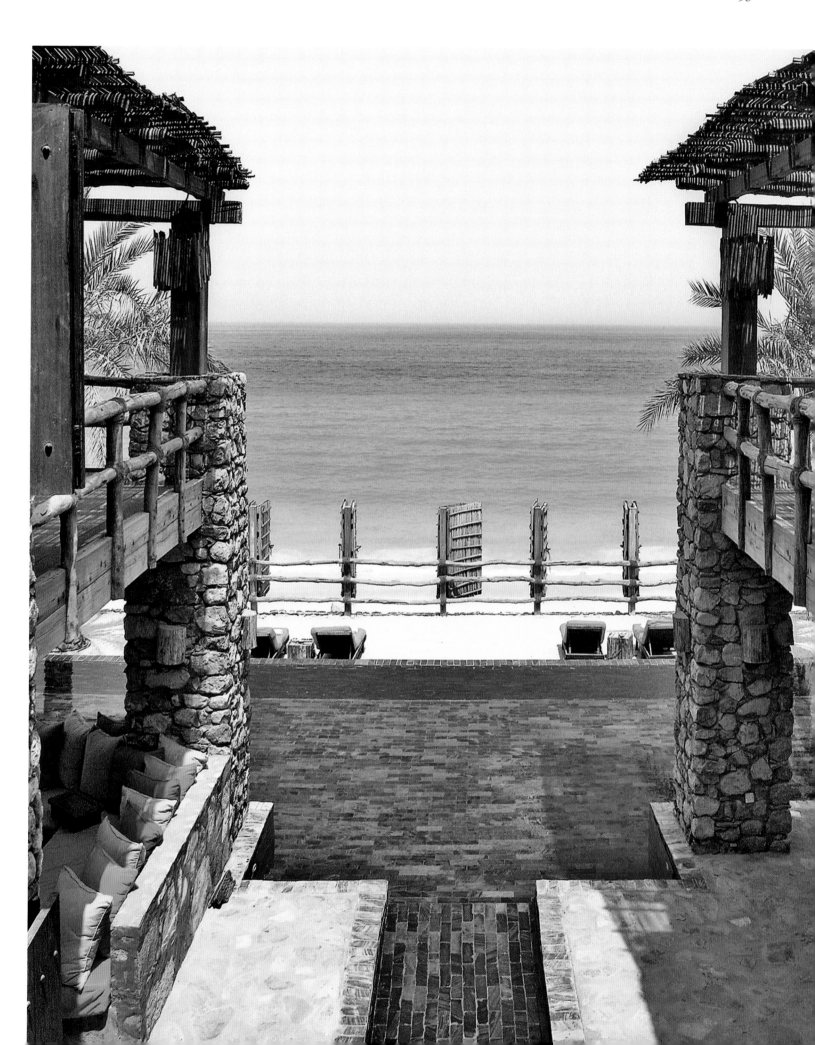

Spa, Health & Other Facilities
Six Senses Spa comprising 9 treatment rooms and 2 hammams, Middle East's only saltwater pool, fitness center, open-air spa pavilion. 3 restaurants, juice bar, Zighy Souk Oman market, private beach, meeting lounge for up to 100 people, library with computer and printer, complimentary Wi-Fi throughout the resort.

Treatments & Services
Asian therapies, bath rituals, body polish and cocoon, daily wellness activities, energy balancing therapies, facial therapies, fitness and wellness consultants, junior journeys, massage therapies, meditation, ready-made packages, sensory therapies, Six Senses treatments, spa beauty, spa journeys, yoga. 24-hour front desk, limousine transfers to and from the airport.

Activities
Biking, bird-watching, canyoning, climbing, cooking classes, cultural tours, cycling, desert and mountain adventures, dhow cruises, scuba diving, fishing, hiking, jogging, kayaking, mountain biking, paraglide and microlight flights, snorkeling, swimming, tennis, wellness seminars, wellness workshops.

Rooms
82 beautifully designed pool villas, available in 1, 2 and 4-bedrooms. 33 beachfront villas. 32,000 square feet (3,000 square meters) 4-bedroom Private Reserve, winner of 2012 Best Hotel Suite/Middle East Hotel Awards.

Located
At the beach of Zighy Bay. 75 miles (120 kilometers) from Dubai.

Musandam Peninsula, PO Box 212
Dibba, Sultanate of Oman
www.sixsenses.com/SixSensesZighyBay

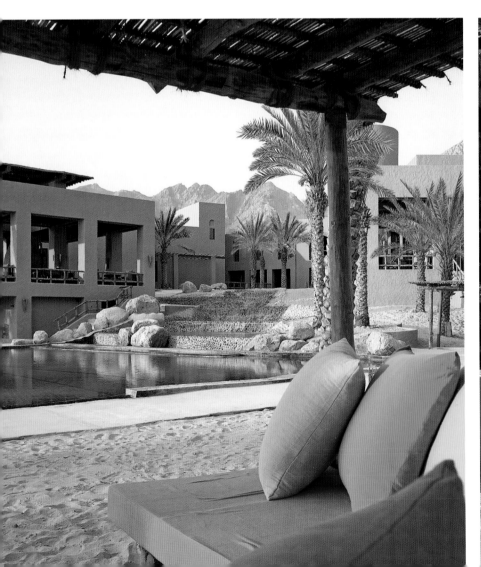
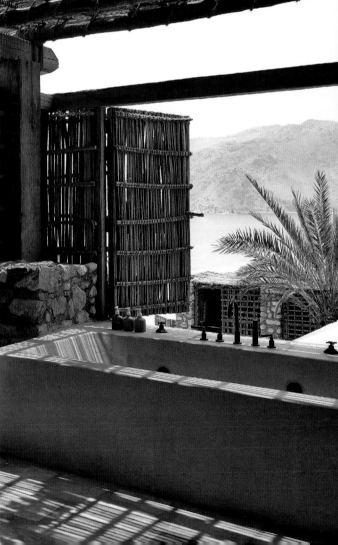

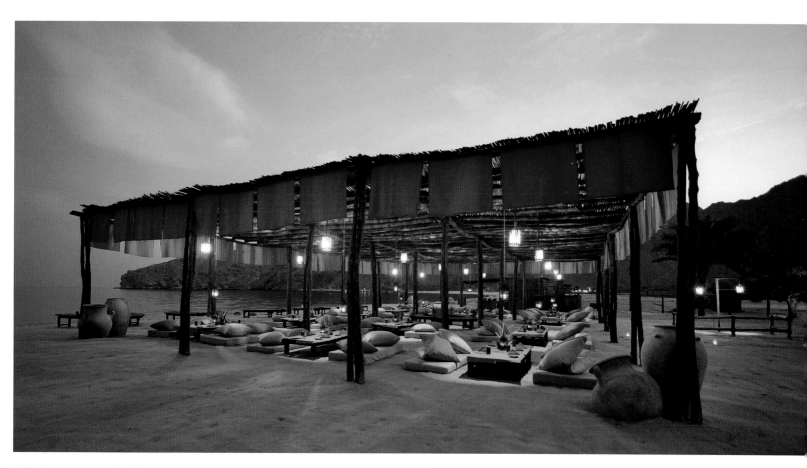

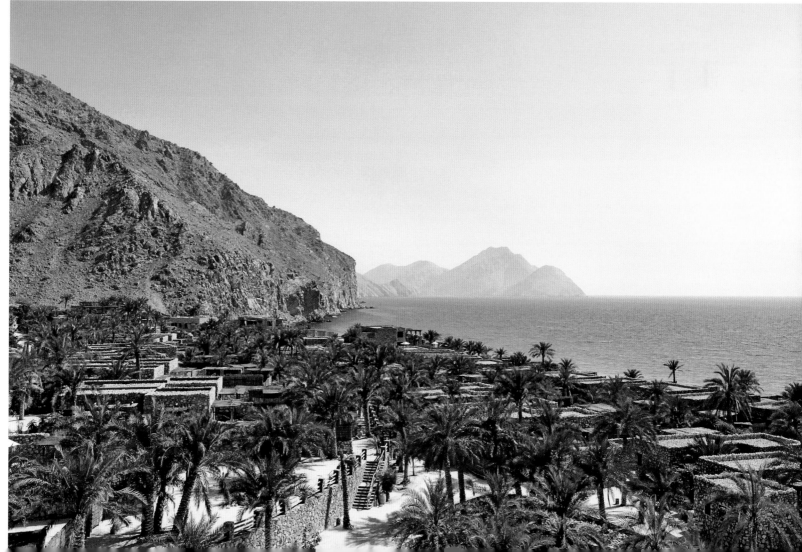

Meditation

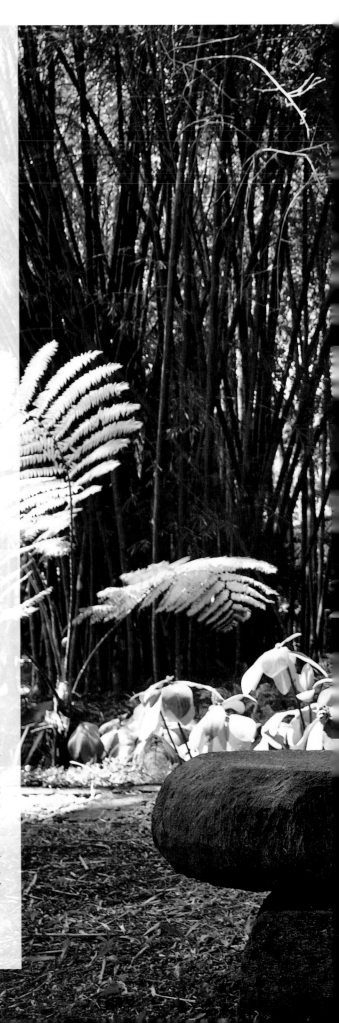

If I had to tell you only one thing about meditation, it would be this: Meditation is your personal experiment, performed in the laboratory of your own mind and body.

Your practice will be inspired by teachers and guided by the practices that the great explorers of meditation have handed down to us. Yet in the end, the form your practice takes is uniquely yours. When you begin your meditation practice you need the structure and direction of an established protocol. Following basic techniques helps you set up the discipline of regular sitting and teaches you how to feel comfortable, how to find inner focus, and keep your mind from running rampant.

As you continue, things will change. You start to catch the meditation current, the inward-flowing slipstream that takes the mind inward. You begin to experience periods of quiet, even contentment. You realize that meditation is actually a natural state and that it will arise on its own if you give it time. In addition, you discover some of the benefits of sitting for meditation—how a practice helps you hold steady in times of emotional turmoil, how creative solutions to problems present themselves naturally when you enter a certain state of quiet.

So, a successful meditation practice requires balancing polarities: focus and letting go, structure and freedom. You need to work with guidelines, but you also need to know when it is time to let go of the "rules" and follow the signals that are coming from your own consciousness. And this requires openness, creativity, and discernment.

One of the best beginning practices is simple mindfulness—paying relaxed attention to the flow of the breathing. Mindfulness of breath is a particularly natural meditation technique, because when you follow the flow of the breath, it automatically causes your mind to turn inside. You can use it not just in seated meditation, but any time you feel the need to feel calmer, more focused, and more relaxed.

Basic Mindfulness of Breath:
Find a time when you can be undisturbed. Sit in a chair or on a cushion, letting your spine be upright but not rigid. If you sit cross-legged, it's important to use a cushion or blankets to support your hips. This will help maintain the upright posture without undue strain on your knees.

With your eyes closed, observe the rise and fall of the breath, noting the coolness of the breath touching your nostrils on the inhalation, and its slight warmth as it touches the nostrils with the exhalation. As you notice thoughts arising, simply note "thinking" and return to your focus on the breath. Another way to practice mindful breathing is by observing the part of your body that moves with it. It might be your upper chest, your diaphragm, or your belly. Instead of trying to "place" the breath, simply observe the breath as it rises and falls.

As you begin a meditation practice, start by sitting for five or ten minutes at a time. If that feels like too long, start with five minutes. Increase your meditation time one minute a day until you've reached twenty minutes. This will gradually create for you a habit of meditating.

Sally Kempton, internationally recognized teacher of meditation
and yoga philosophy and the author of "Meditation for the Love of It"

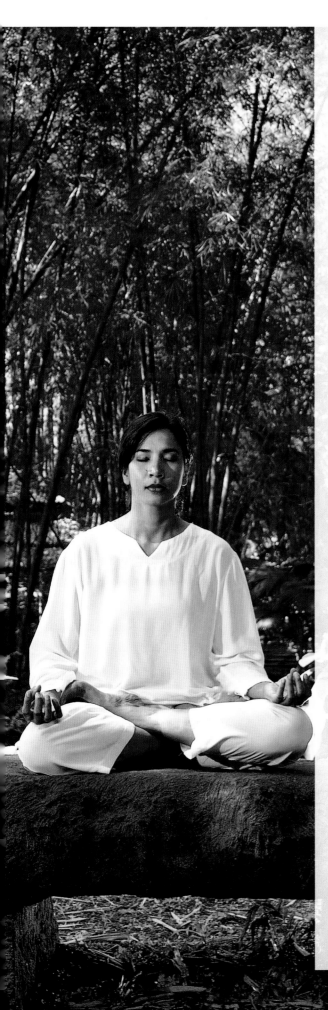

Meditation

Wenn ich Ihnen Meditation in nur einem Satz beschreiben sollte, dann würde er so lauten: Meditation ist Ihr ganz persönliches Experiment, das im Labor Ihres eigenen Geistes und Körpers stattfindet.

Ihre Übungen sind an der Tradition der großen Meister der Meditation orientiert und von Ihren Lehrern inspiriert. Doch letztendlich werden Sie Ihre ganz eigene Meditationsweise finden. Am Anfang brauchen Sie die Struktur bewährter Regeln. Sie werden schnell lernen, sich wohl zu fühlen, sich auf Ihr Inneres zu konzentrieren und nicht gedanklich abzuschweifen.

Im Laufe der Zeit werden sich die Dinge verändern. Sie lassen sich langsam vom Meditationsfluss treiben und spüren den einwärts strömenden Sog, der Ihre Gedanken nach innen richtet. Sie werden Phasen der Ruhe und der Zufriedenheit erfahren. Ihnen wird bewusst, dass Meditation ein natürlicher Zustand ist, der mit Geduld wie von selbst kommt. Die Übungen verleihen Ihnen in Zeiten emotionaler Aufruhr Stabilität, und kreative Lösungen für Probleme zeigen sich in einem Zustand der Ruhe ganz spontan.

Erfolgreiches Meditieren erfordert Gleichgewicht: Konzentrieren und Loslassen, Struktur und Freiheit. Sie brauchen Richtlinien und müssen gleichzeitig wissen, wann der richtige Zeitpunkt gekommen ist, die „Regeln" beiseite zu schieben und den Signalen des eigenen Bewusstseins zu folgen. Dazu bedarf es Offenheit, Kreativität und Urteilsvermögen.

Eine der besten Übungen für Anfänger ist ganz einfach Achtsamkeit. Achten Sie entspannt auf den Rhythmus Ihres Atems. Der Geist richtet sich automatisch nach innen, wenn man sich auf die Atmung konzentriert. Diese Technik können Sie immer und überall üben, wenn Sie das Bedürfnis nach mehr Ruhe, Konzentration und Entspannung verspüren.

Nehmen Sie sich einen Moment ungestörter Zeit. Setzen Sie sich auf einen Stuhl oder ein Kissen und sitzen Sie gerade, aber versteifen Sie sich nicht. Im Schneidersitz ist es wichtig, ein Kissen oder Decken zur Entlastung der Hüften zu Hilfe zu nehmen. Dadurch sitzen Sie weiterhin aufrecht, ohne die Knie übermäßig zu beanspruchen.

Beobachten Sie mit geschlossenen Augen das Ein- und Ausströmen Ihrer Atmung. Dabei werden Sie merken, wie kühl Ihr Atem beim Einatmen ist und wie warm, wenn er beim Ausatmen durch die Nasenlöcher streicht. Sollten sich Gedanken einstellen, nehmen Sie sie einfach nur als „Gedanken" wahr und kehren Sie wieder zur Beobachtung Ihrer Atmung zurück. Ein anderer Weg, um achtsames Atmen zu lernen, ist die Beobachtung des Körperteils, der sich bei der Atmung bewegt. Das kann der Brustkorb, Ihr Zwerchfell oder Ihre Bauchdecke sein. Anstatt die Atmung gezielt an einen bestimmen Ort zu lenken, nehmen Sie ganz einfach das Heben und Senken wahr.

Wenn Sie mit dem Meditieren beginnen, üben Sie zunächst fünf oder zehn Minuten am Stück. Falls Ihnen das zu lange erscheint, meditieren Sie nur fünf Minuten. Meditieren Sie jeden Tag eine Minute länger, bis Sie zwanzig Minuten erreicht haben. Auf diese Weise wird das Meditieren schrittweise zur Gewohnheit.

Sally Kempton, international anerkannte Meditationslehrerin,
Lehrerin für Yoga-Philosophie und Autorin des Buches
„Meditation – Das Tor zum Herzen öffnen"

The Healing Power of Nature

Natur heilt Mensch

Frégate Island Private

As early as the 16th century, pirates took advantage of Frégate Island's tropical paradise when they came here seeking a safe place to rest after their raids. Today, a nature retreat, with its Rock Spa, is located in this pristine region of the Seychelles. The lush, idyllic nature here is a perfect place for stressed souls. Situated on a plateau, surrounded by the island's green landscape and offering marvelous views, the spa provides treatments that are as exotic as they are relaxing. The spa's staff uses fruit, flowers, and spices that you can even pick yourself before they are applied. Like everywhere on the island, the importance of freshness can be felt in the spa. The special treatments depend on nature's seasonal bounty. On Frégate Island, environmental protection and guests' wishes are in perfect harmony. For example, the island offers its guests the chance to adopt a baby Aldabra giant tortoise. During the breeding season, the endangered Hawksbill turtles also come to the island to lay their eggs beneath the blindingly white sand on the beach, trusting that their hatchlings will be safe here.

Schon im 16. Jahrhundert wussten Piraten das Tropenparadies Frégate Island für sich zu nutzen, als sie nach ihren Raubzügen auf der Suche nach Erholung und Schutz hierher kamen. Heute liegt an diesem unberührten Fleckchen Erde auf den Seychellen das Natur-Retreat mit dem Rock Spa. Die heile, reiche Natur ist ein perfekter Ort für gestresste Seelen. Auf einem Plateau mitten im Grün der Insel und mit herrlichem Weitblick bietet das Spa ebenso exotische wie entspannende Behandlungen an. Dazu werden Früchte, Blumen und Gewürze verwendet, die man vor der Anwendung sogar selbst sammeln kann. Wie überall auf der Insel ist auch im Spa die Frische von Bedeutung: Die Spezialanwendungen richten sich nach dem saisonalen Angebot der Natur. Der Schutz der Umwelt und die Wünsche der Gäste stehen auf Frégate Island im Einklang miteinander. So bietet die Insel ihren Gästen zum Beispiel die Möglichkeit, eine Patenschaft für Babys von Aldabra-Riesenschildkröten zu übernehmen. Auch die gefährdete Echte Karettschildkröte kommt während der Brutsaison hierher, um ihre Eier unter dem blendend weißen Sand am Land abzulegen, im Vertrauen darauf, dass die Brut dort sicher ist.

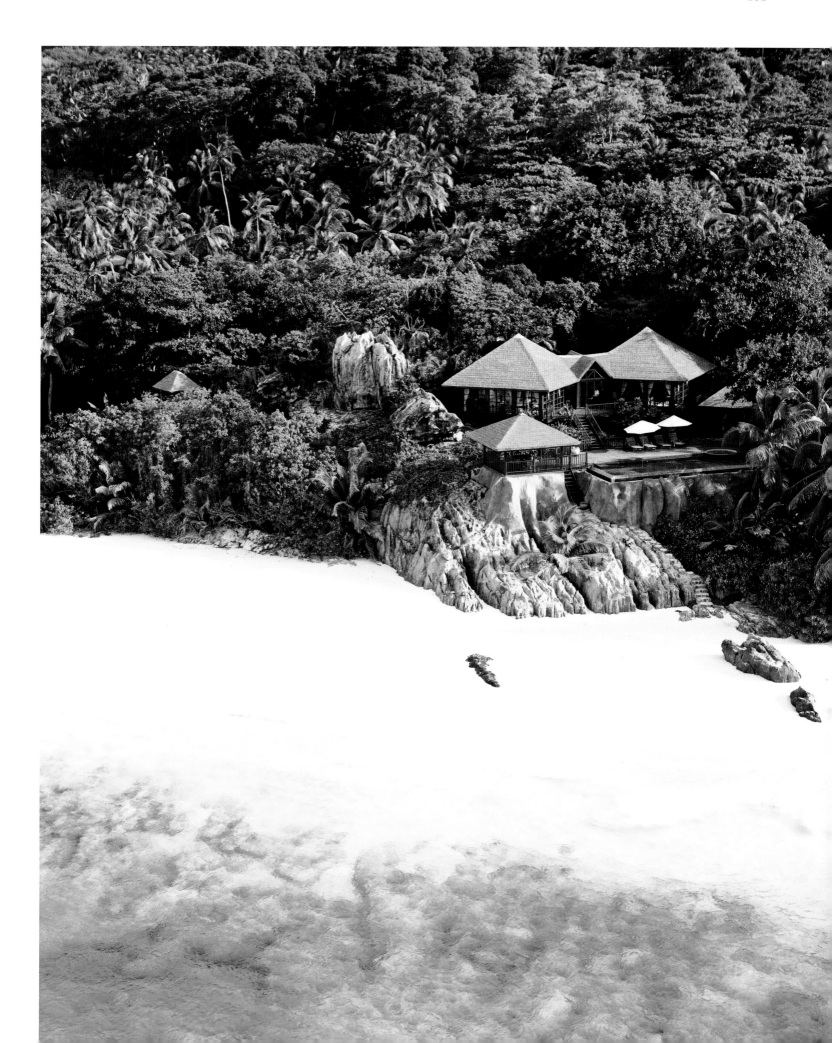

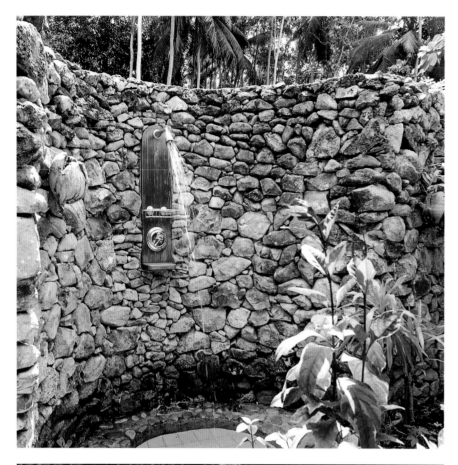

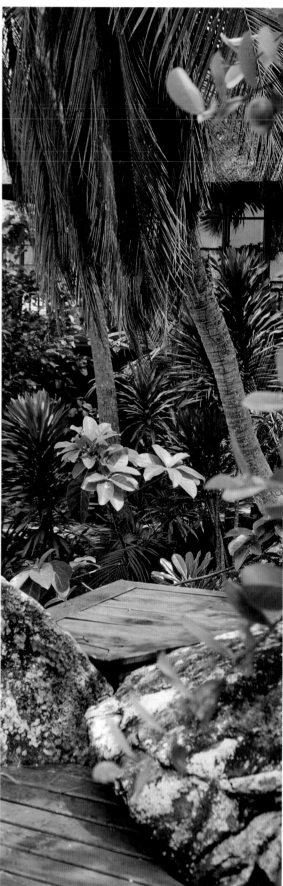

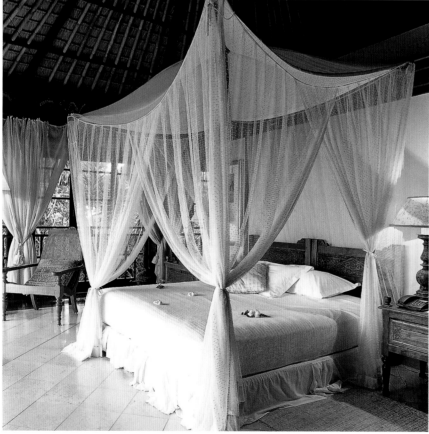

Spa, Health & Other Facilities
The Rock Spa, 2 public pools, gym. Restaurant Frégate House, Plantation House Restaurant, Pirates Bar, Anse Bambous Beach Bar & Restaurant, wine cellar, tree house, private beach limited to 40 guests, tennis court, volleyball/badminton court, golf course, hair salon.

Treatments & Services
Holistic therapies from India, Australia, Polynesia; Mango, papaya, banana, sandalwood body wraps; signature treatments with coconut oil, frangipani, jasmine, papaya massage oils; passionflower, ginger, and lime cleansing wraps; yoga. Babysitting/childcare, private butler service.

Activities
Boccia ball, fishing, golfing, jogging, kayaking, mountain biking, nature excursions, sailing, tennis.

Rooms
16 villas with large infinity pools.

Located
Private island, 20 minutes flight from Mahé.

Frégate Island Private
Mahé Group, Seychelles
www.fregate.com

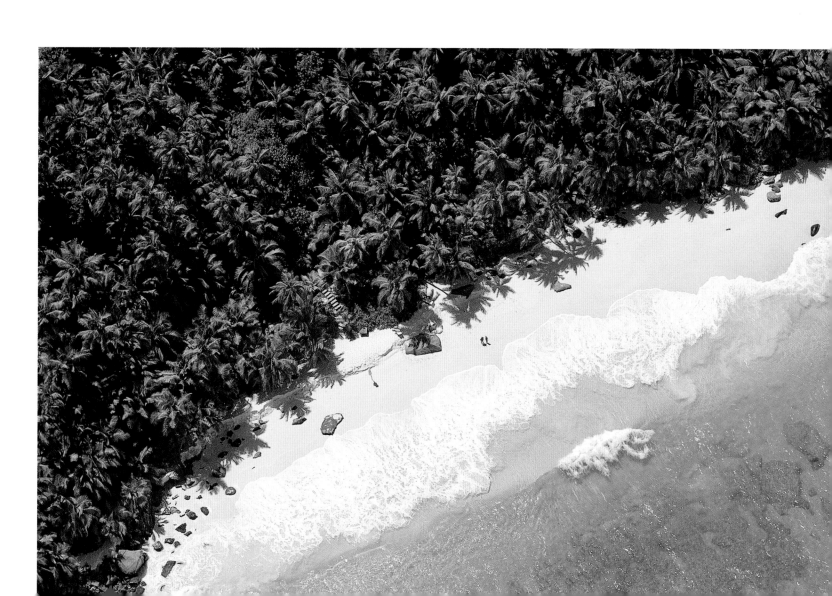

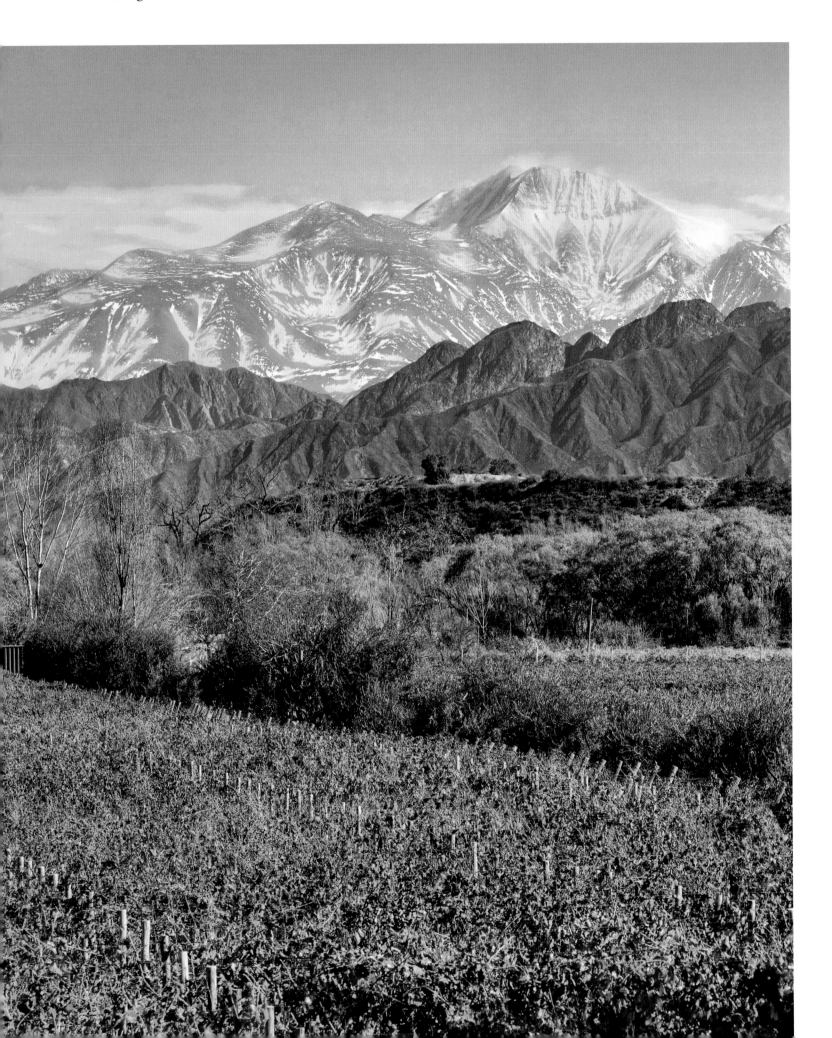

Vistalba, Argentina

The Healing Earth

Wo Erde heilen kann

Entre Cielos

"We looked around and saw the infinite vastness of the land that met a majestic mountain range somewhere in the distance. It was the perfect place to build a resort where people could experience the healing power of nature and connect with their inner selves," explains one of the founders of Entre Cielos. And it was so done. In Mendoza, one of Argentina's best known wine regions, set among vineyards and surrounded by the silhouettes of the Andes, the resort follows the philosophy of "viviendo la vida"—enjoy life with all your senses, see the big picture, touch the sky. One of the guest rooms, the "Limited Edition," is a unique architectonic structure. It is a separate building, mounted on stilts above the vineyard, with gorgeous views of the surrounding area and a skylight that offers a clear glimpse of the star-studded heaven. In keeping with these surroundings, Entre Cielos offers wine therapies that revitalize the body with the phytological power of the grape.

„Wir sahen uns um und erblickten die endlose Weite des Landes, das irgendwo in der Ferne auf eine majestätische Gebirgskette stieß. Der perfekte Ort für ein Resort, in dem Menschen die heilende Kraft der Natur erleben und mit ihrem Selbst in Verbindung treten können", erzählt eine der Gründerinnen von Entre Cielos. Und so geschah es. In Mendoza, einem der bekanntesten Weinanbaugebiete Argentiniens, inmitten von Weinbergen und umgeben von der Silhouette der Anden, lautet die Philosophie: „Viviendo la vida" – das Leben mit allen Sinnen genießen, das große Ganze erkennen, den Himmel berühren. Eine architektonische Besonderheit ist die „Limited Edition", eines der Gästezimmer: ein eigenständiger Bau auf Stelzen über dem Weinberg, der von seiner Terrasse eine herrliche Aussicht auf die Umgebung bietet und durch seine Dachfenster einen unverstellten Blick in den Sternenhimmel freigibt. Passend zu dieser Umgebung bietet das Entre Cielos Weintherapien an, die mit der phytologischen Kraft der Traube eine Neubelebung des Körpers bewirken.

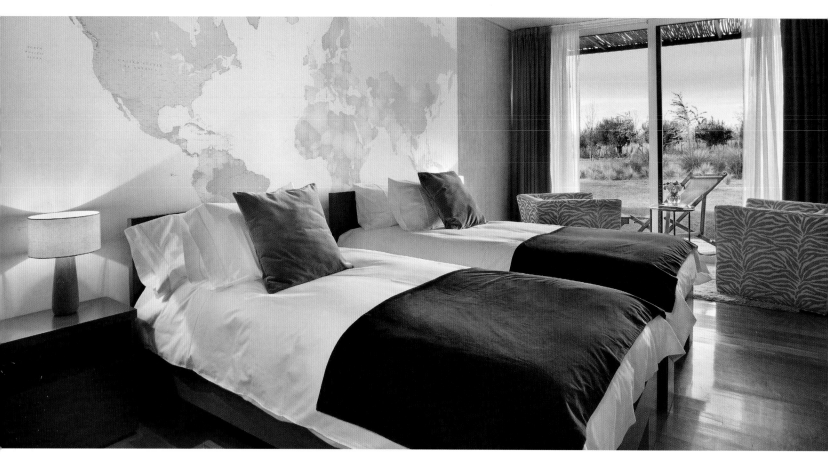

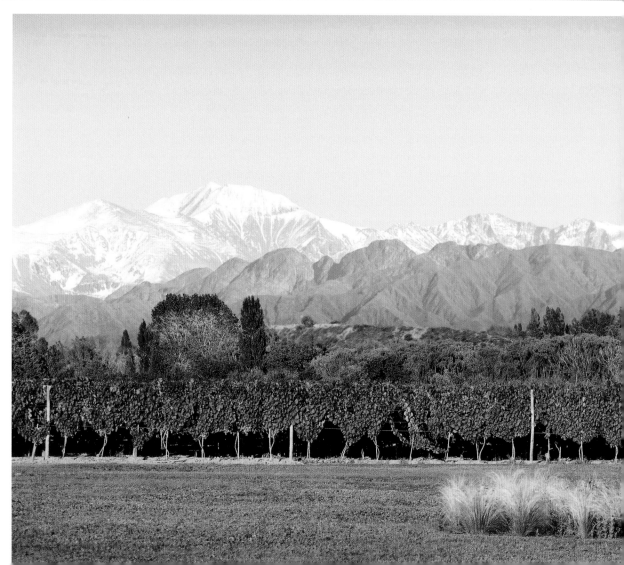

Spa, Health & Other Facilities
Hammam and spa (the first and only in Latin America). Katharina Restaurant, Beef Club, Wine House, Lobby Bar, meeting rooms.

Treatments & Services
Aromatherapy, beauty treatments, hot stone massage, lymphatic drainage, massages, reflexology, Reiki, shiatsu, traditional hammam (6 stages). 24-hour front desk, airport transfer, laundry and ironing service.

Activities
Airplane tours, bird-watching, climbing, fishing, golf, hiking, horseback riding, kayaking, mountain biking, parasailing, rafting, running, skiing (downhill, cross-country), snowboarding, snowshoeing, water-skiing, white water rafting, windsurfing.

Rooms
16 luxury-class rooms.

Located
Luxury Wine Hotel & Spa in the foothills of the Andes in Argentina close to the city of Mendoza.
7 miles (11 kilometers) to Mendoza Airport.

Guardia Vieja 1998
CP. 5509 Vistalba, Mendoza, Argentina
www.entrecielos.com

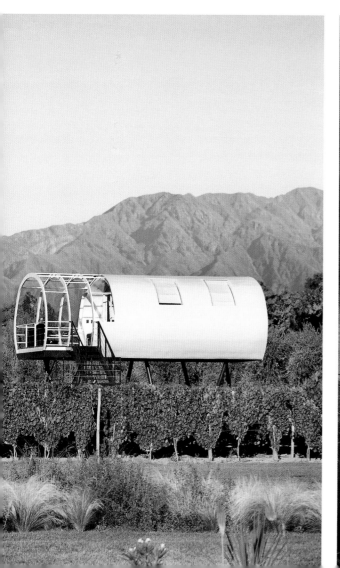

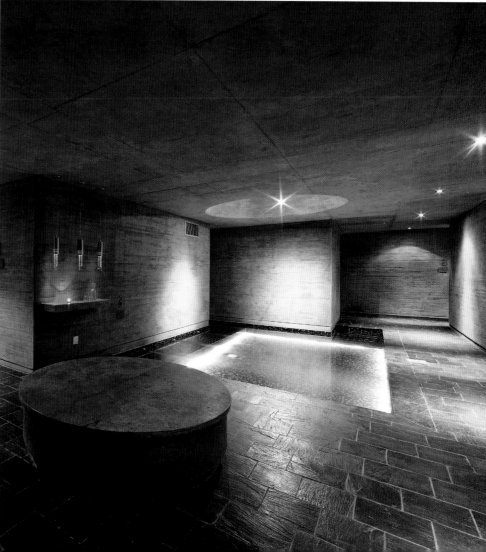

Young Vegetables in Brazil's Oldest Health Spa

Junges Gemüse in Brasiliens ältestem Gesundheits-Spa

Lapinha Spa

Tomatoes that recently hung on the vine and cabbage heads that just came in from the fields now rest on your plate, freshly harvested. Nutrition is an important part of Brazil's first natural health resort, situated in an enchanting landscape. The spa therefore grows vegetables in its own garden—which is visible from the restaurant—without the use of fertilizers or pesticides. Anyone who wants to can help bake bread and make cheese. Every guest receives a personal meal plan, meatless and packed with fiber and vitamins, guaranteeing physical well-being, energy, and a good mood. Special detox and weight loss diets are also available on request. On the farm, surrounded by lush flora, guests learn new, healthy habits and how to adjust their biorhythms. Hydrotherapy by Sebastian Kneipp and natural medicine according to Maximilian Bircher-Benner are additional cornerstones of the 40-year-old health spa. The heat for the resort's main building and pool is generated by renewable resources that come directly from the surrounding fields.

Gerade hingen die Tomaten noch am Strauch und die Kohlköpfe standen auf dem Feld, da liegen sie schon erntefrisch auf dem Teller. Die Ernährung spielt in Brasiliens erstem Naturheil-Resort in traumhafter Lage eine wichtige Rolle. Deshalb wird das Gemüse im eigenen Garten – der vom Restaurant aus sichtbar ist – angebaut, und zwar ohne Dünger oder Pestizide. Wer möchte, kann sogar dabei helfen, das Brot zu backen und den Käse zu machen. Jeder Gast bekommt seinen persönlichen Speiseplan, fleischlos und randvoll mit Ballaststoffen und Vitaminen – ein Garant für körperliches Wohlbefinden, Energie und gute Laune. Bei Bedarf gibt es eine spezielle Diät zum Entgiften oder Abnehmen. Auf der Farm inmitten einer üppigen Pflanzenwelt sollen die Gäste neue, gesunde Gewohnheiten erlangen und ihren Biorhythmus konditionieren. Hydrotherapie nach Sebastian Kneipp und Naturmedizin nach Maximilian Bircher-Benner sind weitere Grundlagen in dem vor 40 Jahren gegründeten Gesundheits-Spa. Die Wärme für das Haus und den Pool der Anlage kommt direkt von den umliegenden Feldern aus nachwachsenden Rohstoffen.

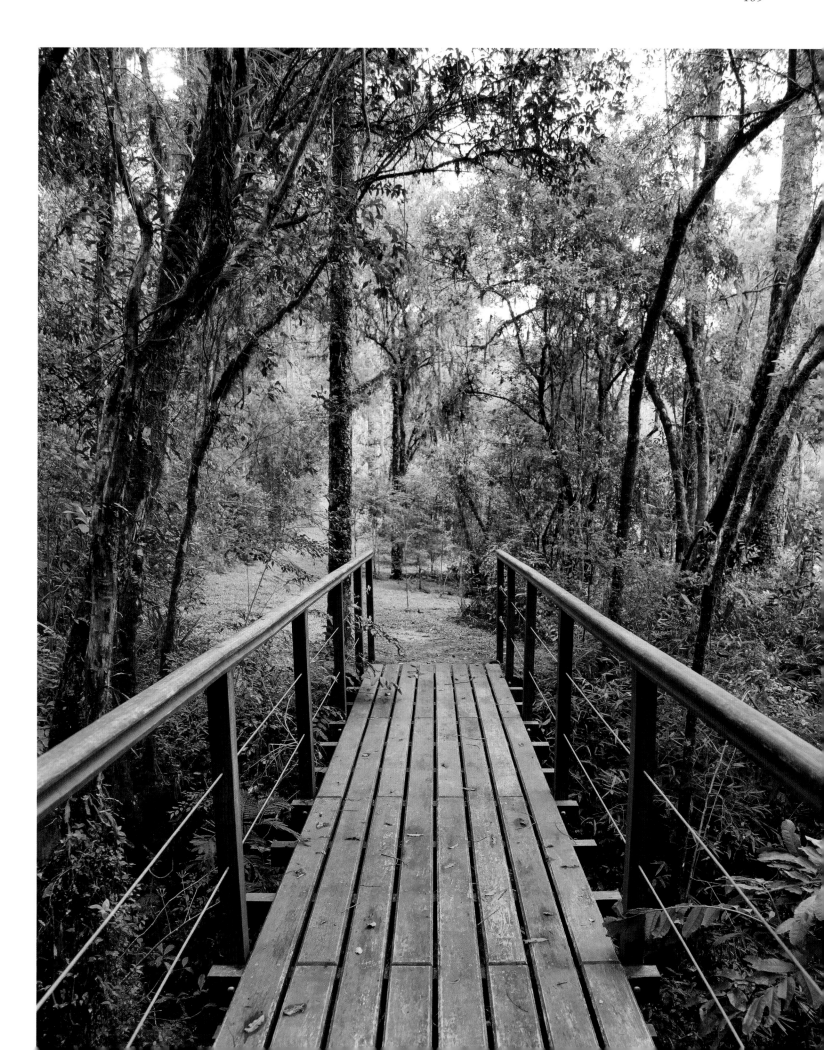

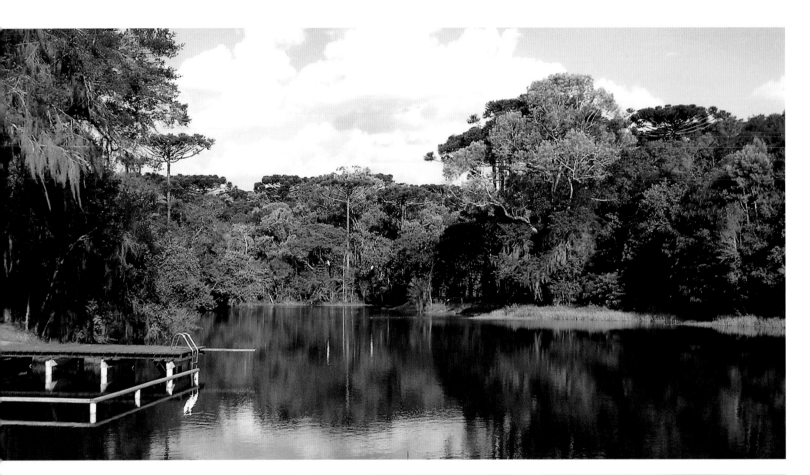

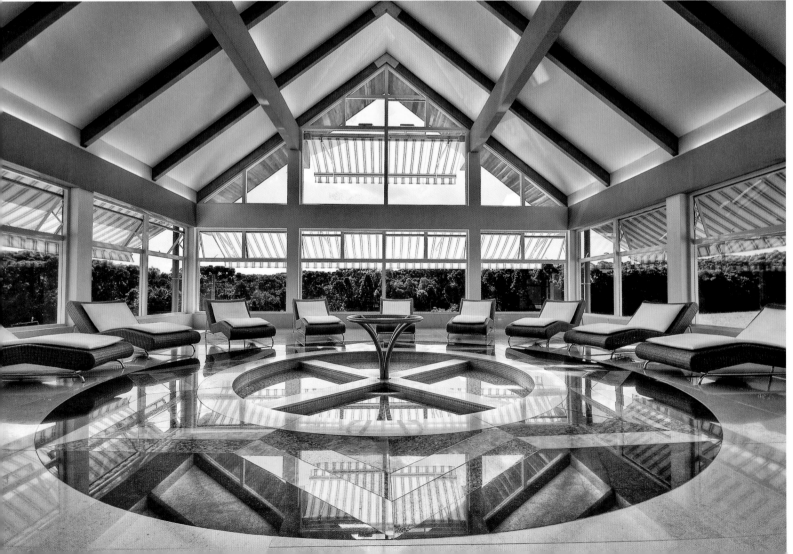

Spa, Health & Other Facilities
The Villa Spa Lapinha offers over 20 private rooms reserved for physical therapy, massotherapy, water therapy, aesthetic and capillary treatments as well as 2 rest areas, sauna, indoor Kneipp tank, relaxation area. Library and reading room, tennis and volleyball court.

Treatments & Services
Anti-stress, burn out, detox, F. X. Mayr, Kneipp, naturopathy, nutritional consultancy, physiotherapy, Pilates, reflexology. Extensive menu of over 50 body and beauty treatments including aromatherapy, hot stone massage, hydrotherapy, Swedish massage, Thai massage, thalasso, Vichy Showers. Airport transfer.

Activities
Biking, cardiovascular circuit, dancing, functional sports, gymnastics, jogging, Lian Gong, Nordic walking, swimming, tennis, volleyball, walking, water aerobics at different levels.

Rooms
38 rooms.

Located
In the rural region of the town of Lapa, 53 miles (85 kilometers) from Curitiba Airport.

Estrada da Lapa – Rio Negro – Km 16
83750-000 Lapa, Brazil
www.lapinha.com.br

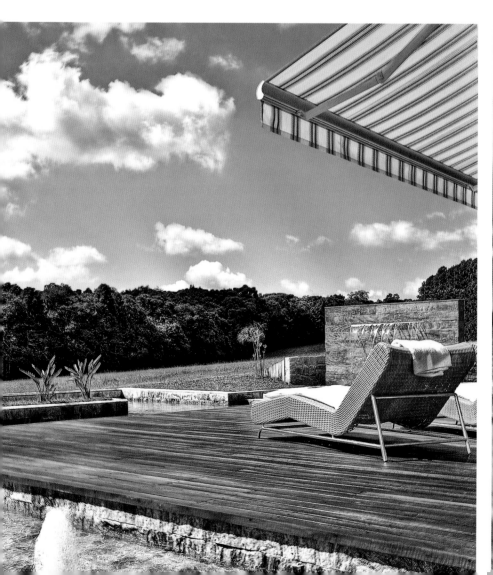

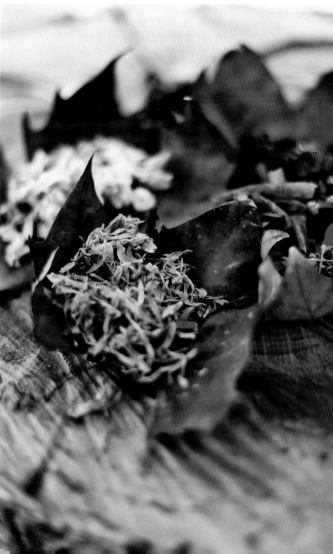

Wellness Pioneers at the Foot of a Sacred Mountain

Wellness-Pioniere am Fuße eines heiligen Berges

Rancho La Puerta

Rancho La Puerta is one of the world's oldest health resorts. For the past 72 years, Deborah Szekely has been pampering her guests with a profound desire to make them feel good in body, mind, and spirit. As early as 1940, Deborah and her husband, Edmond, a pioneer of the fitness, spa, and wellness movement, established this peaceful retreat at the foot of Mount Kuchumaa in Tecate, Baja California, Mexico. Because the resort lies in a sheltered valley, guests benefit from an ideal climate all year round. A citadel of rocky cliffs and fragrant sage, Kuchumaa has been sacred to Kumeyaay tribespeople for thousands of years. Along with organic, semi-vegetarian cuisine of farm fresh, seasonal quality and a world-renowned health and fitness program, which draws visitors from all over the world, the deep spiritual connection with the sacred mountain is what lends the place its positive power.

Rancho La Puerta ist eines der ältesten Gesundheitsresorts der Welt. Seit 72 Jahren hegt und pflegt Deborah Szekely ihre Gäste mit dem umfassenden Wunsch, Wohlbefinden für Geist, Körper und Seele zu bereiten. Schon 1940 gründete sie diesen friedlichen Rückzugsort zusammen mit ihrem Ehemann Edmond, einem Pionier der Fitness-, Spa- und Wellness-Bewegung, am Fuße des Berges Kuchumaa in Tecate, Baja California. Das Resort liegt in einem geschützten Tal, sodass die Gäste das ganze Jahr über von idealen klimatischen Bedingungen profitieren. Für die Stammesmitglieder der Kumeyaay ist der Kuchumaa, eine Zitadelle aus Felsen und duftendem Salbei, seit tausenden von Jahren heilig. Neben teils vegetarischer Bio-Küche mit Zutaten frisch vom Bauernhof und einem weltbekannten Fitness- und Gesundheitsprogramm, das Gäste aus der ganzen Welt anzieht, ist es die tiefe spirituelle Verbindung mit diesem heiligen Berg, die dem Ort seine positive Kraft verleiht.

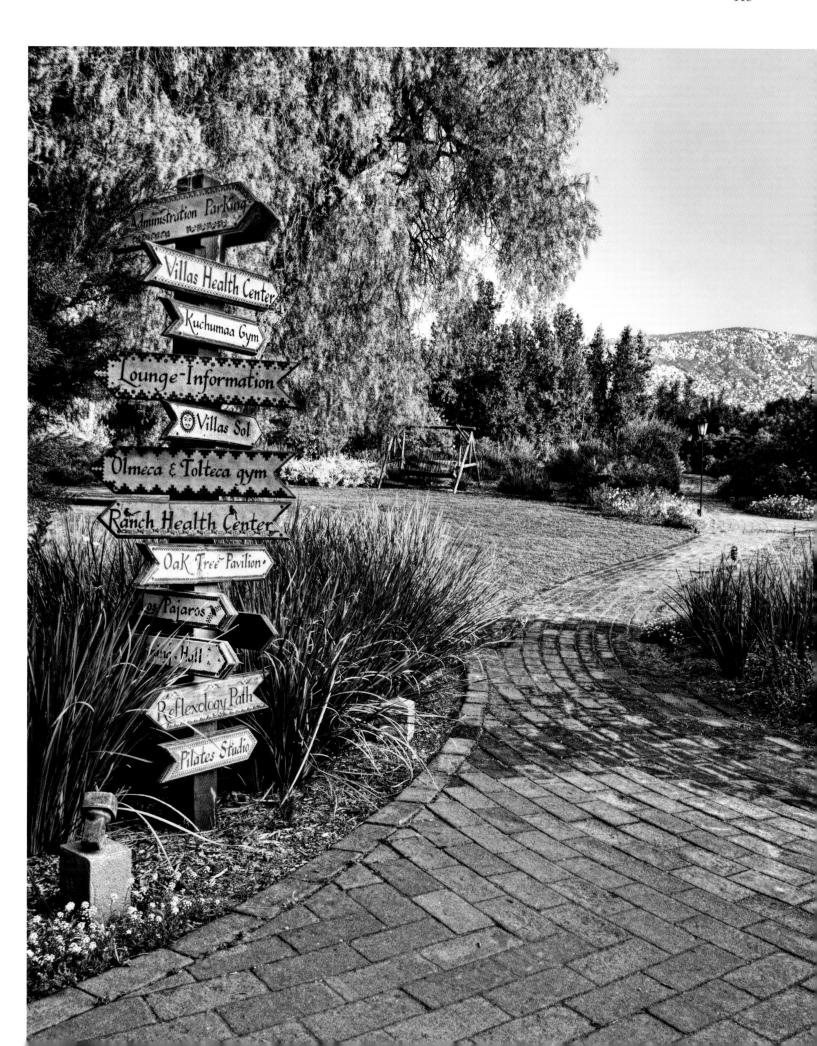

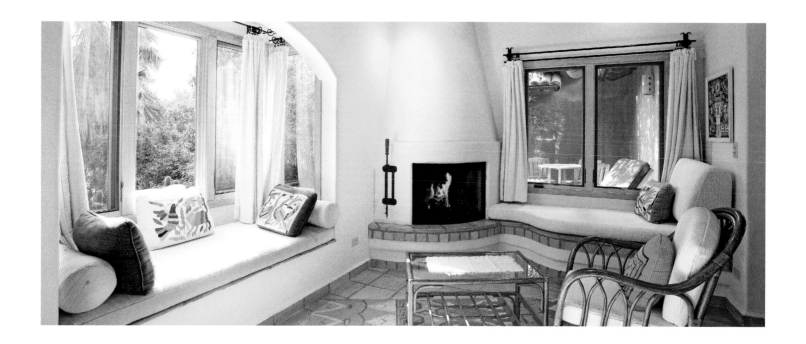

Spa, Health & Other Facilities
3 swimming pools, therapy pool for Watsu, whirpools, saunas, steam rooms, Villa's Health Center, Women's Health Center, Men's Health Center, 11 gymnasiums, health retreats with international leading experts. Meditation rooms, running track, reflexology footpath, meditation labyrinth, tennis courts, volleyball/basketball court. Dining hall and culinary center with 6-acre organic farm.

Treatments & Services
Ayurveda, body wraps, craniosacral, energy work, facials, hot stone massage, hydrotherapy, meditation, Pilates, Qigong, reflexology, Swedish massage, yoga. Cooking classes for health food at La Cocina Que Canta cooking school and culinary center, gourmet meals. Free high-speed Internet access, free parking.

Activities
Bird-watching, culinary tours of Baja California's Valle de Guadalupe Wine Country, garden tours, hiking.

Rooms
83 private "casitas" on a 3,000-acre property – 6 categories: Ranchero Solo, Ranchera, Hacienda, Junior Villa Studio, Villa Studio, 2-bedroom Villa Suite.

Located
In Tecate, Baja California, Mexico. 1 hour from San Diego International Airport.

San Diego, CA 92121, USA
www.rancholapuerta.com

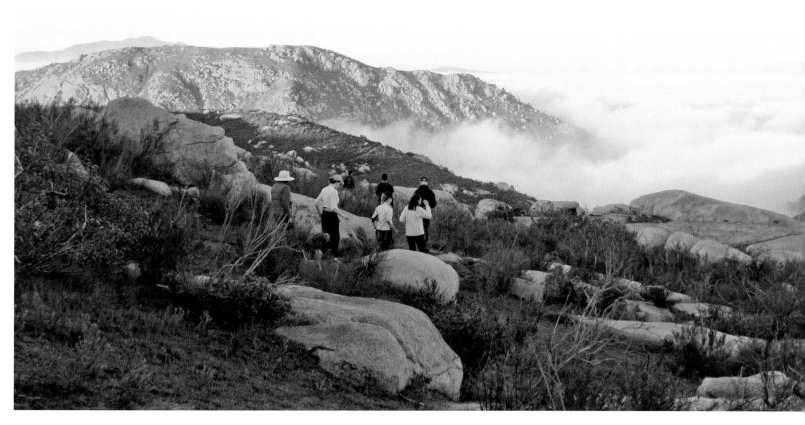

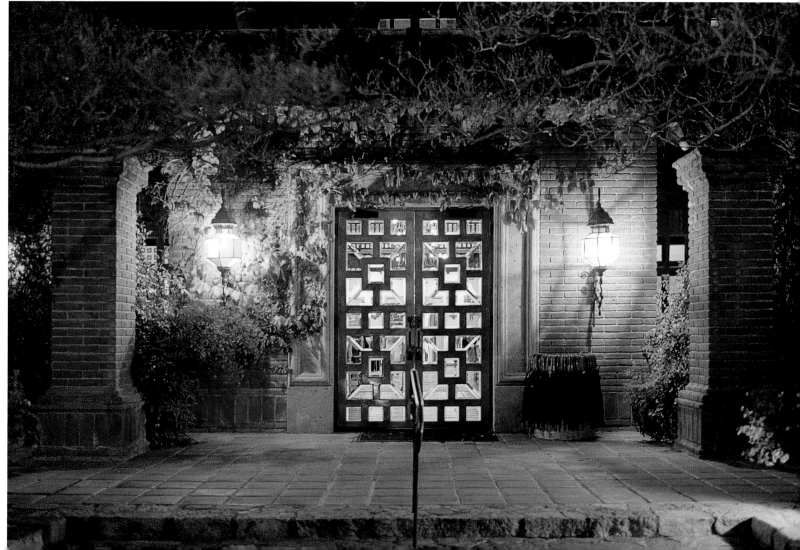

Healthy Sleep

"Heaven has given us humans three things to balance the many travails of life: hope, sleep, and laughter." – Immanuel Kant

Healthy sleep is becoming more and more important these days—and harder and harder to come by. A good night's rest will soon be considered as essential to healthy living as a healthy diet. 90 percent of all processes vital for physical, emotional, and mental healing—such as regeneration, repair, balance, and strengthening the body system—take place while we are sleeping. This means that anyone who wants to live a healthy life should, first and foremost, boost their sleeping experience. Optimal sleep follows naturally if you

1. establish and practice sleep-promoting and sleep-friendly routines and activities (exposure to sunlight, exercise in fresh air, a balanced diet, breaks and relaxation, effective stress management, etc.)
2. use natural, anatomical, orthopedic, climate control bedding that best suits your body (holistic sleeping system)
3. create an interference-free (no electronic smog), neutralized, and harmonic sleeping environment (a personal sleeping island)
4. incorporate and optimize factors that are biologically relevant, such as the earth's magnetic field or the body's grounding in the place of sleep (consult a specialist, if necessary)
5. prepare for sleep both physically and emotionally
6. maintain sleeping rituals for endogenous reversal of stimuli (from the outside to the inside) through relaxation and meditation techniques that help prepare you mentally and emotionally for sleep and attune you to sleep.

When you know the best way to handle sleep, you walk on the sunny side of life.

Dr. med. h. c. Günther W. Amann-Jennson, sleep psychologist and founder of SAMINA Schlafkomfort, author of the books "Schlaf dich gesund" (Sleep Your Way to Health) and "Schlaf Dich jung, fit und erfolgreich" (Sleep Your Way to Youthfulness, Fitness, and Success)

Gesunder Schlaf

> „Der Himmel hat den Menschen als Gegengewicht gegen die
> vielen Mühseligkeiten des Lebens drei Dinge gegeben: die
> Hoffnung, den Schlaf und das Lachen." – Immanuel Kant

Gesunder Schlaf wird in unserer heutigen Zeit immer wichtiger – gleichzeitig aber auch immer seltener. Bald wird die gesunde Nachtruhe den gleichen Wert haben wie sie heute eine gesunde Ernährung hat. 90 Prozent aller für eine körperliche, seelische und geistige Heilung notwendigen Prozesse – wie Regeneration, Reparatur, Ausgleich und Stärkung des Körpersystems – finden im Schlaf statt. Das bedeutet, dass jeder Mensch, der gesund leben möchte, in erster Linie seinen Schlaf optimieren sollte. Gesunder Schlaf ergibt sich durch

1. den Aufbau und die Umsetzung von schlaffördernden, schlaffreundlichen Tagesabläufen und Maßnahmen (Sonnenlicht, Bewegung an frischer Luft, ausgewogene Ernährung, Pausen und Entspannung, effektives Stressmanagement etc.)
2. eine naturkonforme, anatomisch, orthopädisch, bettklimatisch körpergerechte Schlafausstattung (ganzheitliches Schlafsystem)
3. ein störungsfreies, (hinsichtlich Elektrosmog) neutralisiertes und harmonisches Schlafumfeld (persönliche Schlafinsel schaffen)
4. die Berücksichtigung und Optimierung von biologisch relevanten Ordnungsfaktoren wie Erdmagnetfeld, Körper-Erdung am Schlafplatz (evtl. Fachleute zurate ziehen)
5. eine körperlich-seelische Bereitschaft zum Schlafen
6. Einschlafrituale zur endogenen Reizumkehr (von außen nach innen) durch Entspannungs- und Meditationstechniken zur mental-emotionalen Schlafvorbereitung und Schlafeinstimmung.

Wer mit seinem Schlaf optimal umzugehen weiß, steht auf der Sonnenseite des Lebens.

Dr. med. h. c. Günther W. Amann-Jennson, Schlafpsychologe, Gründer von SAMINA Schlafkomfort, Autor der Bücher „Schlaf dich gesund" und „Schlaf Dich jung, fit und erfolgreich"

Room for Caribbean Dreams

Raum für karibische Träume

Jade Mountain

"My aim was to create spaces and experiences that would give guests a spiritual and emotional lift." Indeed, Nick Troubetzkoy, Jade Mountain's architect and owner, exceeded this goal. An heir to the former Russian imperial family, Troubetzkoy has a passion for jade. He has put together an impressive collection of these precious stones in different shapes and sizes. Like a declaration of love to St. Lucia's beauty, the resort that bears the name of this gemstone crowns a cliff high above the sea. Local artisans built an entirely organic establishment in harmony with its natural surroundings. Jade Mountain guests can enjoy relaxing treatments in the spa or in their private rooms. The guest rooms are designed with a special feature: The bedroom, living area, and infinity pool blend smoothly into each other, creating a unique living experience and sense of freedom with rooms that seem to float. All accommodations have a color therapy whirlpool for improving your biorhythm and sense of equilibrium, and they offer an unobstructed panoramic view of the famous Pitons and the Caribbean Sea.

„Mein Ziel war es, Räume und Erfahrungen zu schaffen, die den Gästen einen spirituellen und seelischen Auftrieb geben werden." Dieses Ziel hat Nick Troubetzkoy, Architekt und Eigentümer des Jade Mountain, sogar übertroffen. Er ist einer der Erben der späten russischen Zarenfamilie mit einer Passion für Jade: Troubetzkoy hat eine eindrucksvolle Kollektion des wertvollen Steins in verschiedenen Formen und Größen geschaffen. Wie eine Liebeserklärung an die Schönheit St. Lucias thront das Resort mit dem Namen dieses Steines auf einer Klippe hoch über dem Meer. Im Einklang mit der umgebenden Natur schufen einheimische Handwerker ein rundum organisches Projekt. Gäste vom Jade Mountain können entspannende Behandlungen im Spa-Bereich oder in ihren Privaträumen genießen. Die Besonderheit der Raumkonzeption: Schlafzimmer, Wohnraum und Infinity Pool gehen grenzenlos ineinander über, wodurch ein einmaliges Wohn- und Freiheitsgefühl entsteht – die Räume scheinen zu schweben. Alle Zimmer besitzen einen Farbtherapie-Whirlpool, in dem Biorhythmus und Ausgeglichenheit verbessert werden, und bieten einen unverstellten Panoramablick über die berühmten Pitons und das Karibische Meer.

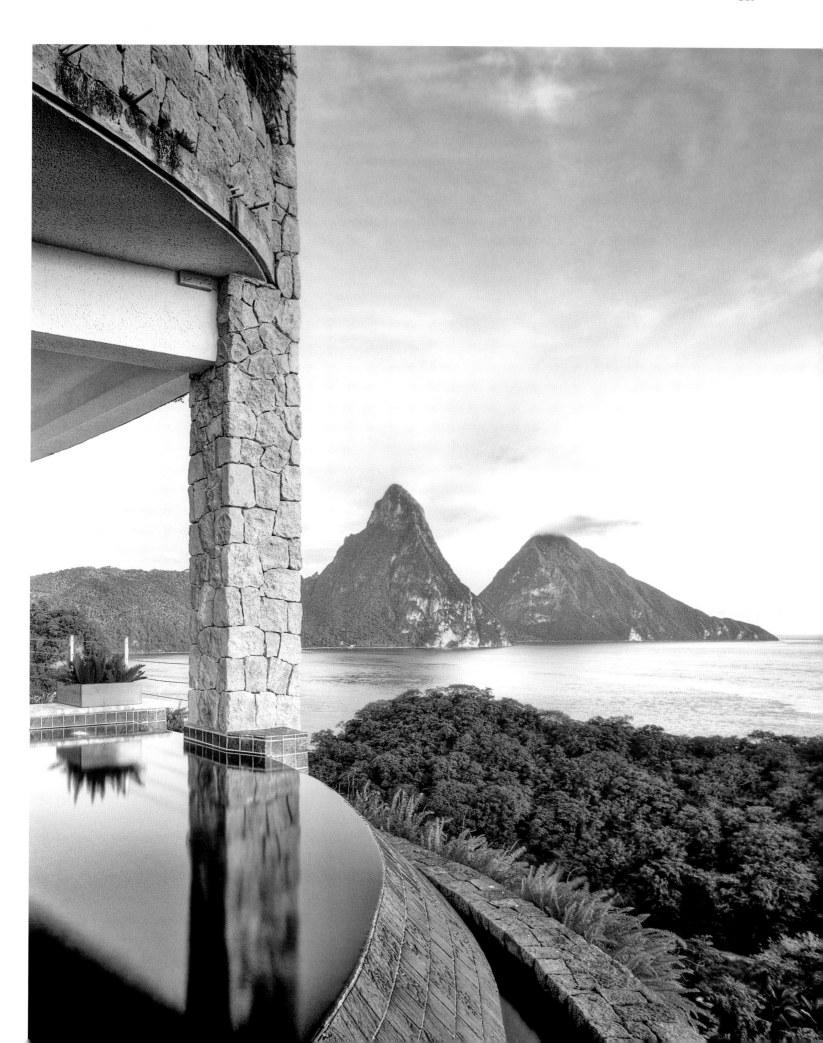

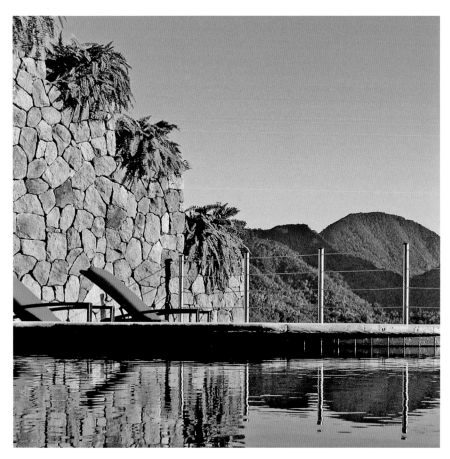

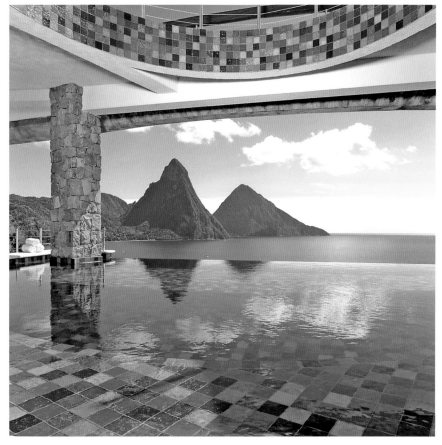

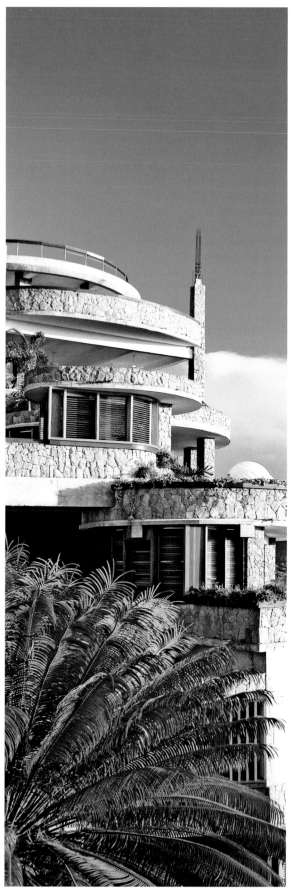

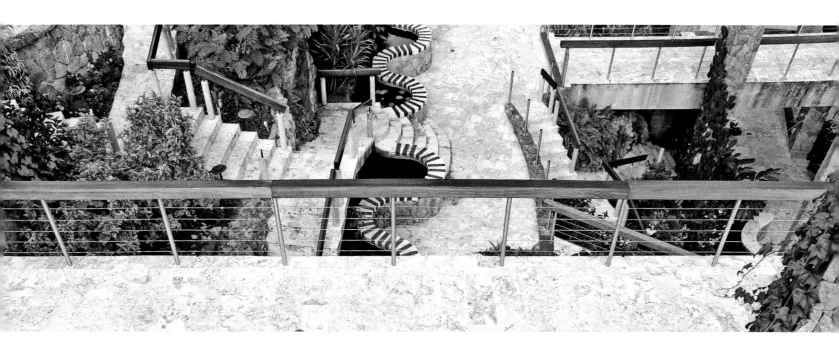

Spa, Health & Other Facilities
Spa and fitness studio Kai en Ciel. 2 soft sandy beaches; scuba, bike, and water sports facilities.
Anse Chastanet's restaurant, bars, poolbar, boutiques, library, art gallery, hair salon.

Treatments & Services
Ayurvedic and holistic services including aromatherapy, Ayurveda, Pilates, reflexology, shiatsu, sunrise
and sunset yoga sessions. Classical body and beauty treatments. Airport transfer, free parking.

Activities
Airplane tours, bicycling, bird-watching, horseback riding, jogging, kayaking,
mountain biking, sailing, snorkeling, swimming, tennis, windsurfing.

Rooms
24 individually designed infinity pool sanctuaries and 5 Jacuzzi suites.
The rooms feature patios with ocean view.

Located
In Soufrière, near Anse Chastanet Beach. 26 miles (43 kilometers) from
Hewanorra International Airport. 2 minutes from a drive-in volcano.

PO Box 4000
Soufrière, St. Lucia
www.jademountain.com

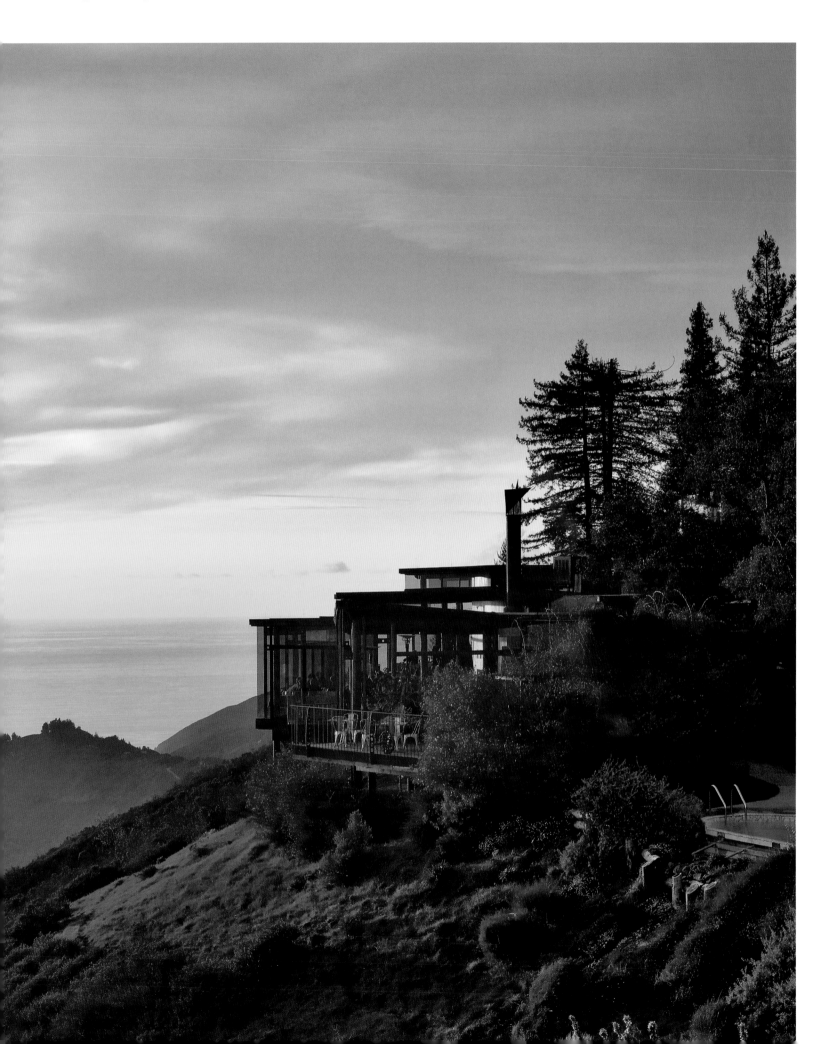

Free as a Bird in the Lap of Nature

Frei wie ein Vogel im Schoße der Natur

Post Ranch Inn

Like a bird's nest, this romantic resort hugs the steep cliffs of a beautiful coast. High above the Pacific Ocean, on the strip of coast known as Big Sur, you feel as safe and close to nature as a small nestling. One is tempted to spread one's wings, take off, and fly away. Each room has a special design that connects guests directly to nature: in the Tree House rooms or a Coast House room, for example, offering a clear view of the vast ocean. The air is free of electrosmog, and the products used are entirely organic. The wellness programs also reunite people with nature. Along with guided nature hikes, yoga, and every conceivable spa treatment, guests can also take a health-giving session with a shaman or observe the night sky through a modern telescope. The sky here is surprisingly dark and starry—for it's a long way to the nearest city.

Wie ein Vogelnest kuschelt sich dieses Resort mit Romantik-Flair in den Fels einer wunderschönen Steilküste. Und so geborgen und naturnah wie kleine Nesthocker fühlen sich die Gäste hier oben, hoch über dem Pazifik am Küstenstreifen Big Sur. Fast möchte man die Flügel ausbreiten, sich fallen lassen und losfliegen. Das besondere Design der Zimmer verbindet die Gäste direkt mit der Natur, etwa in den Baumhauszimmern oder im Coast House, die alle einen unverstellten Blick auf die unendliche Weite des Meeres bieten. Die Luft ist frei von Elektrosmog, die verwendeten Produkte sind rein organisch. Auch die Wellnessangebote bringen Mensch und Natur wieder zusammen. Neben geführten Wanderungen, Yoga und allen denkbaren Spa-Anwendungen können Gäste auf eine heilsame, schamanische Reise gehen oder durch ein modernes Teleskop den Nachthimmel beobachten. Der ist hier überraschend dunkel und sternenklar – denn die nächsten Städte liegen weit entfernt.

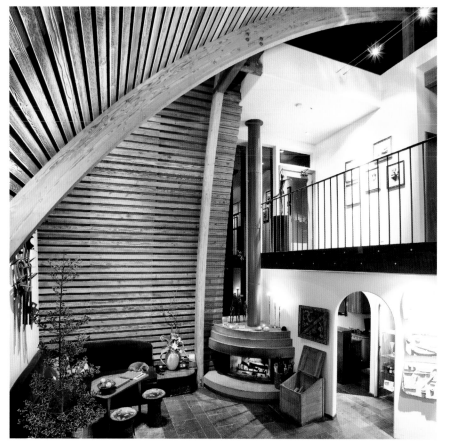

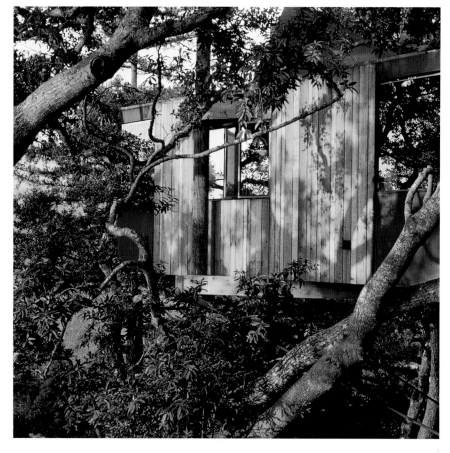

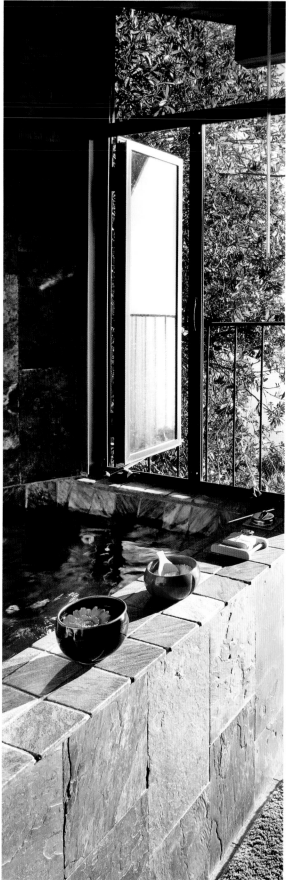

Spa, Health & Other Facilities

2 basking pools with infinity edge, lap swimming pool with mountain views, fitness room.
Sierra Mar restaurant, bar, extensive wine list.

Treatments & Services

Aromatherapy massage, Big Sur jade stone therapy, body wrap, craniosacral therapy, crystal and gemstone therapy, duet massage, exfoliants, facials, lymphatic massage, meditation, Post Ranch massage, prenatal massage, reflexology, Reiki, shaman sessions, Thai massage, therapeutic massage, vibrational resonance, yoga.
24-hour front desk, complimentary valet parking, Internet access and newspapers.

Activities

Guided nature hikes, hiking trails, star gazing with a computerized telescope.

Rooms

40 guest rooms and suites with ocean or mountain views, 2 private houses.
Complimentary minibar nonalcoholic beverages, snacks.

Located

Nestled on the cliffs of Big Sur. 1 hour by car from Monterey Peninsula Airport,
2.5 hours from San Francisco.

Highway 1
Big Sur, CA 93920, USA
www.postranchinn.com

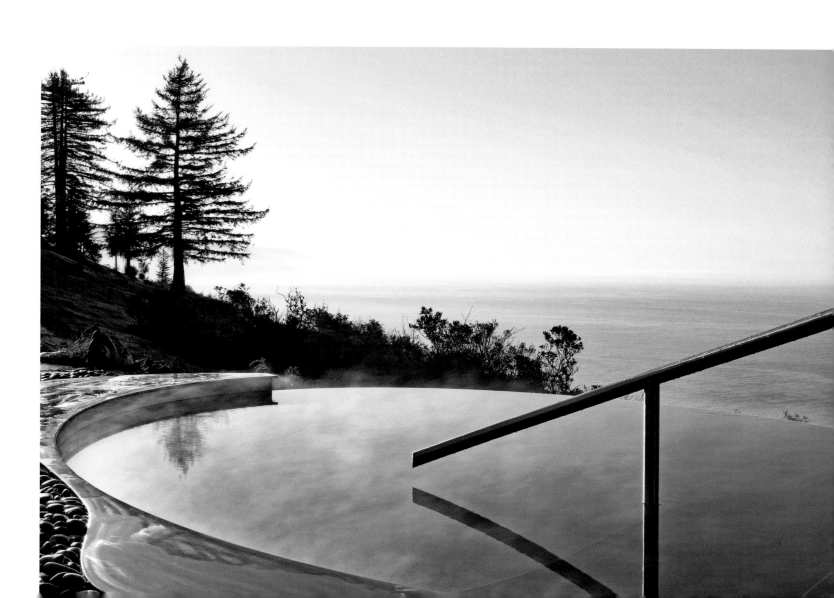

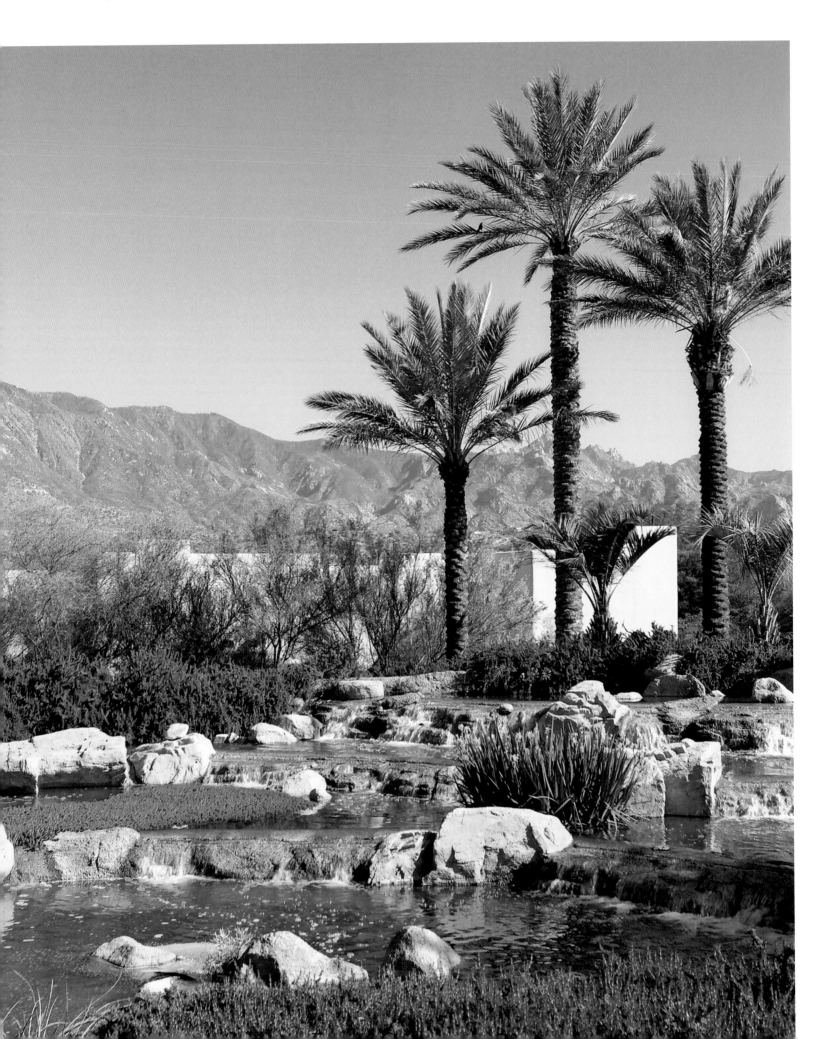

Enjoying the Moment and Learning to Live Better

Das Sein genießen und besser leben lernen

Miraval Resort and Spa

"In everything we do, we encourage our guests to live in the present moment, conscious of the unique intersection of mind, body, and spirit." This is the philosophy and stated goal of the all-inclusive retreat north of Tucson. The resort achieves its objective by offering over 90 activities that are intended to assist every guest on his/her personal journey, including tennis, meditation, various types of yoga and fitness, as well as drumming and mosaic art. In a high ropes course, guests can tackle their fears, while health specialists in the spa provide a deep tissue massage or a "Qi Journey" to promote well-being. Of course, horses are a necessary part of any vacation in cowboy country. In the Equine Experience, these gentle beasts act as therapists rather than serving as a living, breathing piece of sports equipment. A day of energetic exercise comes to a close on your private terrace, where you can watch the sun go down over the Santa Catalina Mountains.

„Mit allem, was wir tun, ermuntern wir unsere Gäste, im Hier und Jetzt zu leben, in dem Bewusstsein des einzigartigen Zusammenspiels von Geist, Körper und Seele" – so lautet die Philosophie und selbstgestellte Aufgabe des All-inclusive-Retreats im Norden von Tucson. Um dies zu erreichen gibt es ein Angebot von über 90 Aktivitäten, die jeden Gast bei seiner individuellen Entwicklung unterstützen sollen. Dazu gehören Tennis, Meditation, Yoga- und Fitness-Variationen ebenso wie Trommeln oder Mosaik-Kunst. Im Hochseilgarten können sich Gäste mit ihren Ängsten konfrontieren, im Spa fördern Gesundheitsspezialisten das Wohlbefinden mit einer „Deep Tissue Massage" oder einer „Qi Journey". Pferde dürfen bei einem Urlaub im Land der Cowboys natürlich nicht fehlen. In den Equine-Programmen nehmen die sanften Vierbeiner die Rolle eines Therapeuten ein, weniger die eines lebenden Sportgeräts. Den aktiven Tag lässt man auf der privaten Terrasse ausklingen, mit Blick auf den Sonnenuntergang über den Santa Catalina Mountains.

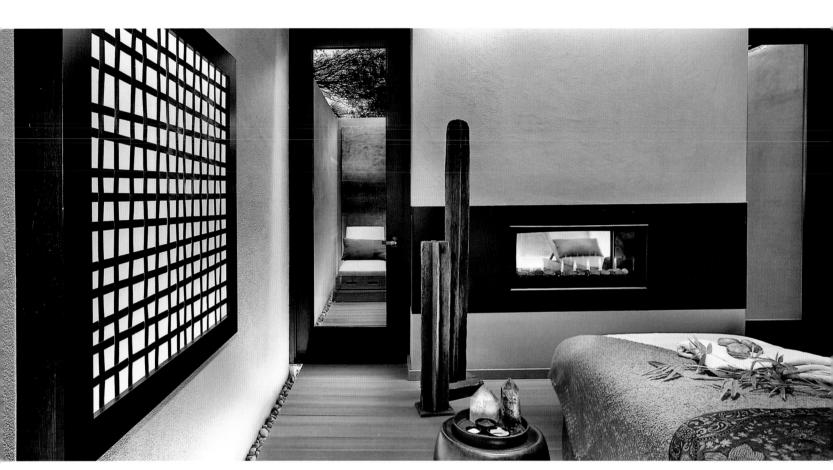

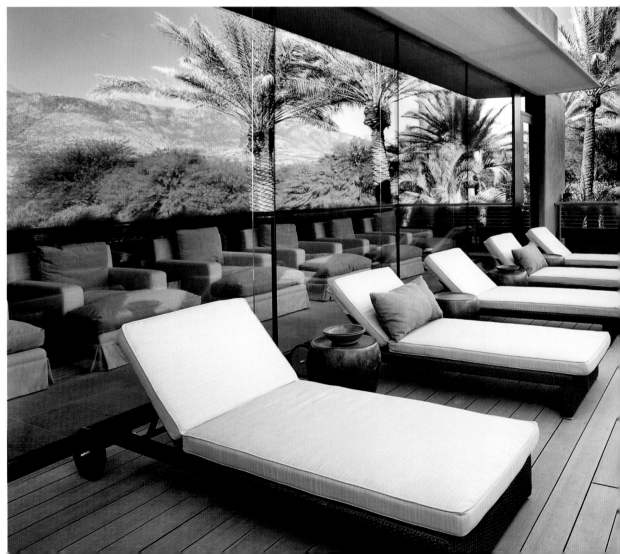

Spa, Health & Other Facilities
World-class spa with outdoor treatment rooms, hot tubs, sauna, and relaxation lounge.
Miraval is a non-tipping resort.

Treatments & Services
Ayurveda, body renewal rituals, energy and oriental bodywork, hand and foot therapies, massages, meditation, outdoor spa treatments, Pilates, skin care, speciality bodywork, yoga. 24-hour front desk, complimentary valet parking, shared shuttle service to Tucson International Airport.

Activities
Biking, cooking demonstration, Equine Experience, fitness classes, golf, high ropes course, hiking, lectures by wellness specialists, mountain biking, rock climbing, tennis.

Rooms
117 luxury rooms and suites, grouped in 6 villages. Private villa accommodations.
Each features sustainable materials.

Located
At the base of the Santa Catalina Mountains, north of Tucson, Arizona.
27 miles (44 kilometers) from Tucson International Airport.

5000 E Via Estancia Miraval
Tucson, AZ 85739, USA
www.miravalresorts.com

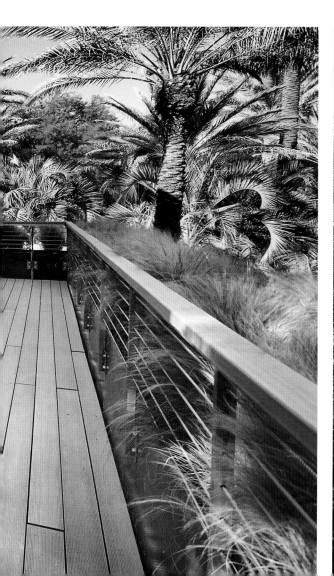
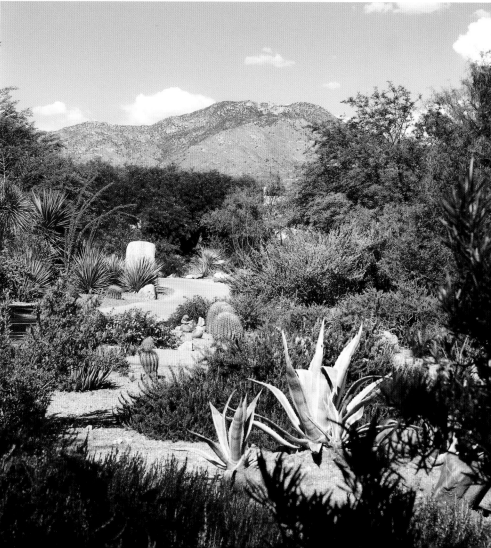

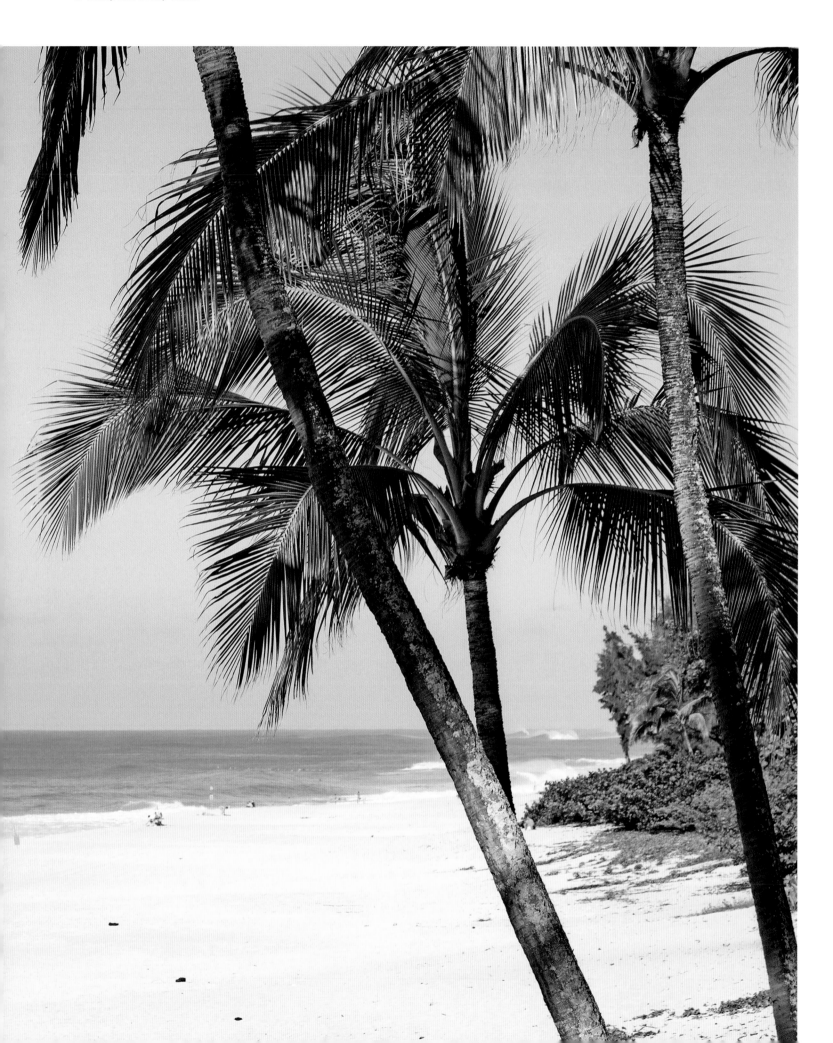

Leaving Negative Thoughts Behind

Den negativen Gedanken entschweben

The Sullivan Estate & Spa Retreat

Aloha and ola loa (Hawaiian for "love and long life"). This breathtaking estate is situated in an extraordinarily beautiful and tranquil location. Featuring only six private rooms, it promises exclusivity and seclusion. The property and amenities meet all the expectations and dreams that people generally associate with Hawaii: beauty, serenity, abundance, and friendliness. Jürgen Klein, the retreat's proprietor, first made a name for himself as a chemist and biologist in the field of natural cosmetics. Since 2003, he has earned a great deal of success in the area of relaxation and stress relief; his spa retreat is one of the world's most progressive anti-stress centers. It is a masterpiece—the epitome of comfort and elegance. The JK7-SPA Sensator, a pool with highly concentrated salt water, is a true innovation. Bathers experience a combination of color, music, and aromatherapy, while their bodies drift about, absolutely weightless. When your brain takes a rest, you have reached the goal: a sense of complete well-being without any disruptive negative thoughts of the past. Along with yoga, meditation, massage, esthetic treatments, and organic vegetarian cuisine, your body, mind, and spirit come into healthy balance and you reconnect with your inner self.

Aloha und ola loa (hawaiianisch für „Liebe und langes Leben")! Das atemberaubende Anwesen in außergewöhnlich schöner, ruhiger Lage mit nur sechs Privaträumen verspricht Exklusivität und Privatheit. Es erfüllt all die Vorstellungen und Träume, die man gemeinhin mit dem Namen „Hawaii" verbindet: Schönheit, Gelassenheit, Fülle, Freundlichkeit. Retreat-Betreiber Jürgen Klein machte sich als Chemiker und Biologe zunächst auf dem Sektor der Naturkosmetik einen Namen. Seit 2003 ist er auf dem Gebiet Entspannung und Stressbeseitigung sehr erfolgreich und bietet mit dem Spa-Retreat eine der weltweit fortschrittlichsten Einrichtungen zur Stressbewältigung. Es ist sein Meisterstück – Komfort und Eleganz einbegriffen. Eine Innovation ist der JK7-SPA Sensator, ein Pool mit hochkonzentriertem Salzwasser, in dem die Badenden eine Kombination aus Farb-, Klang- und Aromatherapie erleben, während der Körper in absoluter Schwerelosigkeit dahintreibt. Wenn das Gehirn abschaltet, ist das Ziel erreicht: ein vollkommenes Wohlbefinden ohne störende negative Gedanken der Vergangenheit. Zusammen mit Yoga, Meditation, Massagen, Schönheitsbehandlungen und einer vegetarischen Bio-Küche finden Körper, Geist und Seele in eine gesunde Ausgeglichenheit und der Mensch kommt sich selbst wieder näher.

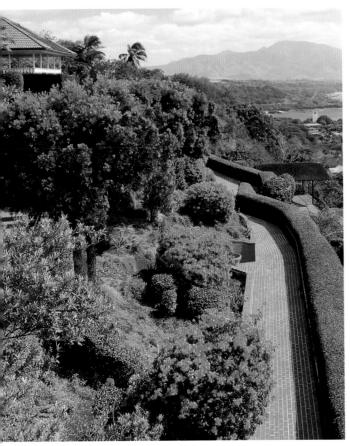
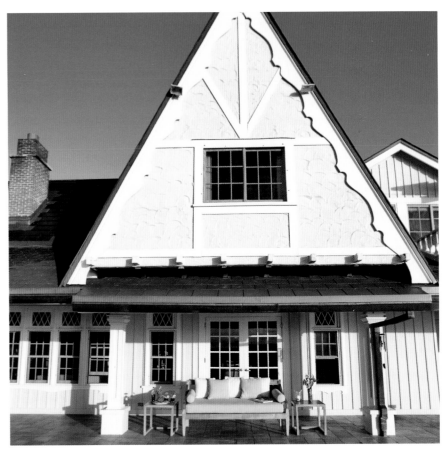
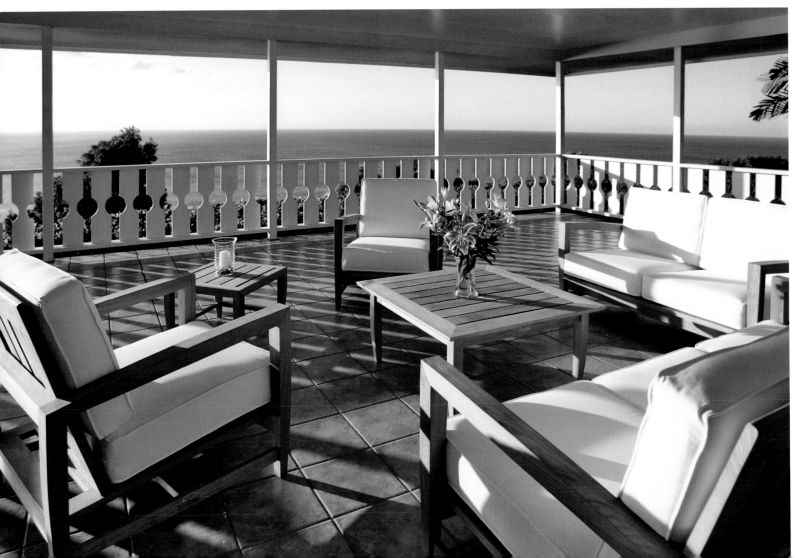

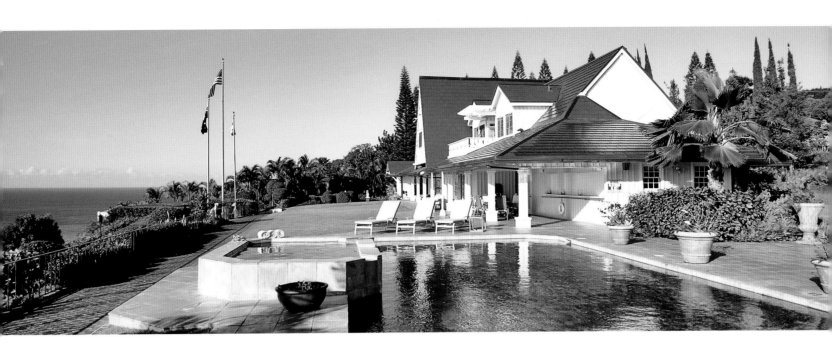

Spa, Health & Other Facilities
Saltwater swimming pool, cold plunge pool, hydro bath tub, Jacuzzi, Finnish and infrared sauna, herbal steam sauna, fitness center, Galileo Power Plate, outdoor relaxation pavilion. Formal dining room, gourmet kitchen,

Treatments & Services
Aromatherapy, body wraps, facials, JK7 OlaLoa Signature Spa Packages, manicures, massages and body therapies, organic body scrubs, pedicures, Slim Legs & Toned Bums, water-body-mind treatments, yoga. Focus on ancient Hawaiian and Ayurvedic treatments. Shuttle service from Honolulu Airport.

Activities
Biking, golf, hiking, horseback riding, reading and relaxing in outdoor lounging areas, surfing, swimming, tennis, whale-watching.

Rooms
Private villa with only 6 bedrooms.

Located
On the North Shore of Hawaii's island of O'ahu. 33 miles (52 kilometers) from Honolulu Airport.

59-338 Wilinau Road
Haleiwa, HI 96712, USA
www.sullivanestate.com

Healthy Aging

Aging is an important part of the human experience—to deny that fact and try to fight aging was to go against nature. Rather than attempting to stop or reverse the aging process, one should focus on aging optimally well by maintaining good health throughout life and limiting inappropriate inflammation.

Chronic inflammation is the main reason for unhealthy aging and the many serious illnesses associated with it, including heart disease, arthritis, and some forms of cancer. A normal inflammatory response is integral to the body's healing system, helping to bring added nourishment and immune activity to sites of injury or infection; when inflammation persists beyond its healing purpose, however, tissue damage and accelerated aging occur.

Factors contributing to chronic inflammation include smoking, a sedentary lifestyle, and persistent psychosocial stress, but dietary choices have a particularly big impact. Learning how specific foods and patterns of eating influence inflammation is the single best strategy for containing the process, thereby reducing the risk of premature aging.

My anti-inflammatory diet represents the nutritional component of a healthy lifestyle and emphasizes whole grains and other slow-digesting carbohydrates; fatty cold-water fish for their anti-inflammatory omega-3 fatty acids; vegetable protein sources such as beans, lentils, and whole soy products that contain healthier fats and fewer toxins than most animal proteins; seeds and nuts; and a variety of brightly colored fresh vegetables and fruit, especially dark berries. Exposure to foods that promote inflammation should be limited by reducing your intake of highly processed foods and fast-digesting carbohydrates; avoiding fast food and products containing partially hydrogenated oils or vegetable shortening; and by reducing the use of polyunsaturated oils such as sunflower, safflower, soy, and corn.

Other components of a healthy aging program include: no smoking; the appropriate use of dietary supplements, such as vitamin D3 and fish oils; regular physical activity; practicing healthy stress management techniques including breath work, meditation, laughter; getting at least seven hours of restorative sleep each night; and maintaining a strong social network.

Growing old need not be synonymous with getting old—the important distinction to be made is between aging well and developing age-related diseases.

Dr. Andrew Weil, M.D., founder and director, Arizona Center for
Integrative Medicine, University of Arizona Health Sciences Center, USA

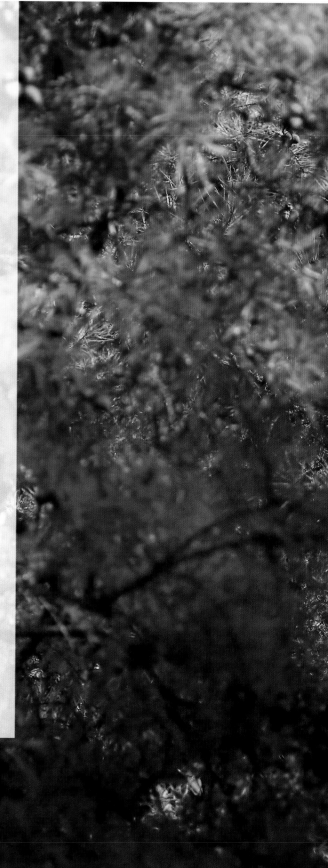

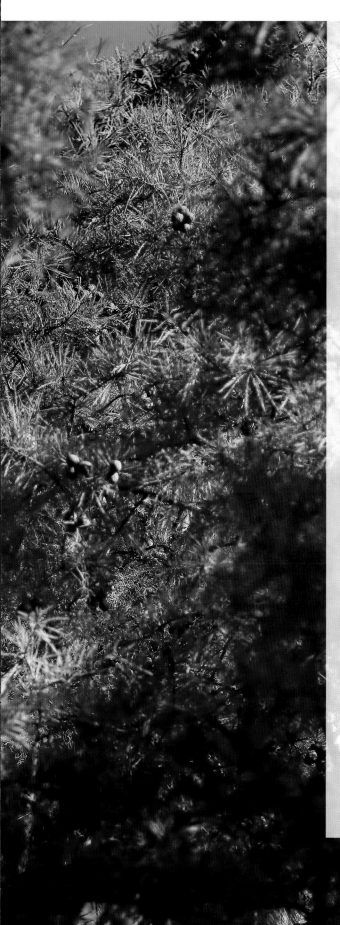

Gesund Altern

Altern ist ein wichtiger Teil der menschlichen Erfahrungswelt. Diese Tatsache zu leugnen und gegen das Älterwerden zu kämpfen, bedeutet, sich der Natur zu widersetzen. Anstatt zu versuchen, den Alterungsprozess aufzuhalten oder umzukehren, sollte man sich lieber darauf konzentrieren, optimal zu altern, indem man die Gesundheit ein Leben lang pflegt und unnötige Entzündungen vermeidet.

Chronische Entzündungen sind der Hauptgrund für ungesundes Altern und für viele, oft im Alter auftretende, schwerwiegende Erkrankungen einschließlich Herzkrankheiten, Arthritis und einiger Krebsarten. Eine normale Entzündungs-reaktion ist für den Heilungsprozess des Körpers von großer Bedeutung, denn verletzte oder infizierte Stellen werden besonders gut versorgt und geschützt. Bleibt die Entzündung jedoch über den Heilungszweck hinaus bestehen, kommt es zu Gewebeschäden und einer Beschleunigung des Alterungsprozesses.

Zu den Faktoren, die chronische Entzündungen begünstigen, gehören: Rauchen, Bewegungsmangel und anhaltender psychosozialer Stress. Auch die Ernährung spielt eine große Rolle. Der Prozess lässt sich am besten aufhalten, wenn man den Einfluss bestimmter Lebensmittel und Essgewohnheiten auf Entzündungen kennt. Dadurch kann das Risiko vorzeitigen Alterns verringert werden.

Die von mir empfohlene entzündungshemmende Kost stellt die Ernährungs-komponente einer gesunden Lebensweise dar und besteht hauptsächlich aus Vollkornprodukten und anderen langsam verdaulichen Kohlenhydraten; fetthaltigem Kaltwasserfisch (aufgrund seiner entzündungshemmenden Omega-3-Fettsäuren); pflanzlichen Proteinquellen wie Bohnen, Linsen und reinen Sojaprodukten, die gesündere Fette und weniger Giftstoffe enthalten als die meisten tierischen Proteine; Samen und Nüssen sowie aus einer bunten Vielfalt an frischen Obst- und Gemüsesorten, insbesondere dunklen Beeren. Der Konsum von entzündungsfördernden Nahrungsmitteln sollte eingeschränkt werden. Vermieden werden sollten darüber hinaus stark verarbeitete Nahrungs-mittel und schnell verdauliche Kohlenhydrate, Fast Food und Produkte mit teilweise gehärteten Ölen oder Pflanzenfetten sowie mehrfach ungesättigten Fetten wie Sonnenblumen-, Distel-, Soja- und Maiskeimöl.

Weitere Aspekte des gesunden Alterns sind Nichtrauchen, angemessene Ein-nahme von Nahrungsergänzungsmitteln wie Vitamin D3 und Fischöle, regelmäßige körperliche Bewegung, Methoden zur gesunden Stressbewältigung einschließlich Atemübungen, Meditation, Lachen, mindestens sieben Stunden erholsamen Schlaf pro Nacht und die Pflege stabiler sozialer Bindungen.

Altern muss nicht Altwerden bedeuten – der entscheidende Unterschied liegt zwischen gesundem Altern und dem Entstehen von altersbedingten Krankheiten.

Dr. med. Andrew Weil, Gründer und Leiter, Arizona Center for
Integrative Medicine, Health Sciences Center der Universität Arizona, USA

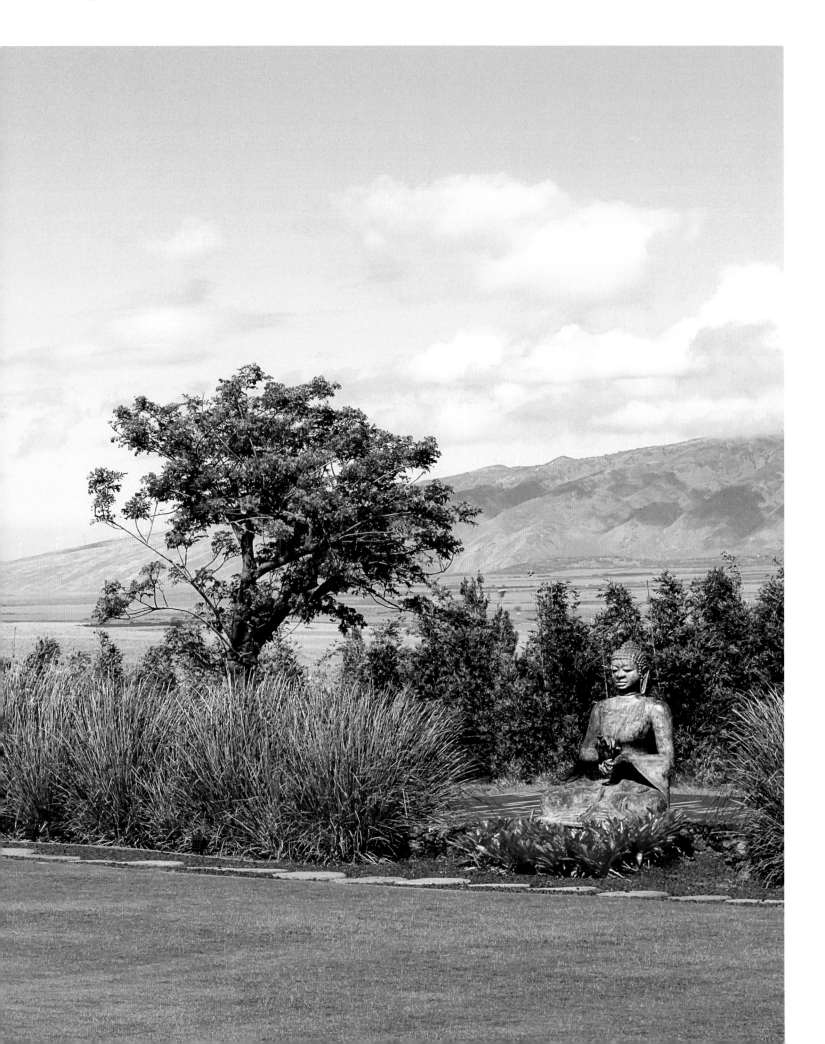

Learning How to Live a Fulfilling Life

Erfülltes Leben lernen

Lumeria Maui

Nature had remarkable things in mind for this part of the world. Lumeria, on the North Shore of Maui, is blessed with lush tropical and edible organic gardens, picturesque sunsets, and countless rainbows. It has always been a place to unplug, rejuvenate, and recalibrate. Built in 1909 as a residence for former sugar cane industry workers, it was later used as a home for World War II veterans and as a college dormitory. Today, Lumeria Maui is an "edventure" retreat—a combination of adventure and education. People come here to connect with themselves and the sacred energy of Maui. Lumeria offers yoga, meditation, and aromatherapy classes as well as gardening seminars that teach participants about the Hawaiians' holistic approach to the fruits of the earth. Wellness treatments such as traditional Hawaiian Lomi Lomi massage go one step further to help guests unwind and recharge body and mind with new ideas and energy.

Mit diesem Fleckchen Erde hat es die Natur besonders gut gemeint. Das Retreat an der Nordküste von Maui ist gesegnet mit seinen üppigen, tropischen Gärten für Bio-Anbau, seinen malerischen Sonnenuntergängen und zahllosen Regenbögen. Seit jeher ist es ein Ort der Ruhe und des Rückzugs: 1909 als Wohnsitz für alte Arbeiter aus der Zuckerrohrindustrie errichtet, diente es später unter anderem als Heim für Kriegsveteranen und als Schlafsaal eines Colleges. Heute ist Lumeria Maui ein „Edventure"-Retreat – ein Mix aus Abenteuer und Lernen. An diesen Ort reisen Menschen, die sich selbst und die spirituelle Energie von Maui bewusst spüren wollen. Dabei helfen Kursangebote wie Yoga, Meditation und Aromatherapie oder auch Seminare zur Gartenbaukunst, die die ganzheitliche Sichtweise der Hawaiianer auf die Früchte der Erde lehren. Wellnessbehandlungen wie die traditionelle hawaiianische Lomi-Massage tun ein Übriges, um abschalten zu können und Körper und Geist mit neuen Ideen und Energie aufzuladen.

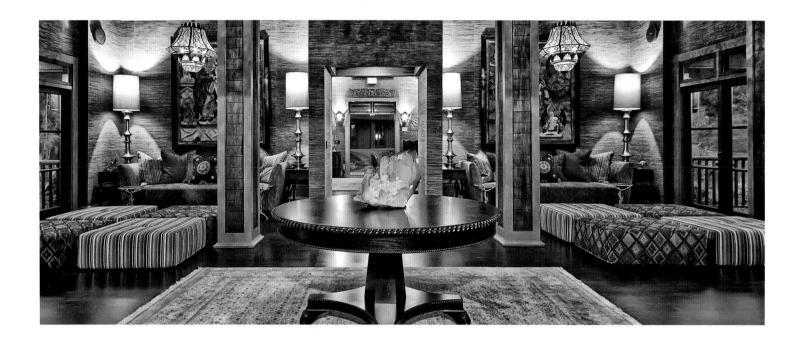

Spa, Health & Other Facilities
Harvest Café, covered and open air lanais, indoor yoga classroom, outdoor yoga platform and 6,000 square feet (560 square meters) lower terrace, tropical and edible organic gardens, meditation gardens, lobby, indoor sanctuary.

Treatments & Services
Aromatherapy, Hawaiian hot stone massage, Hawaiian Lomi Lomi massage, meditation, Reiki, sound healing, yoga.

Activities
Hiking, horseback riding, scuba diving, snorkeling, stand-up paddling, surfing.

Rooms
24 rooms: King Bed Guest Rooms, Double Bed Guest Rooms, and Suites with island and ocean views.

Located
Located between Paia and Makawao on Maui's North Shore, 20 minutes from Kahului International Airport.

1813 Baldwin Ave
Makawao, HI 96768, USA
www.lumeriamaui.com

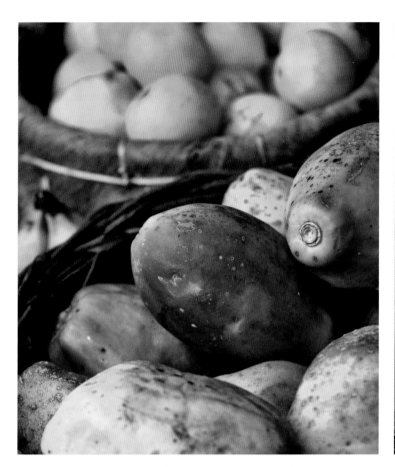

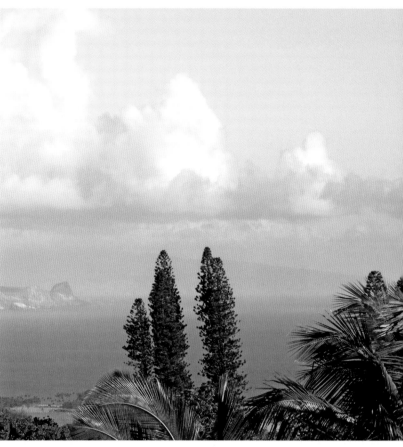

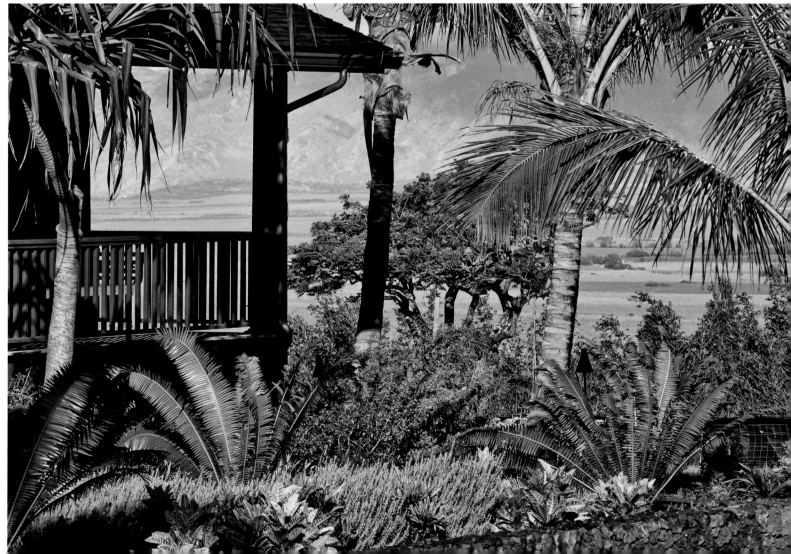

The Holy Grail in Canada's Wilderness

Der Heilige Gral in Kanadas Wildnis

Grail Springs

How did the Holy Grail from medieval Europe end up in the present-day Canadian wilderness? As a symbol of the quest for health, happiness, and eternal life force, the Grail represents the same values as the retreat in Bancroft, Canada's mineral capital. The property is a true place of power: The soil, rich in magnetic quartz, is charged with energy, and the private lake is fed by hundreds of springs. The spa has everything you need for a journey that will transform your life—a journey to yourself aimed at bringing body, mind, and spirit into equilibrium. A labyrinth helps you find your way to a place of reflection, horseback rides invigorate you with the power of nature, and meditation gardens invite you to enjoy moments of stillness. With body treatments, healing therapies, yoga, Qigong, and spiritual life counseling, the staff helps guests release blockages in order to revitalize themselves and feel happy.

Wie kommt der Heilige Gral vom europäischen Mittelalter in die heutige Wildnis Kanadas? Als Sinnbild für das Streben nach Gesundheit, Glück und ewiger Lebenskraft steht der Gral für dieselben Werte wie das Retreat in Bancroft, Kanadas Mineralienhauptstadt. Dieses Anwesen ist ein wahrer Kraftort: Der Boden, reich an magnetischem Quarz, ist energetisch aufgeladen, und der private See wird aus hunderten Quellen gespeist. Alles ist da für eine Reise, die das Leben verändert – eine Reise zu sich selbst, mit der Körper, Geist und Seele ins Gleichgewicht kommen sollen. Ein Labyrinth hilft, den Weg zur Reflexion zu finden, Ausritte stärken mit der Kraft der Natur, Meditationsgärten laden zum Innehalten ein. Mit Körperbehandlungen, Heiltherapien, Yoga, Qigong aber auch spiritueller Lebensberatung helfen die Mitarbeiter den Gästen, Blockaden zu überwinden, um sich wieder lebendig und glücklich zu fühlen.

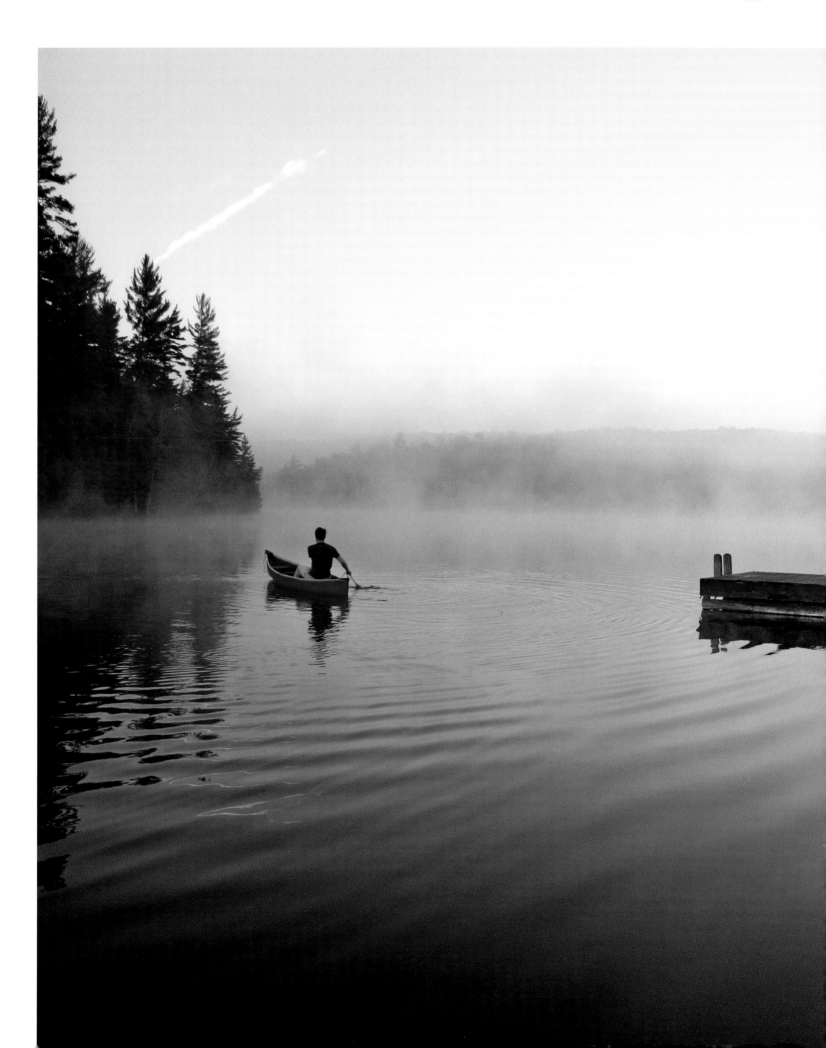

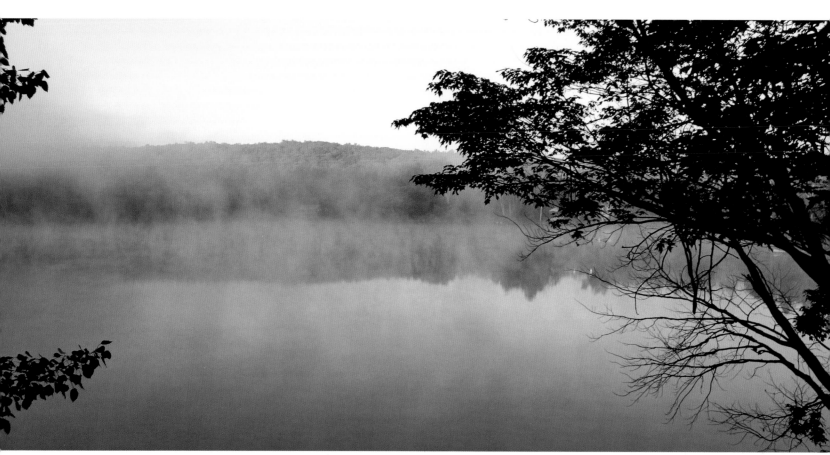

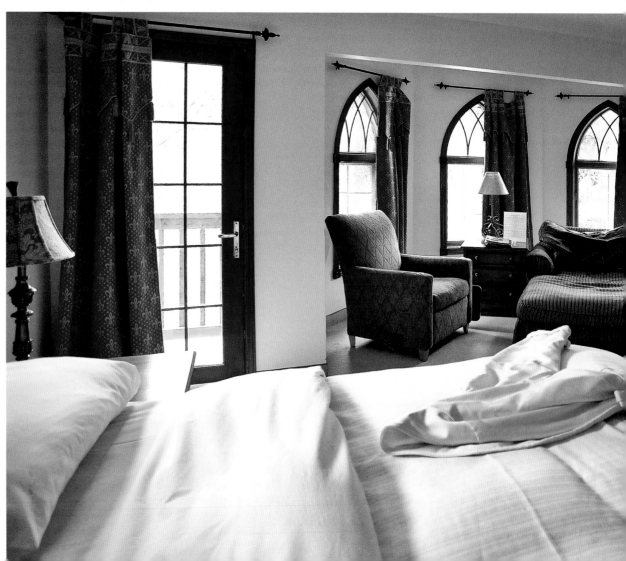

Spa, Health & Other Facilities
Outdoor hot mineral salt soaking tub, cold plunge; infrared, Finnish, and steam sauna;
meditation and yoga studio. Retail shop, locker rooms, creative arts studio.

Treatments & Services
Body wraps, colonics, core cleanse, energy balancing, exfoliants, facials, hands & feet, hair & scalp, massage,
red carpet inch-loss wrap, rituals, water therapy. Gourmet vegetarian cuisine. Airport transfers for guests
booking a stay of 5 nights or longer.

Activities
Beachfront, campfires, canoeing, forest trails, hiking, horseback riding, horse wisdom classes,
labyrinth, meditation gardens, private spring-fed lake, snowshoeing, swimming.

Rooms
13 suites – 4 categories: regular, deluxe, luxury, Spa Loft; 2 eco-forest tabins.

Located
In one of the most magnetically-charged regions of the world.
2.5 hours from Toronto International Airport.

2004 Bay Lake Road Bancroft
K0L 1C0 Bancroft, ON, Canada
www.grailsprings.com

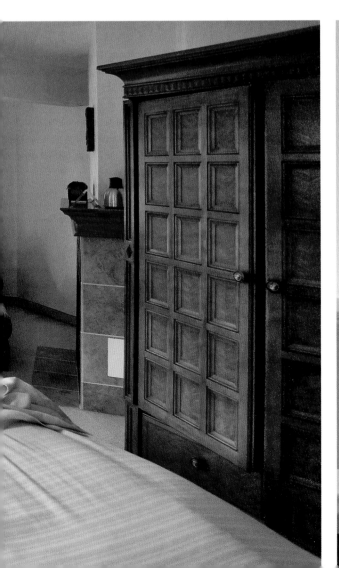
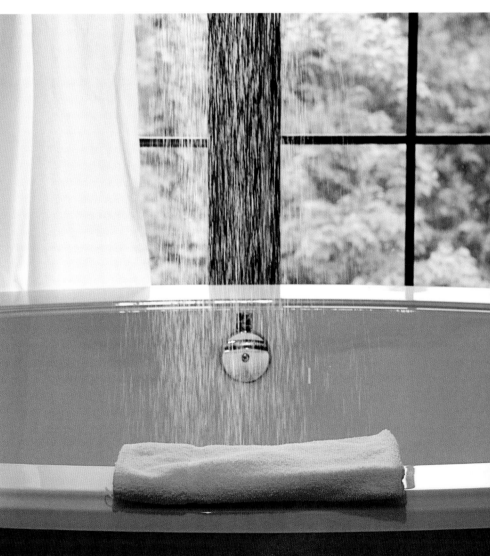

Yoga—the Magic Key

In my daily yoga practice, I work on stabilizing my inner and outer postures.

Through our outer posture, we build strength, become more resilient, and we build a good muscular system early on to ensure fitness in old age.

Inner posture means that I make it my priority to get in touch with my inner self and create a balance between body and soul. My practice on the yoga mat can also help me in my daily life. If I experience a physical impasse on the yoga mat, I cannot break through it by struggling. Instead, I take deep, gentle breaths and try to get past the barrier. The same is true in life. When obstacles arise, I return briefly to my inner self and first take a deep breath. It is important to grasp the whole picture, for the constant effort will unlock the secret to a healthy life.

I started practicing yoga after my first child was born. I suffered from such severe back pain that I could no longer walk. The condition quickly improved through yoga. As I began to practice more intensively, I experienced a deep sense of joy. How is this possible? Yoga is one of humanity's oldest recorded patterns of movement, and it involves, in part, exercises that occur in nature and among babies. When we combine this movement with the breath, we return to our source, a perfect state of bliss.

My daily yoga practice has become a magic key that unlocks my self. Through deep, gentle breathing, you very quickly reach a state of "meditation in motion," which offers infinite blessings.

Ursula Karven, actress, entrepreneur, publisher of the DVDs
"Yoga Everyday" and "Power Yoga"

Yoga – der magische Schlüssel

Bei meiner täglichen Yogapraxis geht es mir um die Stabilisierung der inneren und äußeren Haltung.

Durch die äußere Haltung stärken wir uns, werden widerstandsfähiger und fangen frühzeitig an, ein gutes muskuläres System aufzubauen, um im Alter fit zu sein.

Die innere Haltung bedeutet, dass ich mir selbst Priorität einräume, zu mir selbst zurückfinde und Seele und Körper in Balance bringe. Was ich auf der Yogamatte übe, kann mir auch im Alltag helfen: Wenn ich auf der Yogamatte körperliche Blockaden habe, dann durchbreche ich sie nicht mit Anstrengung, sondern atme sanft durch und versuche, sie auf diese Weise zu lösen. Das Gleiche gilt für das Leben. Wenn Hindernisse auftauchen, dann kehre ich kurz in mich und atme erst einmal durch. Es ist wichtig, zunächst das ganze Bild zu begreifen, damit sich mir durch stetes Bemühen das Leben öffnet.

Yoga begann ich nach der Geburt meines ersten Kindes, als ich so starke Rückenprobleme hatte, dass ich nicht mehr gehen konnte, was sich durch Yoga schnell verbesserte. Als ich dann anfing, intensiver zu praktizieren, stellte sich ein tiefes Glücksgefühl bei mir ein. Wie ist das möglich? Yoga ist die älteste aufgezeichnete Bewegungsform der Menschheit und besteht zum Teil aus Übungen, wie sie in der Natur und bei Säuglingen vorkommen. Wenn wir diese Bewegung zusammen mit dem Atem ausführen, kommen wir zurück zu unserem Ursprung, dem perfekten Zustand von Glückseligkeit.

Meine tägliche Yogapraxis ist ein magischer Schlüssel zu mir selbst geworden: Durch das tiefe, sanfte Atmen findet man sehr schnell zu einer „Meditation in Bewegung", die einem unendlich viel Segen schenken kann.

Ursula Karven, Schauspielerin, Unternehmerin, Herausgeberin der DVDs „Yoga Everyday" und „Power Yoga"

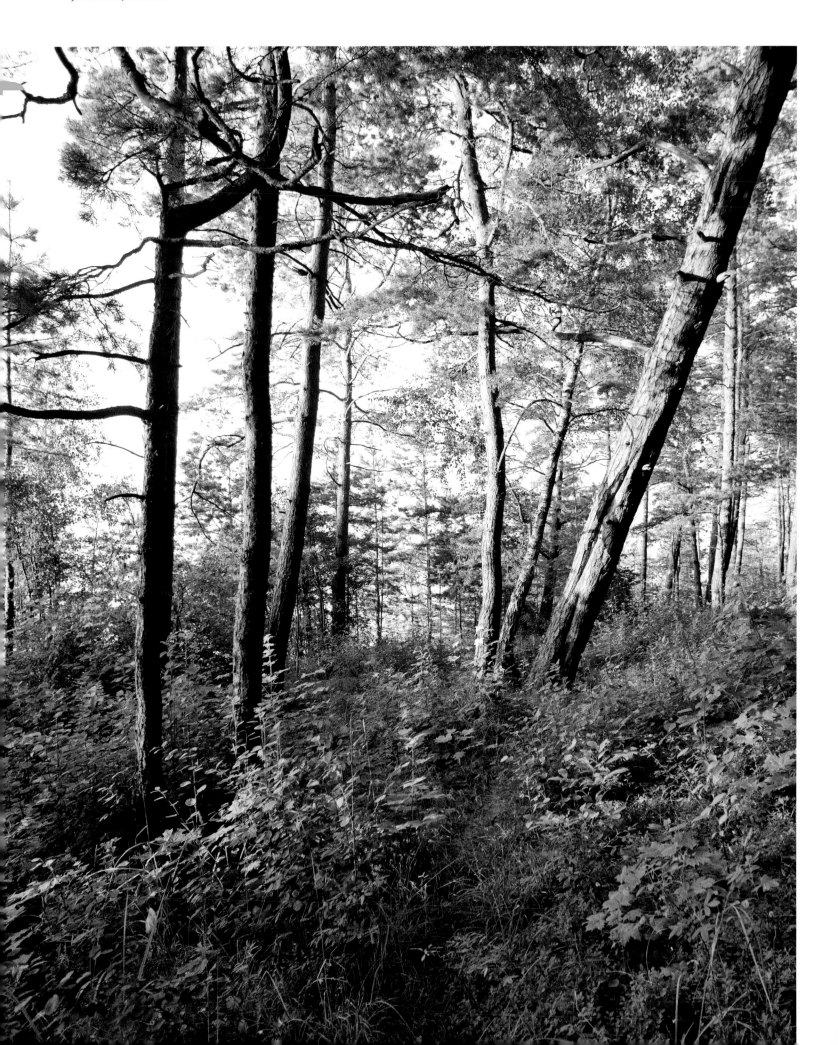

Jūrmala, Latvia

Getting to Know the Latvian Soul

Die tiefe lettische Seele spüren

Amber Spa Boutique Hotel

The sea air carries the scent of pine, the ocean laps gently against the shore, and white sand pampers your feet. The Latvian beach resort of Jūrmala, situated between a pine forest and the seashore, is simply made for restoring your life to its proper balance. Indeed, this healthy environment is one of four factors in the patented "Balans Lifestyle Program" offered by the Amber Spa Boutique Hotel. The program is based on the assumption that everyone is born with a health reserve that is depleted by stressors in the environment. To maintain our health and feel good all around, we have to refill the reservoir at regular intervals. The program includes individual nutrition and fitness plans based on a thorough wellness checkup at the beginning of treatment, along with relaxation phases to achieve emotional equilibrium. Hospitality and modern interpretations of the traditional cuisine enable guests to experience the Latvian soul throughout the hotel.

Die Seeluft duftet nach Kiefern, sanft rauscht das Meer, weißer Sand umschmeichelt die Füße. Der lettische Badeort Jūrmala zwischen Kiefernwald und Küste ist dafür geschaffen, verloren gegangene Lebensbalance wiederzufinden. Genau diese gesunde Umgebung ist einer von vier Faktoren des patentierten „Balans Lifestyle Programms" im Amber Spa Boutique Hotel. Der Ansatz lautet, dass alle Menschen mit einem Vorrat an Gesundheit geboren werden, der von den Stressfaktoren der Umwelt verbraucht wird. Um die Gesundheit zu erhalten und sich rundum wohlzufühlen, muss das Reservoir regelmäßig wieder aufgefüllt werden. Teil des Programms sind individuelle Ernährungs- und Fitnesspläne auf der Basis einer fundierten Anfangs-untersuchung sowie Entspannungsphasen zur emotionalen Ausgeglichenheit. Gastfreundschaft und traditionelle Küche in moderner Zubereitung lassen die Gäste die lettische Seele im ganzen Haus spüren.

Jūrmala, Latvia

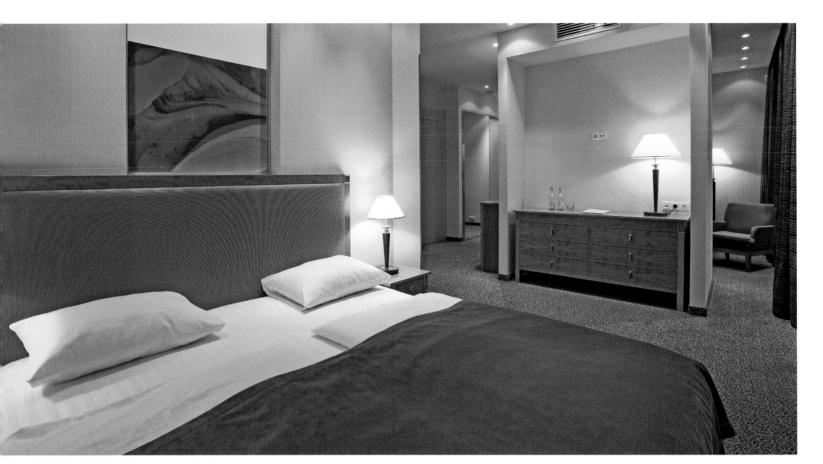

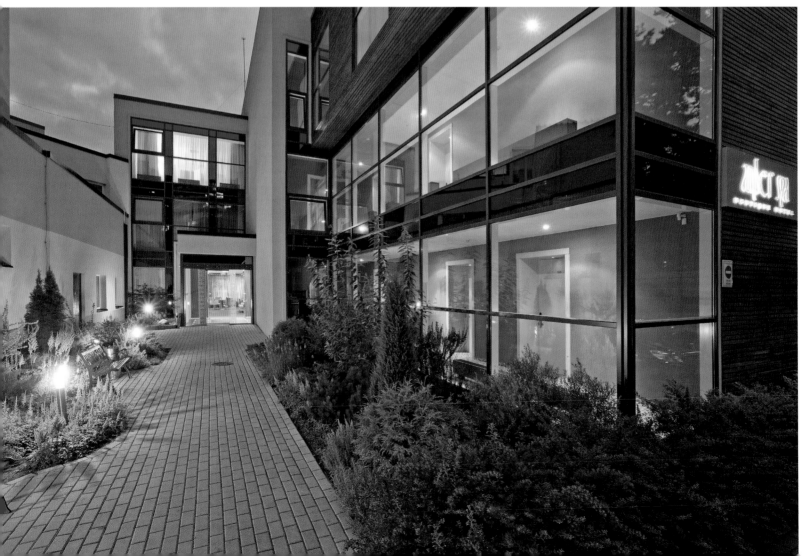

Spa, Health & Other Facilities

Spa & Wellness center, 15 treatment rooms, swimming pool with roof terrace, traditional Russian baths, infrared sauna, fitness studio, gym. Beauty salon, gourmet restaurant and bakery, kids play room, bowling and club lounge, tennis courts, gallery, gift shop, elevator.

Treatments & Services

Acupuncture, aerobics, anti-stress, aqua aerobics, bio-resonance test, burn out, color therapy, craniosacral therapy, detox, emotional balance, facial, fitness diagnostics, holistic health consultations, hydrotherapy, hydrocolon therapy, indigenous healing techniques, kinesiology, lifestyle coaching, Lomi Lomi, lymphatic drainage, manicure, meditation, myostructural massage, nutritional consultation, osteopathy, pedicure, Pilates, reflexology, rehabilitation massage, sleep programs, traditional Russian baths, vacuum massage, yoga. Special diet menues on request, weight loss programs, wellness diagnostics. Babysitting, bicycle rental, hair styling, laundry service.

Activities

Bird-watching, bowling, castle tours, fishing, fitness, golf, guided nature walks, horseback riding on the beach, hunting, Livu water park, picnics, sightseeing in Riga, tennis.

Rooms

21 suites – 1, 2 and 3-bedroom suites, ranging from 431 to 753 square feet (40 to 70 square meters).

Located

15 miles (25 kilometers) from Riga, 15 minutes by car from Riga Airport.

Meža prospekts 49
2010 Jūrmala, Latvia
www.iwcbalans.com

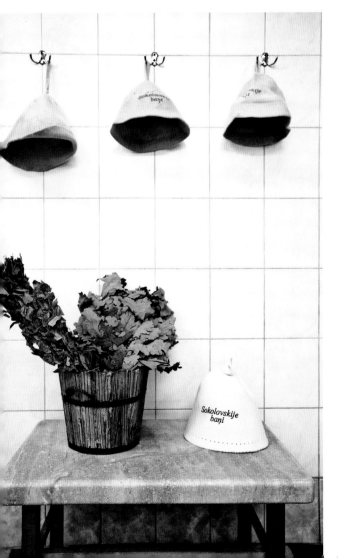

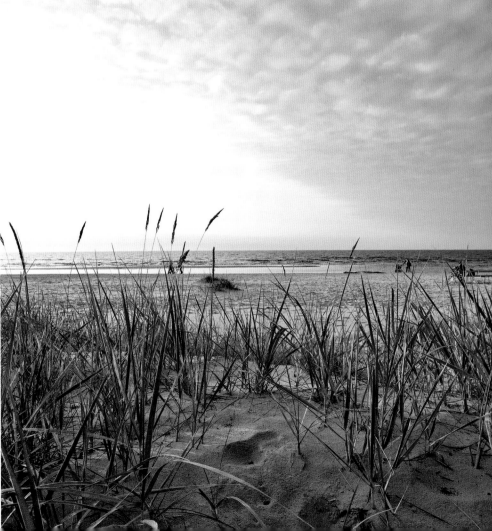

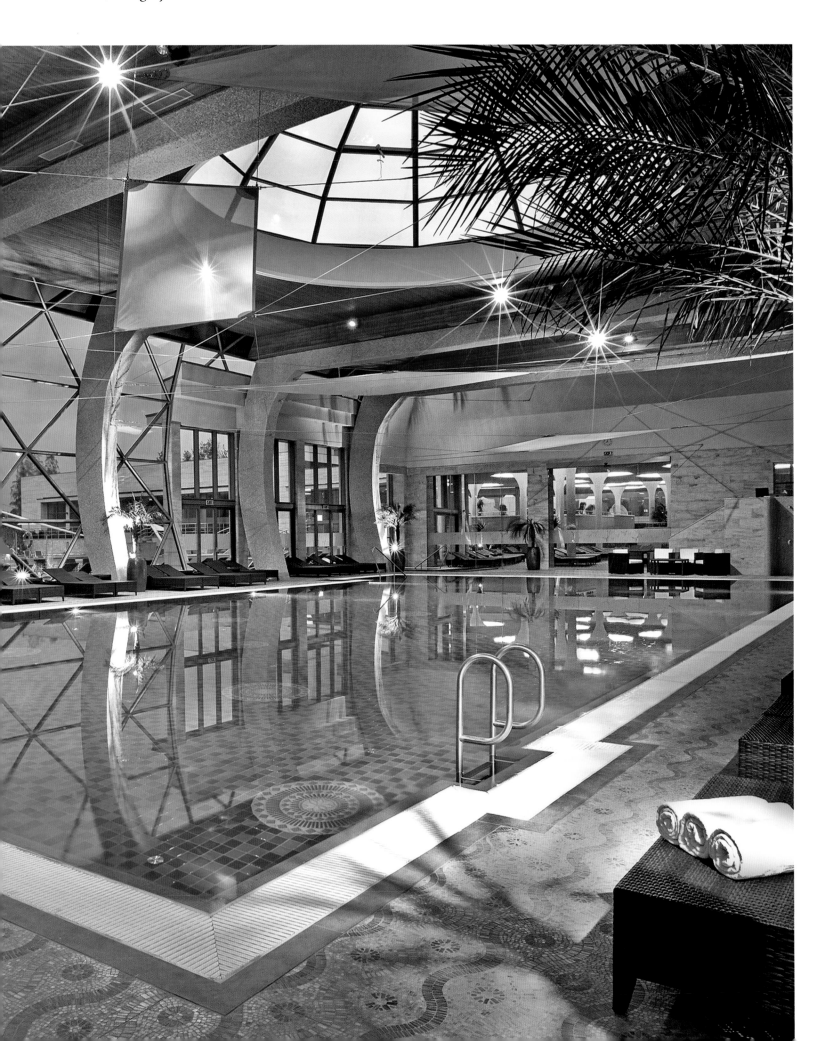

Sárvár, Hungary

Where Health Springs Eternal

An der Quelle der Gesundheit

Spirit Hotel

Like water from a spring, life energy can also bubble up from deep inside of a person—welcome to the fountain of youth for body and soul! The Spirit Hotel, close to the seven lakes of Sárvár, has the good fortune of possessing its own mineral spring. And guests can share in this good fortune, since the Spirit healing water is contained in each of the hotel's pools, which are emptied, cleaned, and refilled daily. After all, in the spa with its numerous pools, everything naturally revolves around water. Most of the wellness programs are based on the warm healing water that bubbles up from depths of more than 3,200 feet. For example, the water is used under a doctor's supervision to treat musculoskeletal system disorders and skin problems. Containing a high concentration of minerals, the water of the Sárvár medicinal crystal bath also has a healing effect. Or one can choose to simply drift about in a thermal pool. For variety, one can listen to underwater music in the swimming pool, relax in the hammam, or be pampered with calming and relaxing treatments. Far from the tourist crowds, the hotel will also invite you to take full advantage of nature's tranquility. Small, natural lakes, lush summer meadows, and peaceful leafy forests await you in the immediate vicinity.

Wie das Wasser aus der Quelle, so kann auch die Lebensenergie wieder aus dem Inneren heraussprudeln. Das Spirit Hotel unweit der sieben Seen von Bad Sárvár hat das Glück, eine eigene Heilquelle zu besitzen. Und Gäste können an diesem Glück teilhaben, denn das Spirit-Heilwasser befindet sich in jedem der hotel-eigenen Heilwasserbecken, die täglich entleert, gereinigt und neu befüllt werden. Auch im Spa-Bereich mit seinen unzähligen Pools dreht sich alles um das feuchte Element. Die meisten Gesundheitsangebote basieren auf dem Heilwasser, das aus über 1 000 Metern Tiefe warm emporsprudelt. Unter ärztlicher Aufsicht wird es zum Beispiel bei Beschwerden des Bewegungsapparates oder Hautproblemen angewendet. Ebenso heilende Wirkung haben die medizinischen Wannenbäder mit Sárvárer Heilkristallsole, die eine hohe Konzentration an Mineralien aufweist. Oder man lässt sich einfach in einem Thermalpool treiben. Zur Abwechslung sollte man im Schwimmbad Unterwassermusik lauschen, im Hamam schwitzen oder sich von beruhigenden und entspannenden Behandlungen verwöhnen lassen. Das Hotel abseits von Touristenströmen lädt darüber hinaus dazu ein, die Ruhe der Natur auszuschöpfen: In unmittelbarer Nähe warten natürliche kleine Seen, saftige Sommerwiesen und stille Laubwälder.

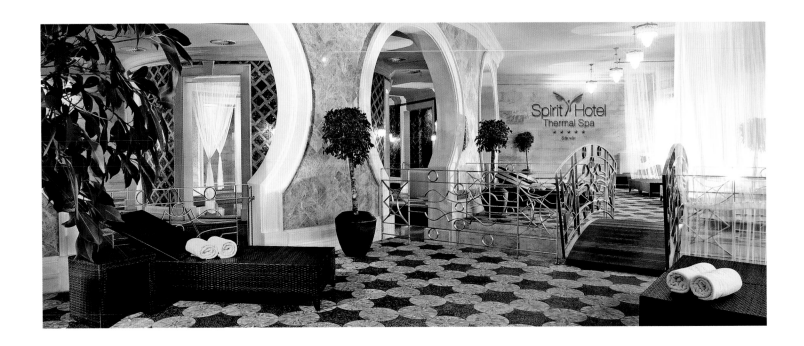

Spa, Health & Other Facilities
22 pools and whirlpools, exclusive outdoor pool area, adventure pool, mineral hot spring pools, steam room, sauna, underwater sound system. Onyx restaurant, Oxygen bar, lobby bar, conference and event center with garden and pool view, fit up to 500 visitors, gift shop, hair salon, library, elevator.

Treatments & Services
Ayurvedic foot massage, Ayurvedic health check, Ayurvedic massage, aromabath, aromamassage, bath for couples, Caracalla Sensation bath, floating, hammam, Kneipp therapy, medical examination, Pharmos Natur Royal treatment, Pharmos Natur VEDA ME purifying massage, rhassoul, Sárvár medical crystal bath, Thali'sens Asia, Thali'sens Orient, Thali'sens Polynesia, therapeutic treatments.

Activities
Biking, bowling, cycling, fishing, fitness, horseback riding, Nordic walking, sightseeing, squash, tennis.

Rooms
271 rooms with balcony.

Located
15 minutes by foot to the center. 2 hours by car to Vienna, 2.5 hours to Budapest.

Vadkert krt. 5
9600 Sárvár, Hungary
www.spirithotel.eu

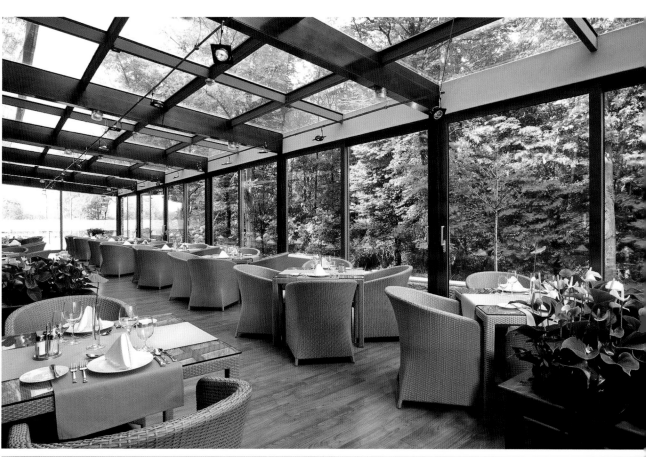

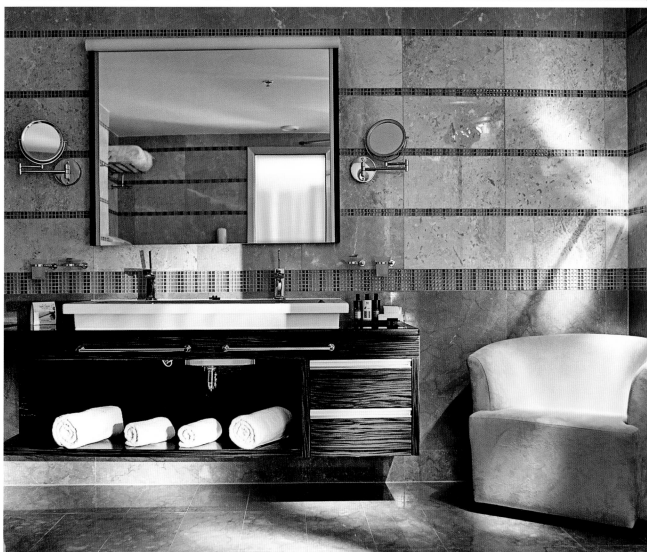

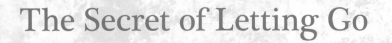

The Secret of Letting Go

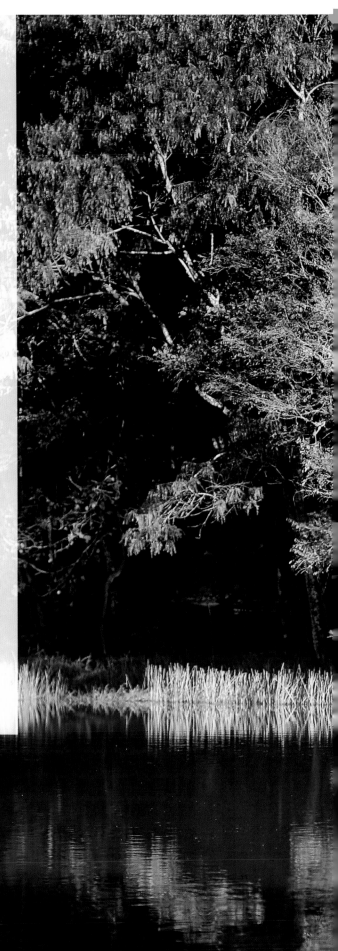

Practicing and realizing mindfulness in ourselves can have tremendous effects on us and our surroundings. Those who practice mindfulness regularly will not only notice that their ability to focus increases, and that they feel more anchored in their daily lives, but also that they remain more relaxed in stressful situations. Those who practice become more attentive—something that we have been exhorted to do since we were children, but which we have lacked the tools to actually achieve.

Concentration is always limited; mindfulness is neutral, and it does not tire us because it is linked to the power that lies in the moment. Being mindful means being free of distractions, both inside and outside. The mind ceases to function as an unwanted commentator that evaluates ourselves and others depending on our mood, that fosters fear, causes us to overreact, and feeds greed, envy, hate, and hostility. When we are mindful, we take a step back from the spontaneous comments we might otherwise make. We react in a more balanced manner and refrain from immediately saying whatever comes to mind; instead, we first reflect out of a neutral position upon our response before we verbalize our thoughts. When we are mindful, we are fully present in every moment and we give our very best. We are no longer dependent on what others think of us, because we have recognized who we really are. That gives us the freedom from which we act instead of clinging to people, things, and ideas.

We meet the words and feelings of others with the serenity necessary for "true" communication to take place. We listen and are heard. The further our development progresses, the less we are entangled in things that do not concern us. When we practice mindfulness, we no longer identify with intellectual attributes ("I am the one who always works the longest," "Why is it always me," "Typical me," "I am always overworked/unchallenged") and we also cease to use these same criteria to judge others. Since each of us is nothing other than clear energy superimposed with thoughts and feelings.

Those who live mindfully approach their true selves. The key to happiness is not found in suppression nor in the realization of what our minds produce in terms of ideas and desires. It is the spark of mindfulness that can ignite the light of understanding in us.

Han Shan, author of "Das Geheimnis des Loslassens" (The Secret of Letting Go), "Wer loslässt hat zwei Hände frei" (Once You Let Go, You Have Both Hands Free), and "Achtsamkeit: Die höchste Form des Selbstmanagements" (Mindfulness: The Highest Form of Self Management)

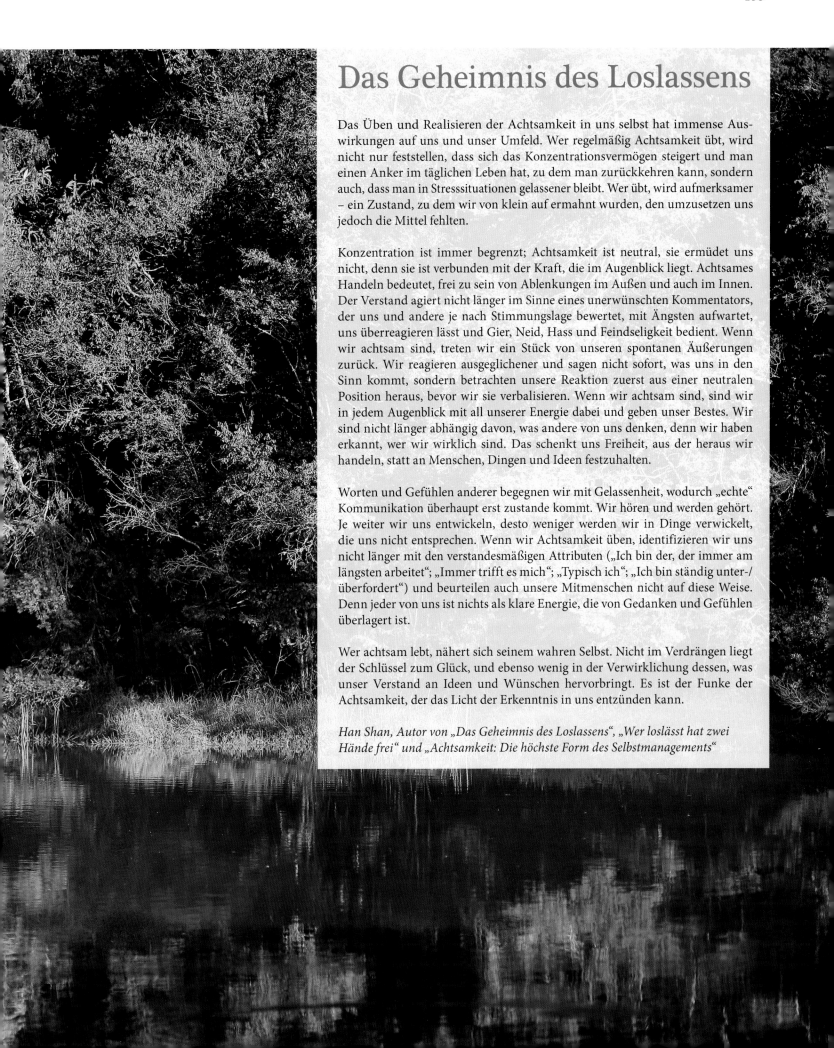

Das Geheimnis des Loslassens

Das Üben und Realisieren der Achtsamkeit in uns selbst hat immense Auswirkungen auf uns und unser Umfeld. Wer regelmäßig Achtsamkeit übt, wird nicht nur feststellen, dass sich das Konzentrationsvermögen steigert und man einen Anker im täglichen Leben hat, zu dem man zurückkehren kann, sondern auch, dass man in Stresssituationen gelassener bleibt. Wer übt, wird aufmerksamer – ein Zustand, zu dem wir von klein auf ermahnt wurden, den umzusetzen uns jedoch die Mittel fehlten.

Konzentration ist immer begrenzt; Achtsamkeit ist neutral, sie ermüdet uns nicht, denn sie ist verbunden mit der Kraft, die im Augenblick liegt. Achtsames Handeln bedeutet, frei zu sein von Ablenkungen im Außen und auch im Innen. Der Verstand agiert nicht länger im Sinne eines unerwünschten Kommentators, der uns und andere je nach Stimmungslage bewertet, mit Ängsten aufwartet, uns überreagieren lässt und Gier, Neid, Hass und Feindseligkeit bedient. Wenn wir achtsam sind, treten wir ein Stück von unseren spontanen Äußerungen zurück. Wir reagieren ausgeglichener und sagen nicht sofort, was uns in den Sinn kommt, sondern betrachten unsere Reaktion zuerst aus einer neutralen Position heraus, bevor wir sie verbalisieren. Wenn wir achtsam sind, sind wir in jedem Augenblick mit all unserer Energie dabei und geben unser Bestes. Wir sind nicht länger abhängig davon, was andere von uns denken, denn wir haben erkannt, wer wir wirklich sind. Das schenkt uns Freiheit, aus der heraus wir handeln, statt an Menschen, Dingen und Ideen festzuhalten.

Worten und Gefühlen anderer begegnen wir mit Gelassenheit, wodurch „echte" Kommunikation überhaupt erst zustande kommt. Wir hören und werden gehört. Je weiter wir uns entwickeln, desto weniger werden wir in Dinge verwickelt, die uns nicht entsprechen. Wenn wir Achtsamkeit üben, identifizieren wir uns nicht länger mit den verstandesmäßigen Attributen („Ich bin der, der immer am längsten arbeitet"; „Immer trifft es mich"; „Typisch ich"; „Ich bin ständig unter-/überfordert") und beurteilen auch unsere Mitmenschen nicht auf diese Weise. Denn jeder von uns ist nichts als klare Energie, die von Gedanken und Gefühlen überlagert ist.

Wer achtsam lebt, nähert sich seinem wahren Selbst. Nicht im Verdrängen liegt der Schlüssel zum Glück, und ebenso wenig in der Verwirklichung dessen, was unser Verstand an Ideen und Wünschen hervorbringt. Es ist der Funke der Achtsamkeit, der das Licht der Erkenntnis in uns entzünden kann.

Han Shan, Autor von „Das Geheimnis des Loslassens", „Wer loslässt hat zwei Hände frei" und „Achtsamkeit: Die höchste Form des Selbstmanagements"

Healing from the Depth of the Mountains

Heilung aus der Tiefe der Berge

Grand Park Hotel

Restful nights are a key to well-being. The Grand Park Hotel has an in-house sleep lab where guests get the opportunity to have their sleeping patterns analyzed and to learn how to get more rest. Yet, it would be a big mistake to sleep away the entire stay amid the mountains and hot springs of the beautiful Gastein Valley. Thanks to the hotel's wellness program, which integrates both indoor and outdoor therapies, everyday life will seem very far away. What shouldn't be missed are the health packages based on the renowned Gasteiner healing water, which was prized even by the ancient Romans, or on the Gasteiner Heilstollen (a curative cave gallery). Pleasant heat and health-giving radon pampers guests as they bathe in the hot springs and when entering the gallery—an effective and natural treatment for ailments such as joint pain.

Erholsame Nächte sind ein Schlüssel zum Wohlbefinden. Deshalb kann man im hoteleigenen Schlaflabor des Grand Park Hotels sein Schlummer-Verhalten analysieren lassen und lernen, besser zur Ruhe zu kommen. Den Aufenthalt zwischen Bergen und Quellen im wunderschönen Gasteinertal allerdings komplett zu verschlafen, wäre ein großer Fehler. Dank des Wellnessangebots im Haus und in der freien Natur rückt der Alltag nämlich in weite Ferne. Gesundheitspakete rund um das berühmte Gasteiner Heilwasser, das schon die alten Römer schätzten, und den Gasteiner Heilstollen dürfen dabei nicht fehlen. Angenehme Wärme und heilsames Radon verwöhnen die Gäste beim Baden im Thermalwasser und bei der Einfahrt in den Stollen – eine wirksame und natürliche Behandlung, zum Beispiel von Gelenkleiden.

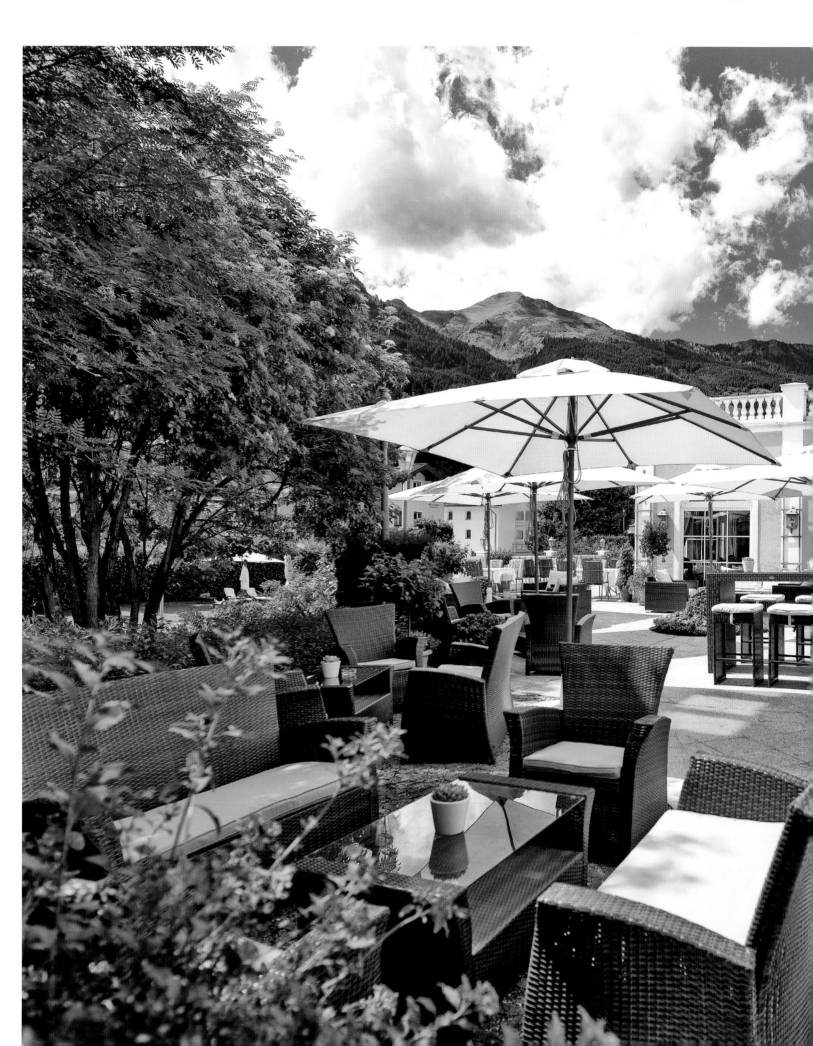

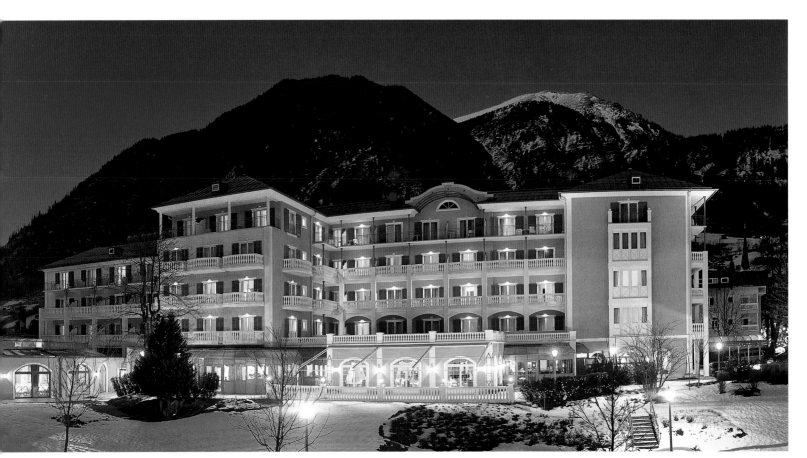

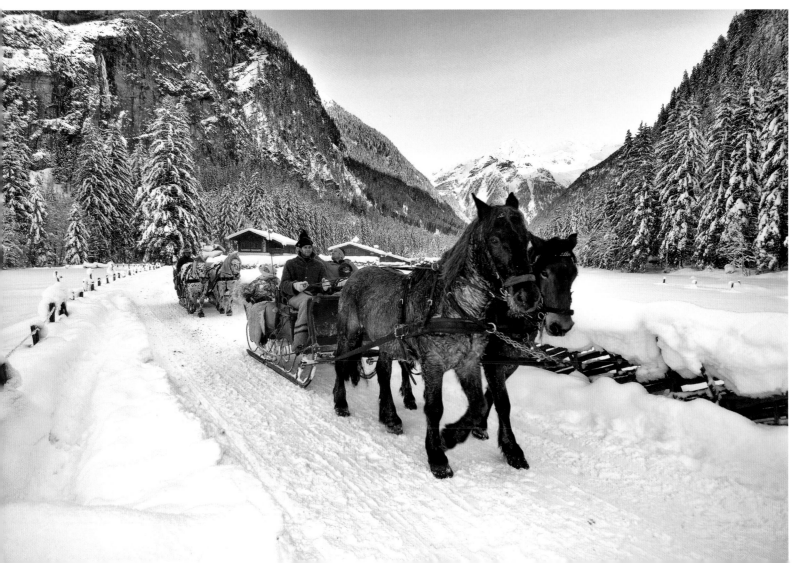

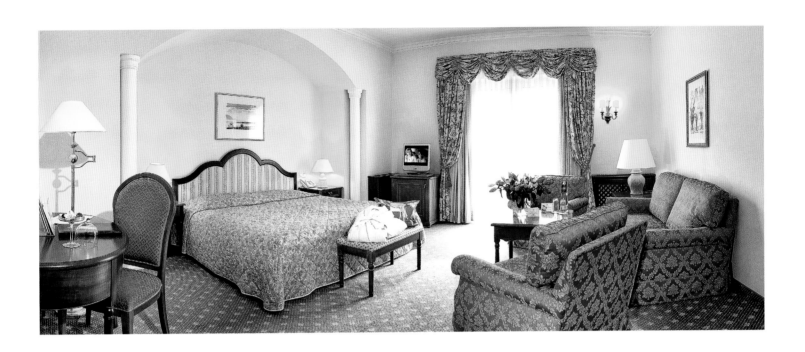

Spa, Health & Other Facilities
Thermal indoor pool, 2 whirlpools, gym. Grand Park Spa: rose quartz steam bath, aromatic steam grotto, snail adventure showers, circular shower, sole inhalation grotto, laconium, tepidarium, ice igloo, Finnish sauna, aromatic sauna, bio-herb sauna, circular cliff shower, heat bench retreat, Kneipp footpath, room of silence.
A la carte and half-board restaurant, Grand Park & Grand Spa Cuisine, bar/ lounge, conference rooms for groups up to 50 people.

Treatments & Services
Aromatherapy, body treatments and baths, La Stone Therapy, manual lymphatic drainage; packages for rheumatism, arthritis and arthrosis, fibromyalgia, and Bekhterev's disease; reflexology, Swedish massage.
24-hour front desk, free parking, multilingual staff, transfer service from the airport.

Activities
Climbing, golf, hiking, jogging, mountain biking, Nordic walking, outdoor program, ski, swimming, tennis.

Rooms
89 rooms and suites. Each room features a balcony.

Located
56 miles (90 kilometers) from Salzburg Airport. The next train station is Bad Hofgastein.

Kurgartenstraße 26
5630 Bad Hofgastein, Austria
www.grandparkhotel.at

Traditional Values of Natural Simplicity

Traditionelle Werte natürlicher Einfachheit

Hotel Post

In earlier times, people knew what was good for them—living in harmony with nature, making do with the essentials of life, and maintaining an awareness of quality and authenticity. Too often today, people lose sight of these values. Fortunately, there is a place where they've been preserved: the Hotel Post in the picturesque Bregenz Forest. Clarity, style, and warmth blend to perfection, while purist architecture and unfussy design meet delicious, top-rated cuisine and a prize-winning spa. Everyday stress evaporates in the hotel's various saunas or is rinsed away in the open-air whirlpool and outdoor saltwater pools under the open sky. Run by the Kaufmann family for generations, the hotel near Lake Constance is already an established tradition. Susanne Kaufmann owns and manages the Hotel Post, which is known for its remarkable TCM program. Under the direction of Dr. Brigitte Klett, the program focuses on active stress reduction, healthy sleep, burnout recovery, pain relief, and weight regulation. The hotel has its own line of cosmetics based on regional, plant-derived agents, which are used in the Susanne Kaufmann Spa. At the Hotel Post, health means living in harmony.

Früher wussten die Menschen noch sehr genau, was ihnen gut tut – ein Leben im Einklang mit der Natur, die Beschränkung auf das Wesentliche, ein Bewusstsein für Qualität und Wahrhaftigkeit. Heute gehen solche Werte jedoch viel zu oft unter. Zum Glück gibt es einen Ort, an dem sie gewahrt sind – das Hotel Post im idyllischen Bregenzerwald. Klarheit, Stil und Wärme sind hier perfekt kombiniert: Puristische Architektur und schnörkelloses Design treffen auf eine ausgezeichnete Haubenküche und ein mehrfach ausgezeichnetes Spa. Hier schmilzt der Alltagsstress in diversen Saunen dahin, oder er wird im Open-Air-Whirlpool oder Außen-solebecken unter freiem Himmel fortgespült. Seit Generationen von der Familie Kaufmann betrieben, hat das Hotel nahe dem Bodensee bereits Tradition. Susanne Kaufmann ist die Inhaberin und Leiterin vom Hotel Post, das für seine bemerkenswerten TCM-Programme unter der Leitung von Dr. Brigitte Klett bekannt ist und folgende Schwerpunkte hat: aktiven Stressabbau, gesunden Schlaf, Burnout-Rehabilitation, Schmerzlinderung und Gewichtsregulierung. Es gibt eine eigene Kosmetiklinie, die auf pflanzlichen Wirk-stoffen aus der Region basiert und im Susanne Kaufmann Spa verwendet wird. Gesundheit heißt hier in Harmonie leben.

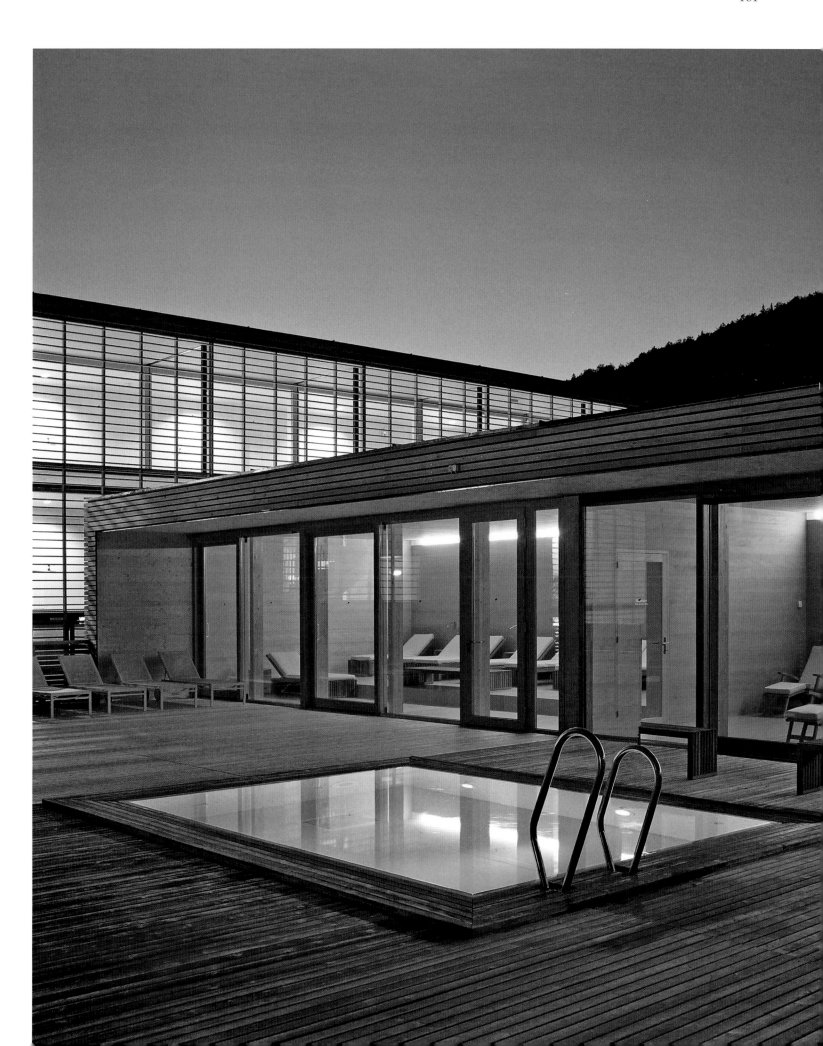

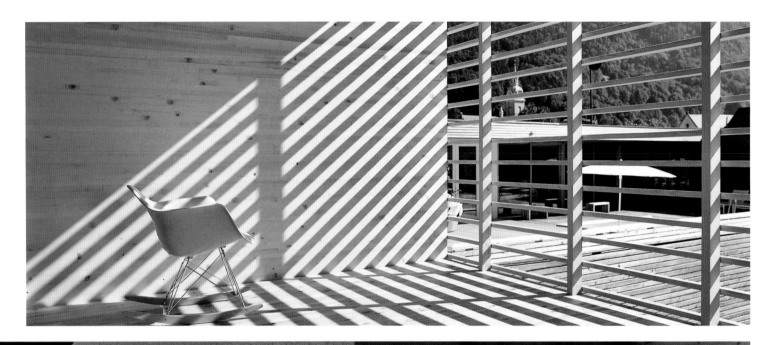

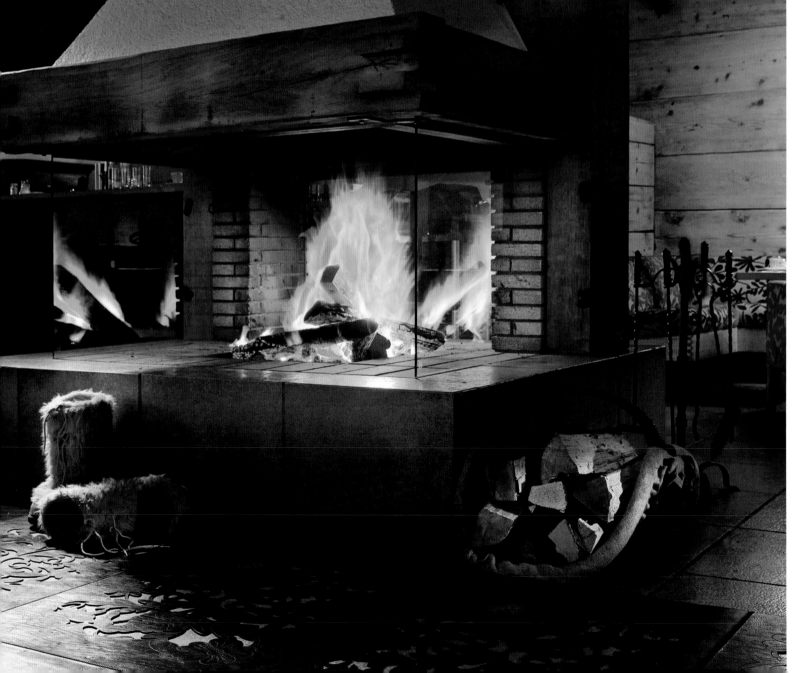

Spa, Health & Other Facilities
Indoor pool, outdoor saltwater pool, open-air Jacuzzi, Susanne Kaufmann Spa, 15 treatment rooms and multi-functional cabins, bath house, Finnish sauna, bio sauna, steam bath, garden sauna, gym, sun deck, relaxation rooms, Samina power sleeping room. Business center. Detox cuisine.

Treatments & Services
Beauty, body, and individual treatments, natural anti aging, personal training, Pilates, Qigong, TCM medical treatments, yoga. Use of the own cosmetic line (www.susannekaufmann.com). Free parking.

Activities
Cross-country skiing, golf, hiking, mountain biking, Nordic walking, Skiing, snowshoeing, tennis.

Rooms
54 rooms and 4 suites.

Located
Bregenzerwald, close to the German and Swiss border. 44 miles (70 kilometers) from Friedrichshafen Airport, 93 miles (150 kilometers) from Zurich Airport, 155 miles (250 kilometers) from Munich Airport.

Brugg 35
6870 Bezau, Austria
www.hotelpostbezau.com

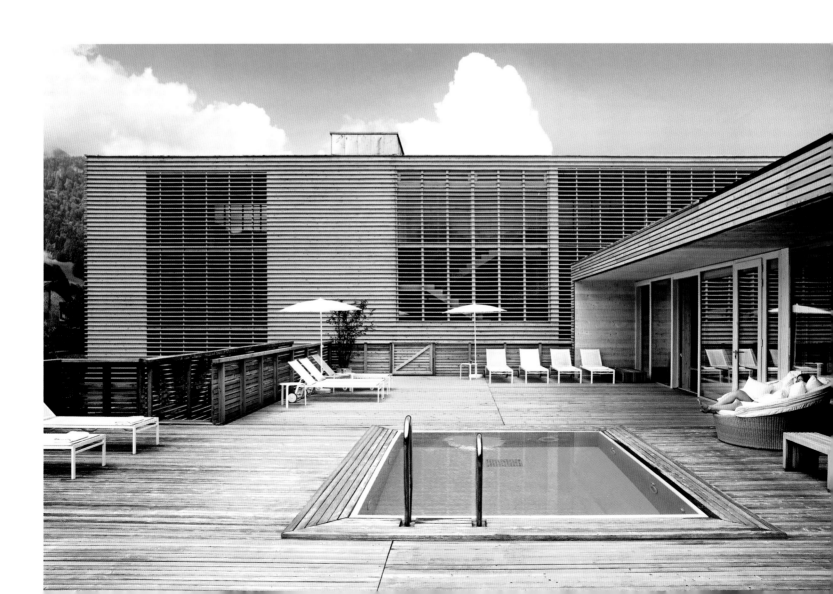

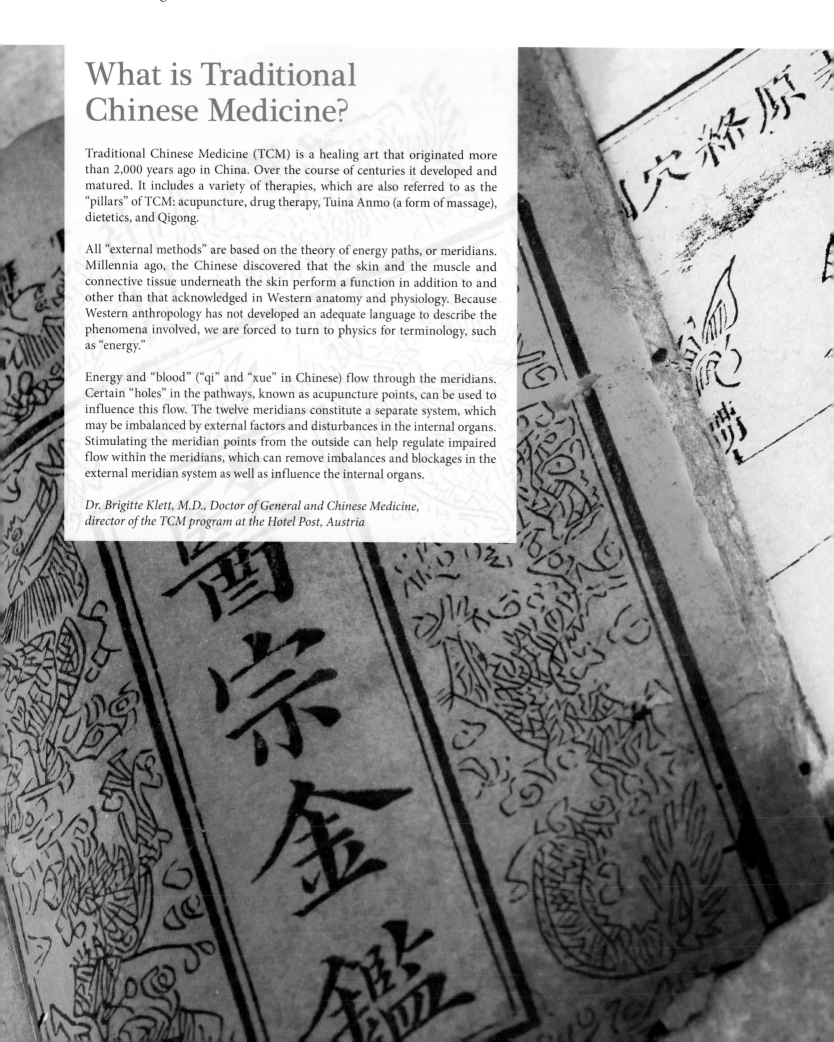

What is Traditional Chinese Medicine?

Traditional Chinese Medicine (TCM) is a healing art that originated more than 2,000 years ago in China. Over the course of centuries it developed and matured. It includes a variety of therapies, which are also referred to as the "pillars" of TCM: acupuncture, drug therapy, Tuina Anmo (a form of massage), dietetics, and Qigong.

All "external methods" are based on the theory of energy paths, or meridians. Millennia ago, the Chinese discovered that the skin and the muscle and connective tissue underneath the skin perform a function in addition to and other than that acknowledged in Western anatomy and physiology. Because Western anthropology has not developed an adequate language to describe the phenomena involved, we are forced to turn to physics for terminology, such as "energy."

Energy and "blood" ("qi" and "xue" in Chinese) flow through the meridians. Certain "holes" in the pathways, known as acupuncture points, can be used to influence this flow. The twelve meridians constitute a separate system, which may be imbalanced by external factors and disturbances in the internal organs. Stimulating the meridian points from the outside can help regulate impaired flow within the meridians, which can remove imbalances and blockages in the external meridian system as well as influence the internal organs.

Dr. Brigitte Klett, M.D., Doctor of General and Chinese Medicine, director of the TCM program at the Hotel Post, Austria

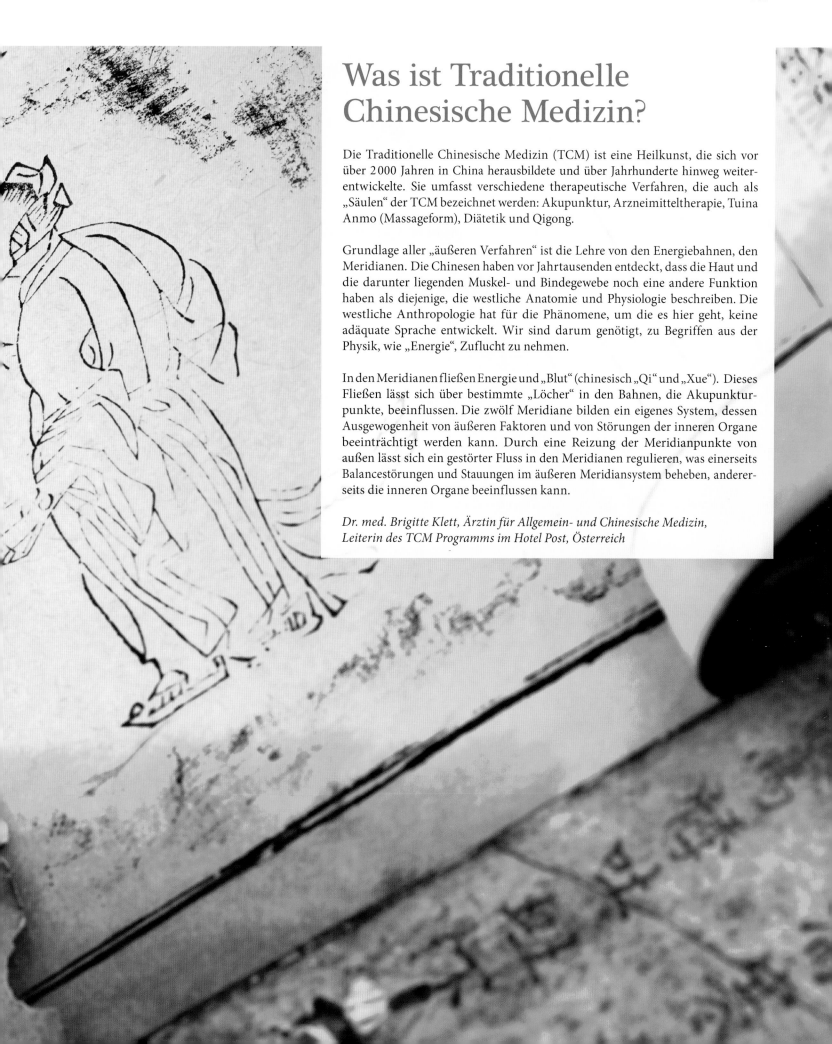

Was ist Traditionelle Chinesische Medizin?

Die Traditionelle Chinesische Medizin (TCM) ist eine Heilkunst, die sich vor über 2000 Jahren in China herausbildete und über Jahrhunderte hinweg weiterentwickelte. Sie umfasst verschiedene therapeutische Verfahren, die auch als „Säulen" der TCM bezeichnet werden: Akupunktur, Arzneimitteltherapie, Tuina Anmo (Massageform), Diätetik und Qigong.

Grundlage aller „äußeren Verfahren" ist die Lehre von den Energiebahnen, den Meridianen. Die Chinesen haben vor Jahrtausenden entdeckt, dass die Haut und die darunter liegenden Muskel- und Bindegewebe noch eine andere Funktion haben als diejenige, die westliche Anatomie und Physiologie beschreiben. Die westliche Anthropologie hat für die Phänomene, um die es hier geht, keine adäquate Sprache entwickelt. Wir sind darum genötigt, zu Begriffen aus der Physik, wie „Energie", Zuflucht zu nehmen.

In den Meridianen fließen Energie und „Blut" (chinesisch „Qi" und „Xue"). Dieses Fließen lässt sich über bestimmte „Löcher" in den Bahnen, die Akupunkturpunkte, beeinflussen. Die zwölf Meridiane bilden ein eigenes System, dessen Ausgewogenheit von äußeren Faktoren und von Störungen der inneren Organe beeinträchtigt werden kann. Durch eine Reizung der Meridianpunkte von außen lässt sich ein gestörter Fluss in den Meridianen regulieren, was einerseits Balancestörungen und Stauungen im äußeren Meridiansystem beheben, andererseits die inneren Organe beeinflussen kann.

Dr. med. Brigitte Klett, Ärztin für Allgemein- und Chinesische Medizin, Leiterin des TCM Programms im Hotel Post, Österreich

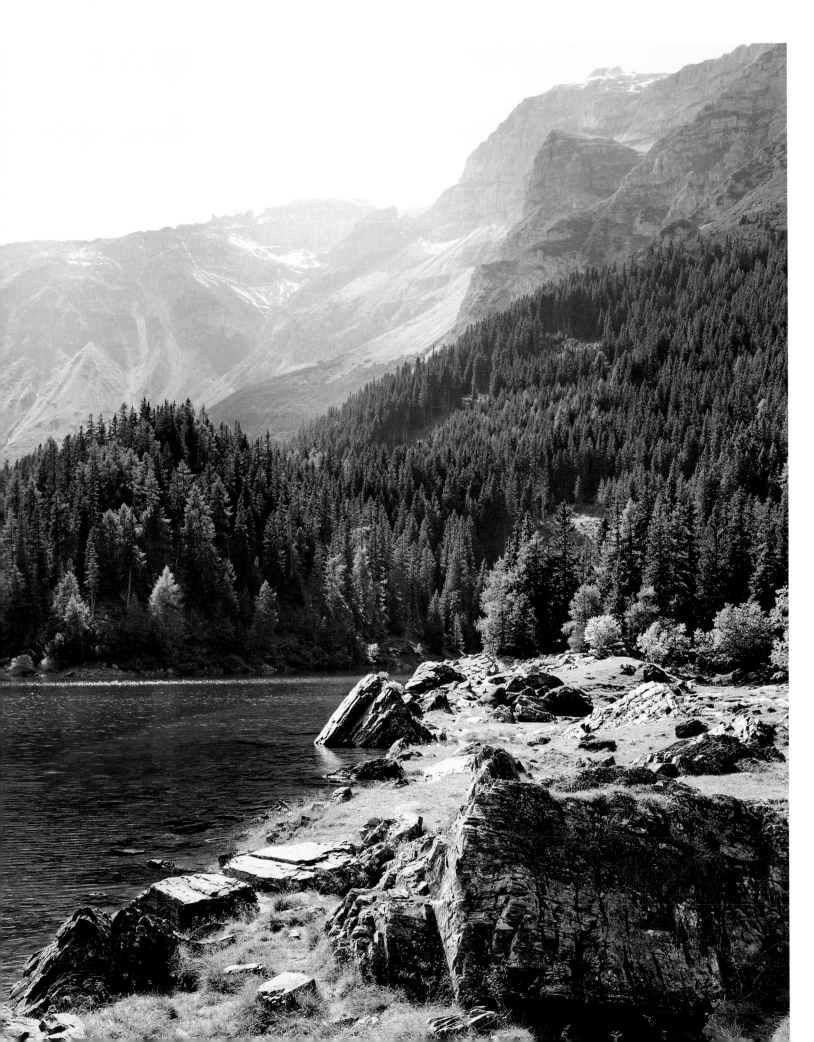

Lans, Austria

The Philosophy of Holistics

Philosophie der Ganzheit

Lanserhof

"How can the mind, spirit, and consciousness best influence human health?" The Lanserhof posed this question as many as three decades ago. The holistic LANS Med Concept was developed on the basis of Modern Mayr Medicine. LANS Med practitioners consider every way to sustainably help, heal, and revitalize patients. The concept combines top international medical knowledge with traditional naturopathic healing methods, so that every patient can rely on a sensitive system of measurably successful diagnoses and therapies. This includes detox treatments, innovative body and movement therapies, vital aging diagnosis and therapy, mental and emotional regeneration assistance, life coaching, and a scientifically based skin, beauty, and esthetics program. In addition, the Lanserhof offers a balanced, healthy, and delicious diet known as Energy Cuisine. Even the Lanserhof's architecture promotes a sense of well-being. Flowing shapes, open spaces, light, air, and transparency stimulate the spirit and support relaxation.

„Wie können Geist, Seele und Bewusstsein die Gesundheit des Menschen optimal beeinflussen?", fragte man sich im Lanserhof vor nunmehr drei Jahrzehnten. Aufbauend auf der Modernen Mayr-Medizin wurde das ganzheitliche LANS Med Concept entwickelt. Es zieht jede Möglichkeit in Betracht, um nachhaltig zu helfen, zu heilen, zu revitalisieren. Internationale Spitzenmedizin ist mit traditionellen naturheilkundlichen Heilverfahren kombiniert, sodass jedem Gast ein sensibles System an messbar erfolgreichen Diagnose- und Therapieformen zur Seite steht. Dazu gehören Detox-Behandlungen, innovative Körper- und Bewegungs- therapien, Vital Aging-Diagnostik und -Therapie, mental-emotionale Regenerationsbegleitung, Life Coaching und ein wissenschaftlich fundiertes Haut-, Beauty- und Ästhetikprogramm. Hinzu kommt eine ausgewogene, gesunde und genussvolle Ernährung: die Energy Cuisine. Selbst die Architektur des Lanserhofs fördert schon das Wohlbefinden: Fließende Formen, weite Flächen, Licht, Luft und Transparenz stimulieren den Geist und unterstützen die Entspannung.

Spa, Health & Other Facilities
14 treatment rooms, 10 massage rooms, 5 medical consultation rooms, foot care room, fitness room, movement room, seminar room, library, fireside room, swimming pool, sauna, sanarium. Energy Cuisine, dining room, tea bar, 2 sun terraces, parking spaces, garage.

Treatments & Services
LANS Med Concept. Anti-stress, burn out, dermatherapy, detox, emotional balance, energy therapy, F. X. Mayr, graceful aging, holistic health consultancy, Kneipp, life executive coaching, medical checks, meditation, mind and mental health programs, naturopathy, nutritional consultancy, physiotherapy, Pilates, Qigong, reflexology, shiatsu, sleep medicine, Tai Chi, vital aging, weight loss, yoga.

Activities
Biking, cross-country skiing, golf, jogging, Nordic walking, skiing, swimming.

Rooms
62 rooms and 90 beds, individually designed, equipped with wooden furniture.

Located
At the foot of the Patscherkofel (7,369 feet), on the outskirts of town. 8 miles (12 kilometers) from Innsbruck Airport, 124 miles (200 kilometers) from Munich Airport. The next train station is Innsbruck Central Station.

Kochholzweg 153
6072 Lans, Austria
www.lanserhof.com

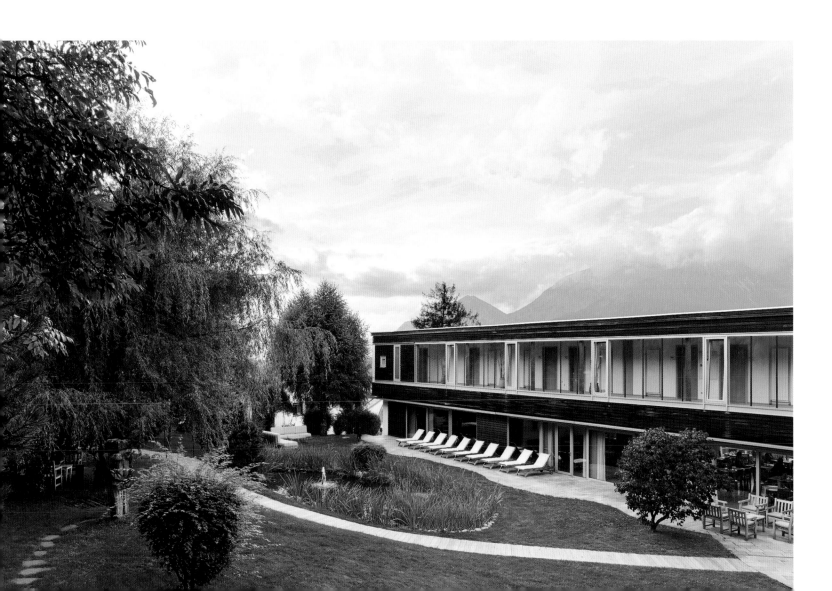

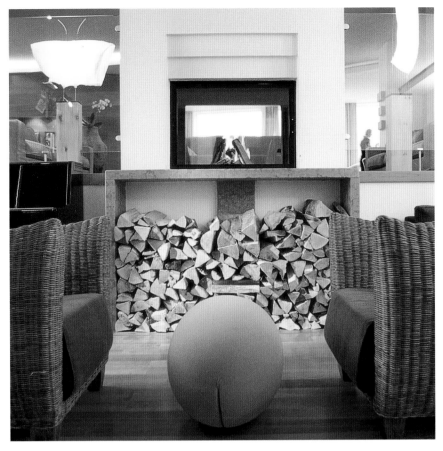

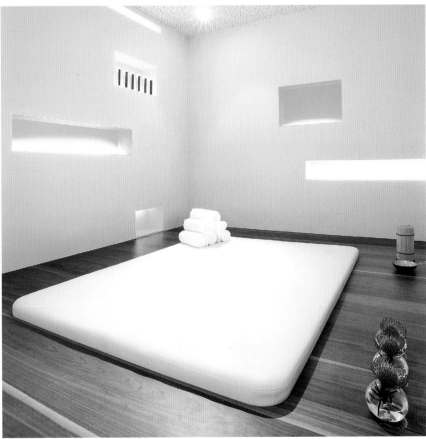

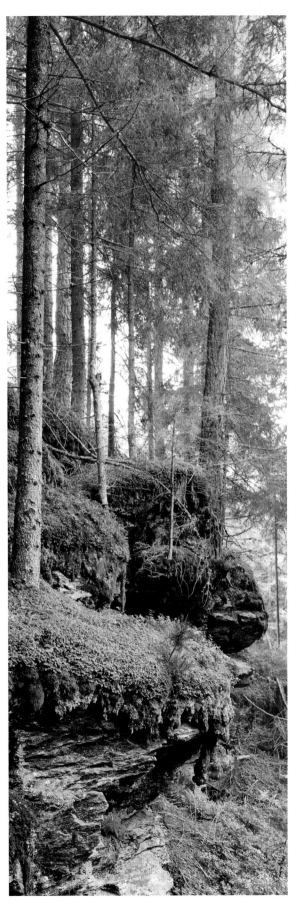

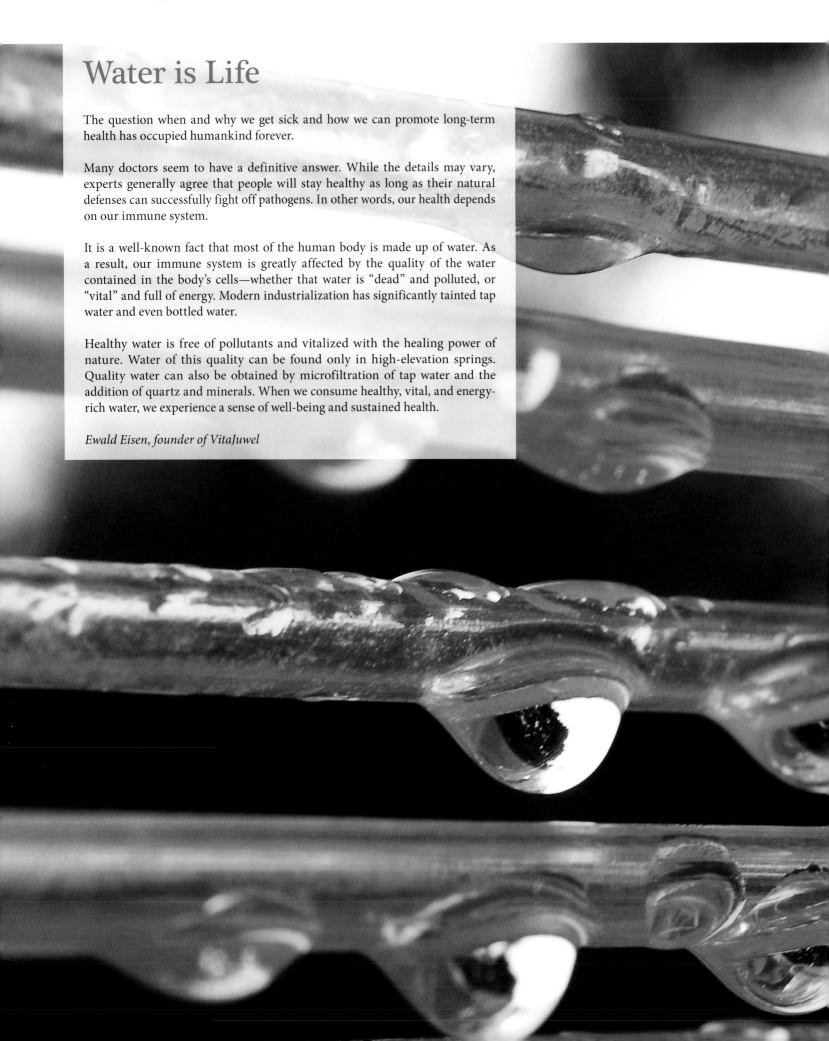

Water is Life

The question when and why we get sick and how we can promote long-term health has occupied humankind forever.

Many doctors seem to have a definitive answer. While the details may vary, experts generally agree that people will stay healthy as long as their natural defenses can successfully fight off pathogens. In other words, our health depends on our immune system.

It is a well-known fact that most of the human body is made up of water. As a result, our immune system is greatly affected by the quality of the water contained in the body's cells—whether that water is "dead" and polluted, or "vital" and full of energy. Modern industrialization has significantly tainted tap water and even bottled water.

Healthy water is free of pollutants and vitalized with the healing power of nature. Water of this quality can be found only in high-elevation springs. Quality water can also be obtained by microfiltration of tap water and the addition of quartz and minerals. When we consume healthy, vital, and energy-rich water, we experience a sense of well-being and sustained health.

Ewald Eisen, founder of VitaJuwel

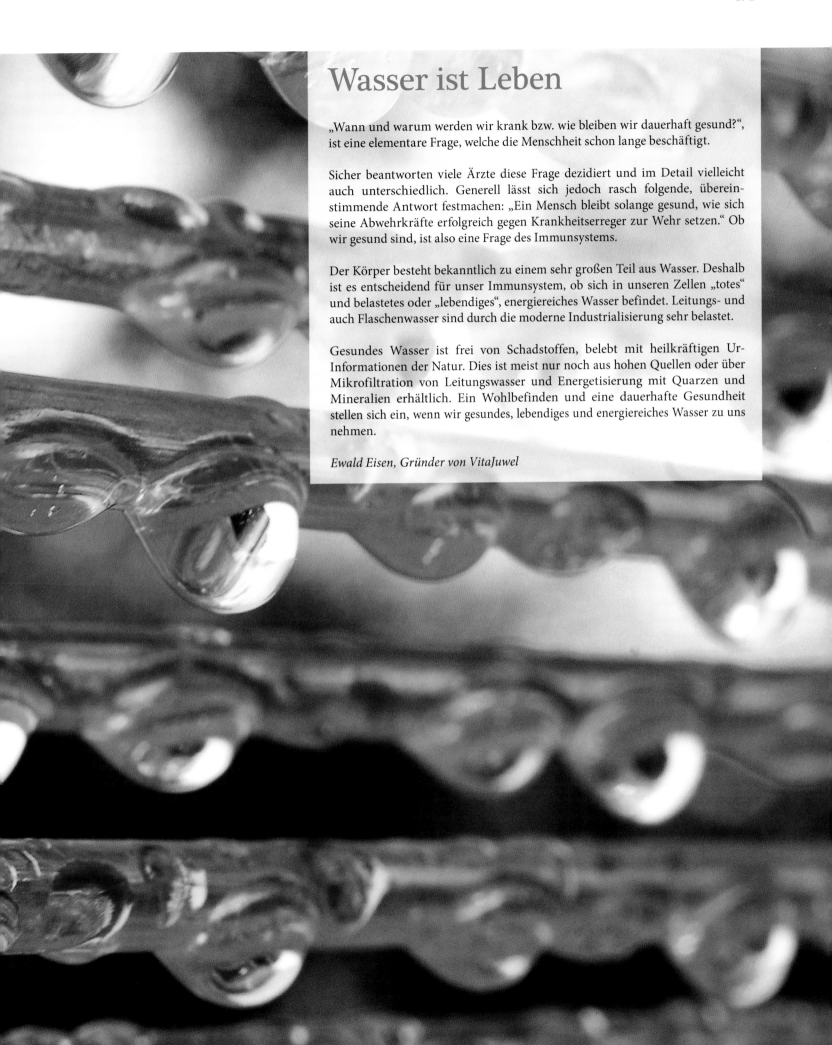

Wasser ist Leben

„Wann und warum werden wir krank bzw. wie bleiben wir dauerhaft gesund?", ist eine elementare Frage, welche die Menschheit schon lange beschäftigt.

Sicher beantworten viele Ärzte diese Frage dezidiert und im Detail vielleicht auch unterschiedlich. Generell lässt sich jedoch rasch folgende, übereinstimmende Antwort festmachen: „Ein Mensch bleibt solange gesund, wie sich seine Abwehrkräfte erfolgreich gegen Krankheitserreger zur Wehr setzen." Ob wir gesund sind, ist also eine Frage des Immunsystems.

Der Körper besteht bekanntlich zu einem sehr großen Teil aus Wasser. Deshalb ist es entscheidend für unser Immunsystem, ob sich in unseren Zellen „totes" und belastetes oder „lebendiges", energiereiches Wasser befindet. Leitungs- und auch Flaschenwasser sind durch die moderne Industrialisierung sehr belastet.

Gesundes Wasser ist frei von Schadstoffen, belebt mit heilkräftigen Ur-Informationen der Natur. Dies ist meist nur noch aus hohen Quellen oder über Mikrofiltration von Leitungswasser und Energetisierung mit Quarzen und Mineralien erhältlich. Ein Wohlbefinden und eine dauerhafte Gesundheit stellen sich ein, wenn wir gesundes, lebendiges und energiereiches Wasser zu uns nehmen.

Ewald Eisen, Gründer von VitaJuwel

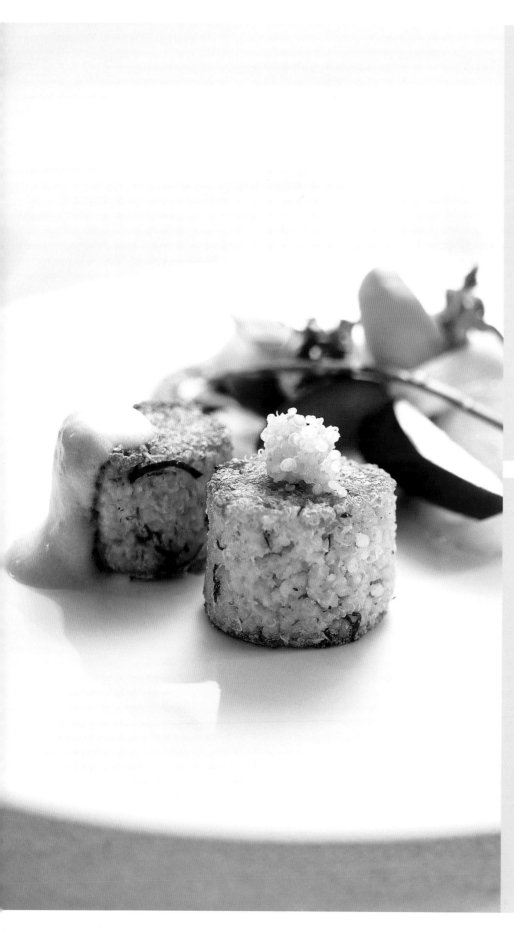

Patties:
- › 200 g whole grains (quinoa, millet, or buckwheat)
- › 120 g vegetable cubes (carrots, celery, fennel, leeks), finely chopped
- › 1 egg yolk
- › 80 g tofu, strained
- › fresh herbs to taste
- › Himalayan salt
- › nutmeg

Vegetables:
- › 500 g mixed seasonal vegetables (asparagus, carrots, fennel, bell peppers, zucchini, etc.)
- › 60 g scallions
- › 2 tbsp fresh herbs to taste
- › 2 tbsp cold-pressed oil (olive, almond, or sesame oil)
- › Himalayan salt

Serves 4

Laibchen:
- › 200 g Getreide (Quinoa, Hirse oder Buchweizen)
- › 120 g Gemüsewürfel (Karotte, Sellerie, Fenchel, Lauch), fein geschnitten
- › 1 Eigelb
- › 80 g Tofu, passiert
- › frische Kräuter nach Belieben
- › Himalayasalz
- › Muskatnuss

Gemüse:
- › 500 g gemischtes Gemüse nach Saison (Spargel, Karotten, Fenchel, Paprika, Zucchini usw.)
- › 60 g Frühlingszwiebeln
- › 2 EL frische Kräuter
- › 2 EL kaltgepresstes Öl (Oliven-, Mandel- oder Sesamöl)
- › Himalayasalz

Für 4 Personen

Whole Grain Patties on a Colorful Bed of Mixed Vegetables

Method

Cook the whole grains in approximately twice the volume of liquid. Briefly steam the vegetable cubes and mix with the grain. Stir in the egg and tofu. Season to taste with Himalayan salt and fresh herbs, such as parsley, marjoram, garlic, or thyme. Add grated cheese (optional) to refine the grain mixture. Form small patties and fry on both sides in a pan with a small amount of olive oil until golden brown.

Wash the vegetables and cut into the shape of leaves, sticks, or diamonds, as desired. Steam in a steamer basket, keeping in mind that some of the vegetables will take less time to cook than others. Season to taste with Himalayan salt, fresh herbs, and quality oil. Serve with the whole grain patties.

Health benefits

Fresh, crunchy, and highly aromatic. Sun-ripened, organic fruit and vegetables are an important source of micronutrients, fiber, and phytochemicals.

Free of pesticides and genetic manipulation, organic fruit and vegetables are preferred over conventionally farmed produce, even if they are less attractive to the eye. However, visual appearance has nothing to do with quality. Choose locally grown, fresh fruits and vegetables in season, ideally from your own vegetable garden or directly from the farm. If this is not possible, a farmer's market will be a good place to purchase high quality food.

Getreidelaibchen auf buntem Gemüseallerlei

Zubereitung

Das Getreide in ungefähr der doppelten Menge Flüssigkeit dünsten. Die Gemüsewürfel kurz dämpfen und unter das Getreide mengen. Als Bindemittel Ei und Tofu unterrühren. Mit Himalayasalz und frischen Kräutern, z. B. Petersilie, Majoran, Knoblauch oder Thymian, nach Belieben würzen. Zusätzlich kann die Getreidemasse noch mit geriebenem Käse verfeinert werden. Zu kleinen Laibchen formen und in einer Pfanne mit etwas Olivenöl goldbraun von beiden Seiten braten.

Für das Allerlei das Gemüse waschen und nach Belieben in Blätter, Stifte oder Rauten schneiden. Im Dampfgarer dämpfen, dabei die Garzeiten der unterschiedlichen Gemüsesorten beachten. Mit Himalayasalz, frischen Kräutern und einem feinen Öl abschmecken. Gemeinsam mit den Getreidelaibchen anrichten.

Gesundheitlicher Nutzen

Frisch, knackig und hocharomatisch: Sonnengereiftes, biologisches Gemüse und Obst sind eine wichtige Quelle von Vital-, Ballast- und sekundären Pflanzenstoffen.

Frei von Pestiziden und gentechnischer Veränderung ist Bio-Gemüse und -Obst herkömmlich angebauten Produkten vorzuziehen, auch wenn es oft weniger ansprechend für das Auge ist. Die Optik spricht jedoch nicht für die Qualität. Bevorzugen Sie regionale, saisonale, frische Obst- und Gemüsesorten, idealerweise aus dem eigenen Gemüsegarten oder direkt vom Bauernhof. Ist dies nicht möglich, sind Wochen- und Bauernmärkte eine gute Gelegenheit, hochwertige Lebensmittel zu kaufen.

Everything Flows, Everything Changes

Alles fließt und bleibt im Wandel

Grand Resort Bad Ragaz

Heraclitus put it in a nutshell: "Everything flows." Of course, he wasn't thinking about the healing power of the thermal springs in Bad Ragaz. And yet had he bathed in these springs, he would certainly have experienced his philosophy of eternal creation and change right up close, and he would have emerged again feeling like a new person. The water of the thermal spring, with its balanced blend of minerals, is the healing force behind this Swiss town. The spring in the Tamina Gorge has been bubbling forth and filling the pools of the 36.5° Wellbeing & Thermal Spa since the Middle Ages. At a temperature of 97 degrees Fahrenheit, you can get away from it all and let yourself drift, recharge your batteries, and focus on your sense of feeling good. Resort guests will also find professional guidance in the areas of nutrition, rehabilitation, sports medicine, and maintaining healthy skin and teeth. Soothing treatments, health programs, and numerous sports opportunities provide a unique combination of well-being, health, and comfort.

Heraklit brachte es auf den Punkt: „Alles fließt." Natürlich dachte er dabei nicht an das heilkräftige Thermalwasser von Bad Ragaz. Doch hätte er ein Bad darin genommen, hätte er sicher das ewige Werden und Wandeln hautnah gespürt und wäre wie neugeboren wieder aufgetaucht. Das Thermalwasser mit seinen ausgewogenen Mineralien ist die heilende Kraft des Schweizer Ortes. Seit dem Mittelalter entspringt die Quelle der Taminaschlucht und füllt die Becken des 36.5° Wellbeing & Thermal Spa. Bei 36,5 Grad Celsius kann man sich dort treiben lassen, abschalten, neue Energie gewinnen und sich auf sein Wohlbefinden konzentrieren. Daneben finden die Gäste des Resorts fachgerechte Anleitung in Sachen Ernährung, Rehabilitation, Sportmedizin oder Haut- und Zahngesundheit. Verwöhnbehandlungen, Gesundheitsprogramme sowie zahlreiche Sportmöglichkeiten bieten eine einmalige Kombination aus Wellbeing, Gesundheit und Komfort.

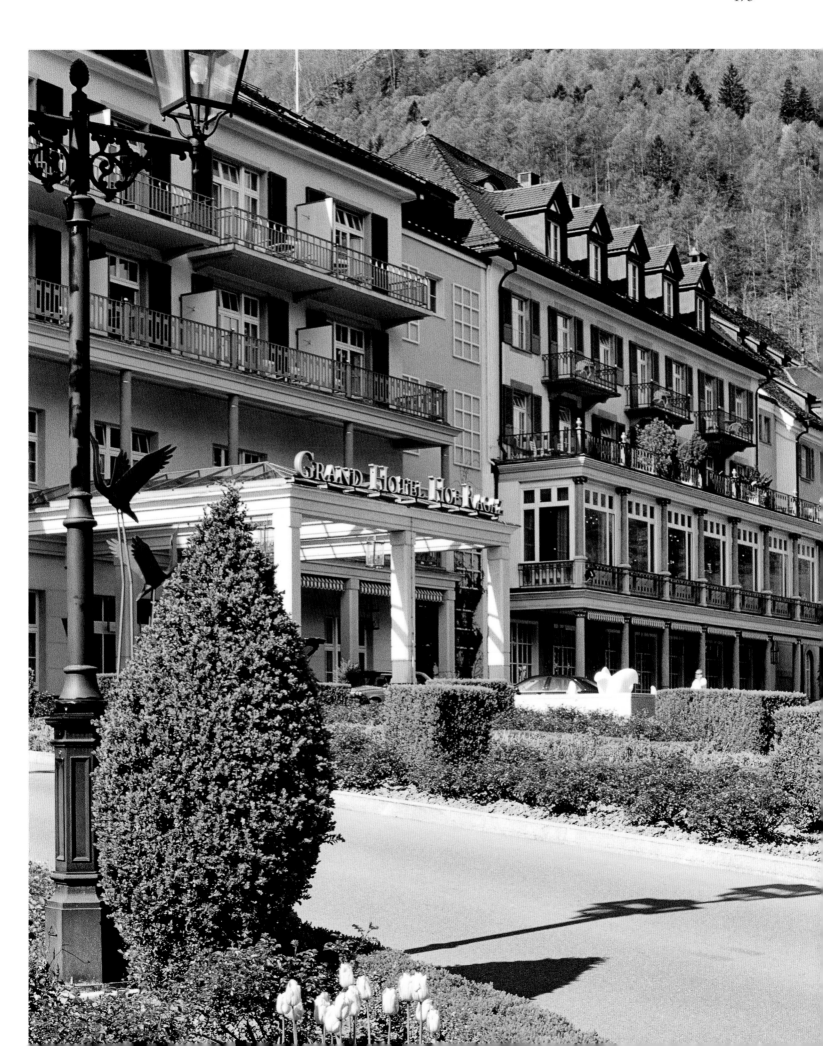

Spa, Health & Other Facilities
138,000 square feet (12,800 square meters) 36.5° Wellbeing & Thermal Spa area, Medical Health Center.
8 restaurants, tennis court, golf, outdoor pool, parking lot, casino, rooms for disabled.

Treatments & Services
Wide range of wellness and medical treatments. 24-hour front desk, car rental.

Activities
Wide range of indoor and outdoor sports. Artistic, culinary, cultural, and musical events,
summer and winter activities in the picturesque Heidiland region.

Rooms
290 elegant rooms and suites.

Located
62 miles (100 kilometers) from Bodensee Airport, Friedrichshafen, and Zurich Airport.

7310 Bad Ragaz, Switzerland
www.resortragaz.ch

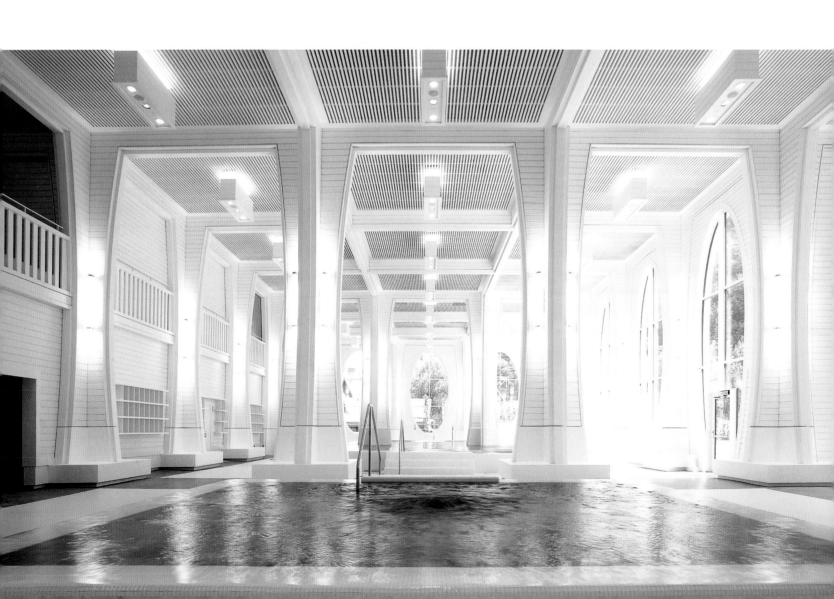

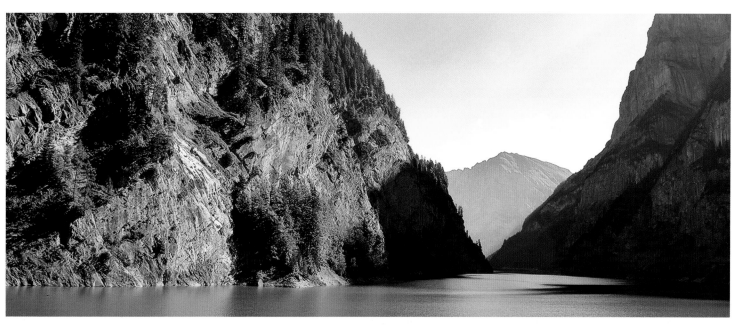

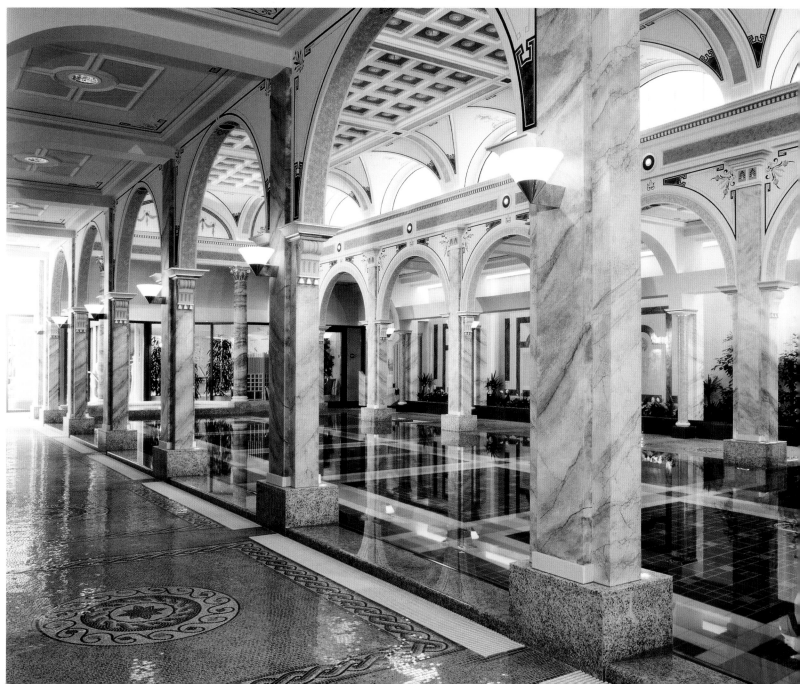

Energy in All Forms

Energie in jeglicher Form

Hubertus Alpin Lodge & Spa

It smells like earth, wood, and fire—almost like in an alpine chalet. Nature and architecture form a harmonious whole. Natural building materials such as untreated white pine and ancient rock shape the foundation of the Alpine Spa. It is the hotel's energy center, and pretty much everything here revolves around energy. The family-run lodge takes care to make guests forget that they are staying in a hotel: It is comfortable with a sense of warmth and security. And yet, absolutely nothing here is quite like it is at home. Innovative, effective spa treatments with sonorous names like "AlpYurveda" and "Alpine Urkraft" (primal force) reflect Asian and local healing methods as well as a combination of the two. The health services include energy treatments, health checks, consultations, and pain relief programs. At an elevation of over 3,200 feet, the healing forces of nature can be felt at first hand.

Es duftet nach Erde, Holz und Feuer – fast wie in einer Almhütte. Natur und Architektur formen hier ein harmonisches Ganzes. Natürliche Baustoffe, wie unbehandelte Weißtanne und sehr altes Gestein, bilden die Grundlagen des Alpin Spa. Es ist das energetische Zentrum des Hotels, und um Energie dreht sich hier so ziemlich alles. Das familiengeführte Haus sorgt zwar dafür, dass man sich bloß nicht wie in einem Hotel fühlt: Es ist gemütlich und strahlt Geborgenheit aus. Und doch ist hier gerade gar nichts so wie zu Hause. Innovative, effektive Spa-Anwendungen mit klangvollen Namen wie AlpYurveda und Alpine Urkraft erzählen von asiatischen und einheimischen Heilmethoden und der Kombination aus beidem. Zu den Gesundheitsangeboten gehören Energiebehandlungen, Gesundheitschecks und -beratungen sowie Programme zur Schmerzlinderung. Hautnah spürt man hier oben auf 1 000 Metern Höhe die heilenden Kräfte der Natur.

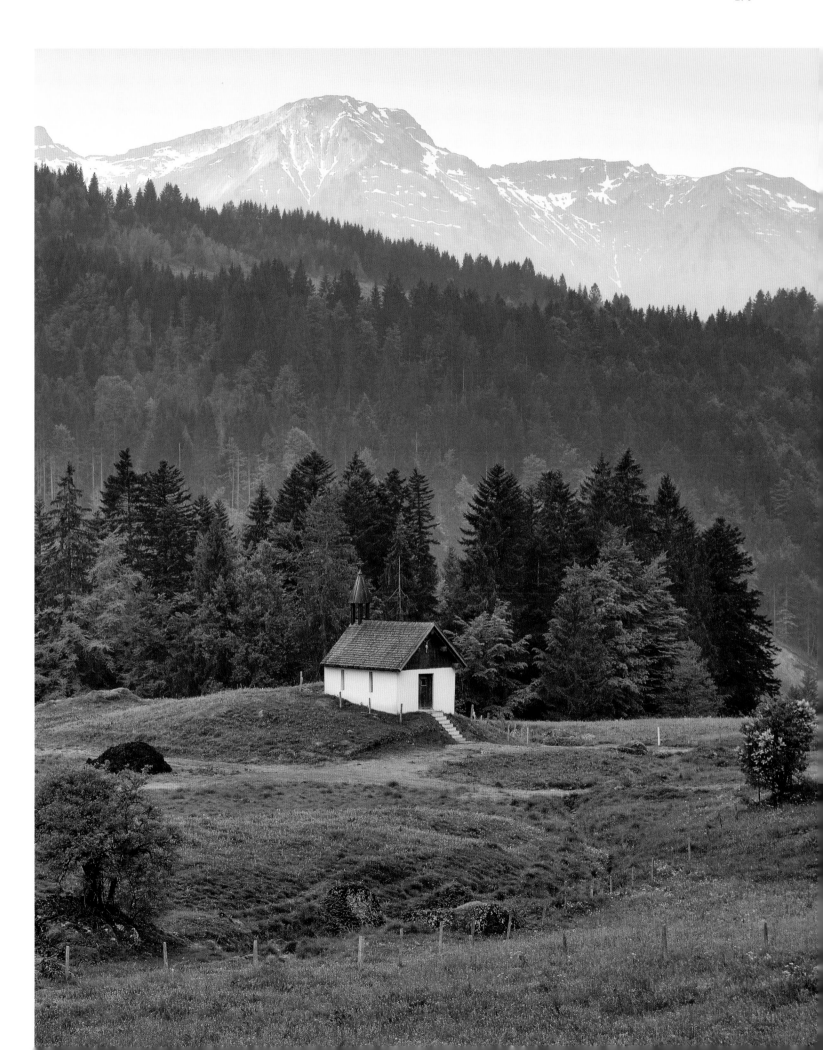

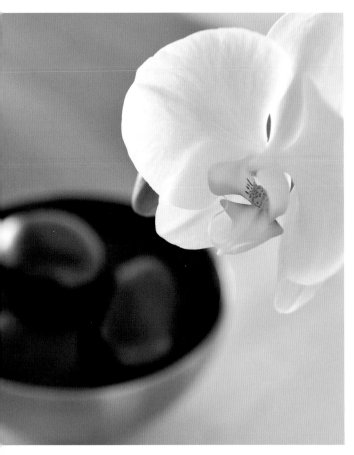

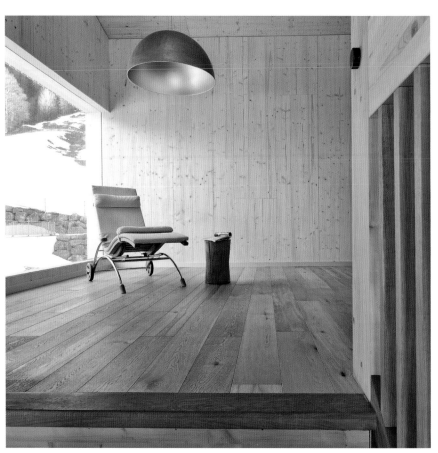

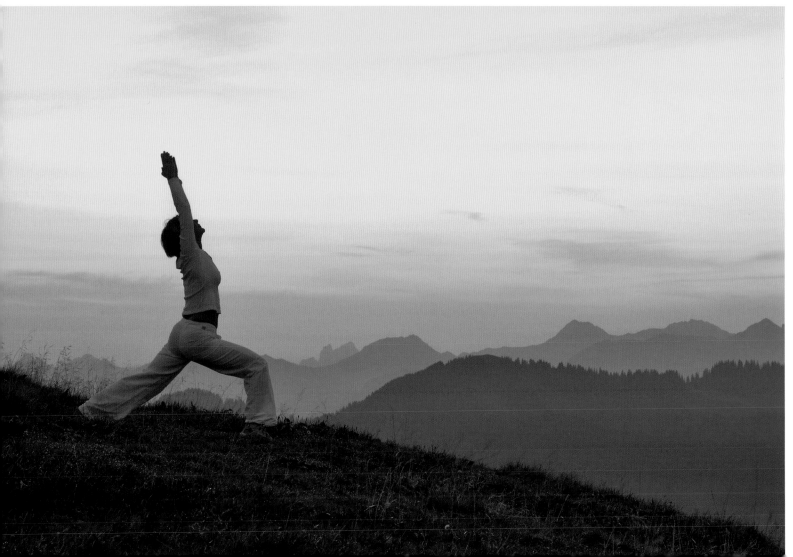

Spa, Health & Other Facilities

21,500 square feet (2,000 square meters) spa area comprising outdoor pool, 12 treatment rooms, foot reflexology path ("Via Sensus"), herbal sauna, Alpin sauna, Finnish sauna, steam bath, relaxation rooms, fitness lounge with cardio equipment, geomantic force fields. 7 different dining rooms, elevator.

Treatments & Services

Beauty treatments for face and body, energy therapy, fitness programs, massages, natural healing, personal coaching. Free parking, hotel safe.

Activities

Climbing, cross-country skiing, golf, hiking, mountain biking, Nordic walking, skiing, snowshoeing.

Rooms

60 rooms and 6 suites. Each room features a balcony.

Located

2 hours from Munich, Stuttgart, and Zurich. The next airport is Memmingen Airport.

Dorf 5
87538 Balderschwang, Germany
www.hotel-hubertus.de

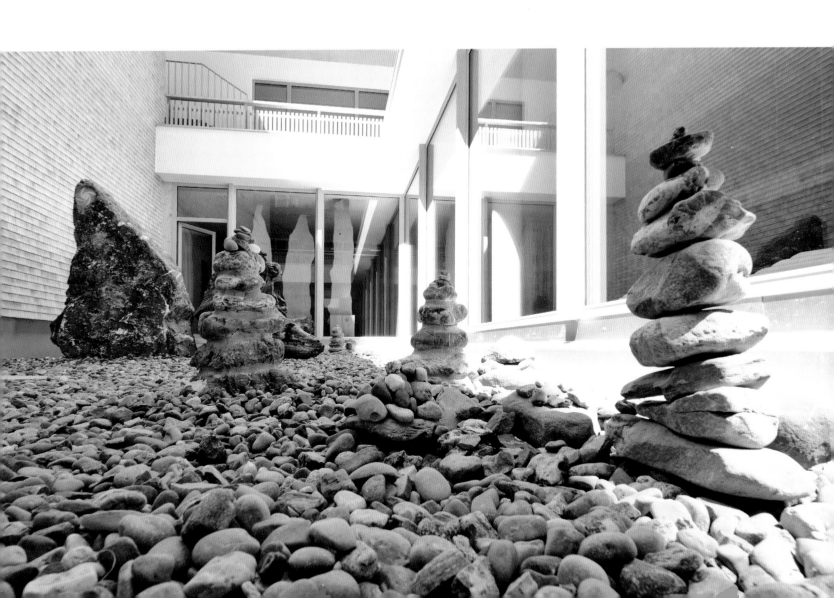

Beauty on Königsallee

Für die Schönheit auf die Kö

Breidenbacher Hof, A Capella Hotel

The Königsallee in Düsseldorf is where you go to shop or to see and be seen—but who would suspect that people go there for relaxation and health? That sounds unusual. And yet, the luxury hotel Breidenbacher Hof, one of the oldest in Germany and situated right on Königsallee, offers an oasis of beauty and well-being. Leaving the hustle and bustle of the city's historic center behind, visitors immediately find themselves enveloped by a pleasant stillness in the elegant ambiance of the Schnitzler Beauty Lounge. The Schnitzler's underlying philosophy is to establish harmony between body and spirit through personalized health treatments. Those who want to check and improve their health in an exclusive atmosphere can enjoy the comfort of a luxury guest room or suite and take advantage of its private access to the in-house health clinic. The "Preventicum" is run by leading experts in the field of preventive medicine as well as internationally recognized cardiologists. Among other things, the clinic provides internal medical examinations.

Auf die Düsseldorfer Königsallee geht man zum Shoppen oder zum Sehen und Gesehenwerden – aber der Entspannung und Gesundheit halber? Das klingt ungewöhnlich. Und doch, in einem der ältesten Grandhotels Deutschlands, dem Luxushotel Breidenbacher Hof direkt an der Kö, versteckt sich eine Oase für Schönheit und Wohlergehen. Nachdem der Besucher den Trubel der Altstadt hinter sich gelassen hat, umfängt ihn im eleganten Ambiente der Schnitzler Beauty Lounge sofort eine angenehme Stille. Schnitzlers grundlegende Philosophie ist es, die Harmonie zwischen Körper und Geist mittels einer individuellen Anwendung herzustellen. Wer noch dazu in exklusiver Atmosphäre seine Gesundheit checken lassen und verbessern will, der kann den Komfort der großzügigen Gästezimmer oder Luxussuiten genießen und den privaten Zugang zur hauseigenen Klinik in Anspruch nehmen. Das „Preventicum" wird von führenden Experten auf dem Gebiet der Präventivmedizin sowie international anerkannten Kardiologen geleitet und bietet unter anderem internistische Untersuchungen an.

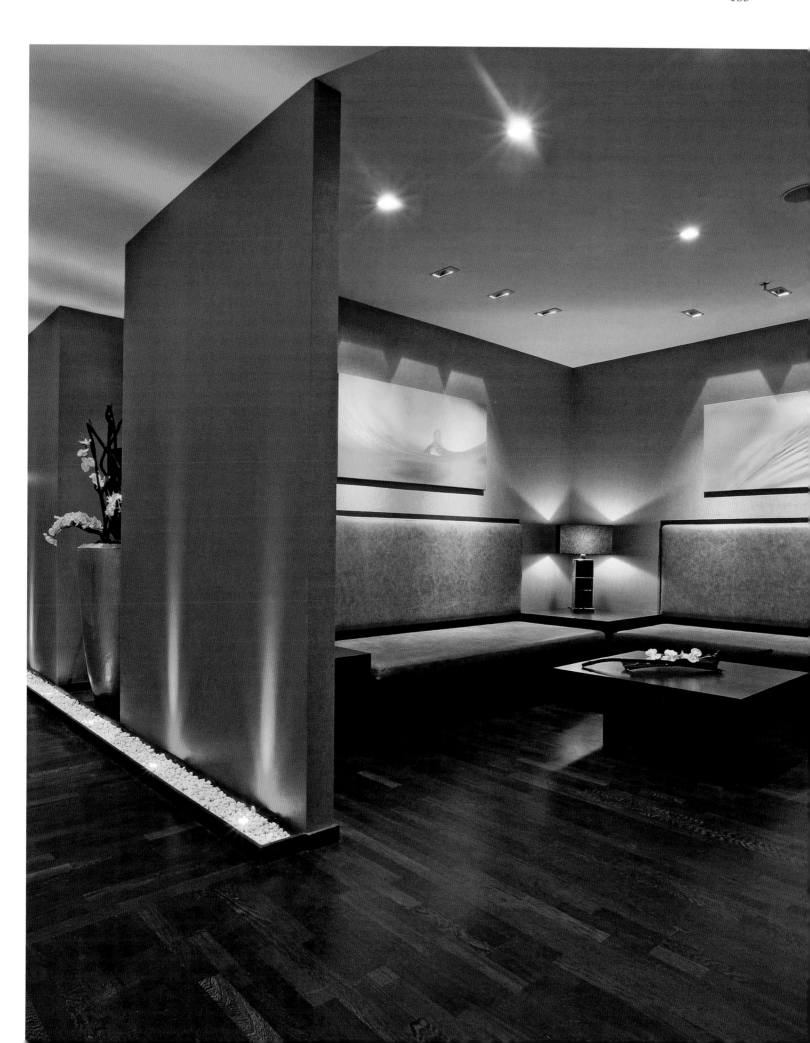

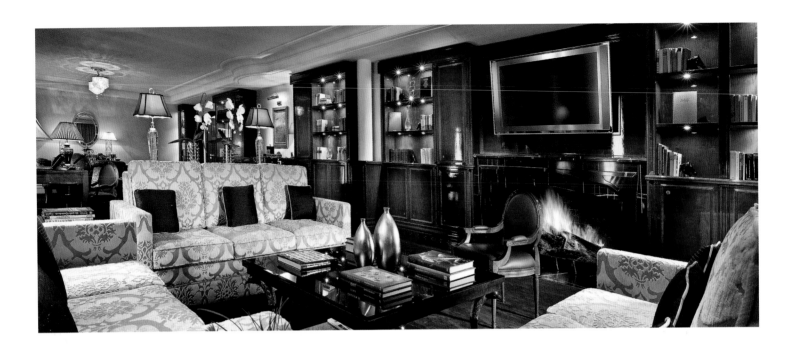

Spa, Health & Other Facilities
Schnitzler Beauty Lounge, 24-hour Technogym fitness area. Brasserie "1806", Capella Bar & Cigar Lounge, Lobby Lounge, Capella Living Room, signature stores, refreshment center.

Treatments & Services
24-hour in-room dining and beverage service, flexible check-in and check-out times, free Wi-Fi and iPads, nightly turndown service, service of personal assistants.

Activities
Biking, city tours, explorations of the Old Town and the Medienhafen (Media Harbor), hiking, shopping and dining on Königsallee.

Rooms
79 spacious rooms and 16 elegant suites.

Located
Centrally located on the Königsallee. 6 miles (9 kilometers) from Düsseldorf Airport. The next metro station is Heinrich-Heine-Allee, 1 mile (2 kilometers) to Düsseldorf Central Station.

Königsallee 11
40212 Düsseldorf, Germany
www.capellahotels.com/dusseldorf

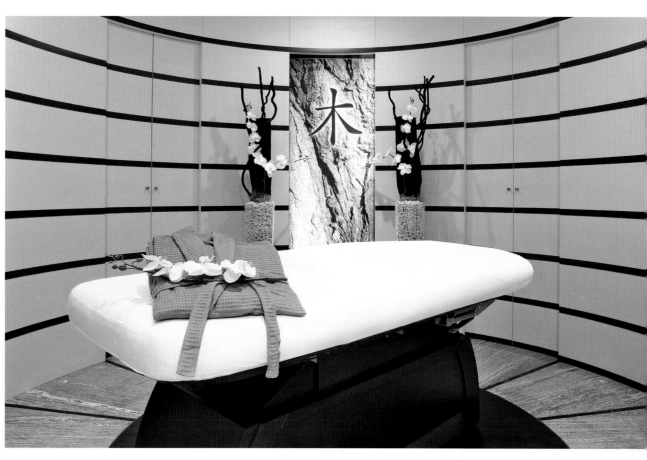

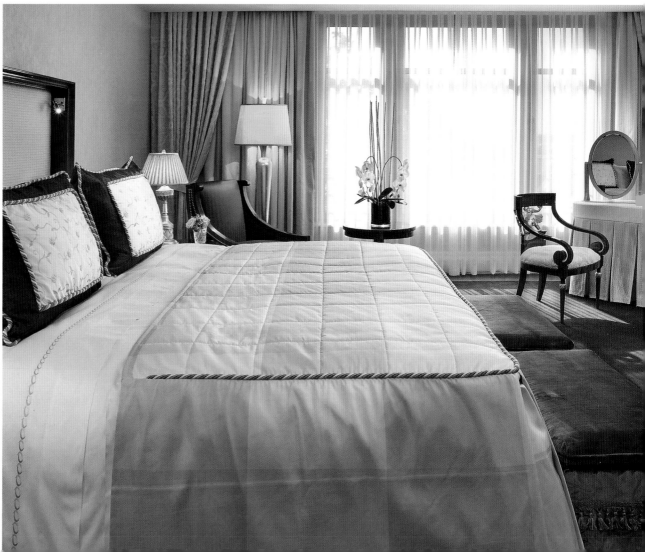

Relaxing while You Travel

Flights, time differences, taxis, meetings, too little sleep—frequent travelers are often under a lot of stress. Life without stress is impossible—and unnecessary. The important thing is for a stressful phase to be followed by a relaxing one, so that your body can recover. Therefore, you should make sure that you get the necessary balance while being on a business trip.

Active recreation, for example through the balancing effect of exercise, is the best way to do your body good. It's enough to simply swim a lap, take a walk, or go for an easy jog. However, it is important to enjoy the exercise. Forcing yourself to do something only because you think it is good for you just creates more stress. Yoga, meditation, and Qigong are also helpful. Indulging in a massage or making use of the wellness zone can be recuperative as well.

In addition, a visit to a museum can take your mind off things and do you a world of good. At mealtimes, choose foods that are not too spicy and that contain light ingredients, which means eating plenty of fruit and vegetables. When you are stressed, coffee and alcohol tend to have a negative effect on your state of health. It is better to drink a lot of water or juice spritzers.

Prof. Dr. Dietrich Baumgart, M.D., Preventicum private practice at Breidenbacher Hof, Düsseldorf, Germany

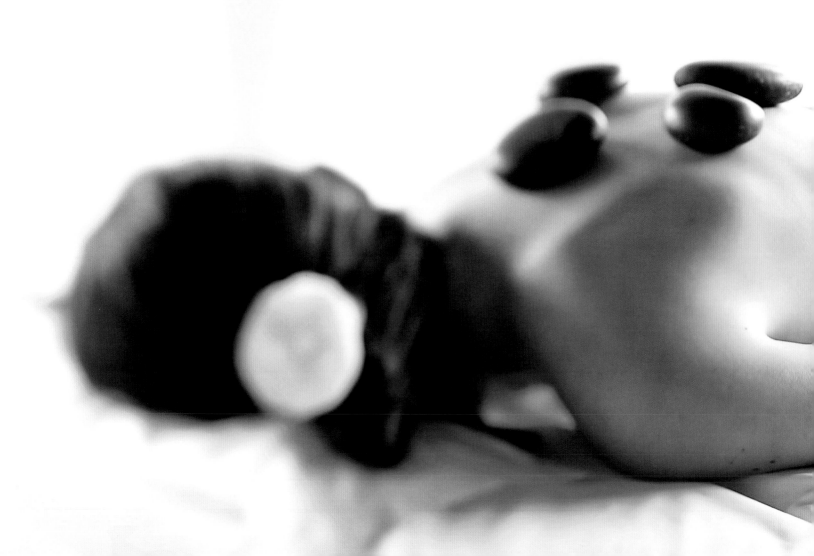

Entspannen auf Reisen

Flug, Zeitverschiebung, Taxi, Meetings, wenig Schlaf – gerade wer viel unterwegs ist, ist häufig gestresst. Ein Leben ohne Stress ist nicht möglich und auch nicht nötig. Es ist nur wichtig, dass auf eine Phase der Anspannung eine Phase der Entspannung folgt, sodass sich der Körper erholen kann. Daher ist es ratsam, zum Beispiel während der Geschäftsreise auf den nötigen Ausgleich zu achten.

Um dem Körper etwas Gutes zu tun, ist eine aktive Entspannung, etwa durch ausgleichende Bewegung, am besten. Spazieren gehen, locker joggen oder eine Runde schwimmen kann dabei schon ausreichen. Wichtig ist der Spaß an der Bewegung. Wenn man sich wieder zu etwas zwingt, nur weil es vermeintlich gut ist, bedeutet das neuen Stress. Hilfreich sind darüber hinaus Yoga, Meditation oder Qigong. Erholsam ist es auch, sich eine Massage zu gönnen oder Angebote im Wellnessbereich zu nutzen.

Ein Besuch im Museum kann ebenfalls guttun und dabei helfen, auf andere Gedanken zu kommen. Beim Essen sollte darauf geachtet werden, dass es nicht zu scharf ist und leichte Zutaten enthält, das heißt viel Obst und Gemüse. Kaffee und Alkohol wirken sich bei Stress eher negativ auf das Befinden aus. Besser ist es, viel Wasser oder Fruchtsaftschorlen zu trinken.

Prof. Dr. med. Dietrich Baumgart, Privatpraxis Preventicum
im Breidenbacher Hof, Düsseldorf, Deutschland

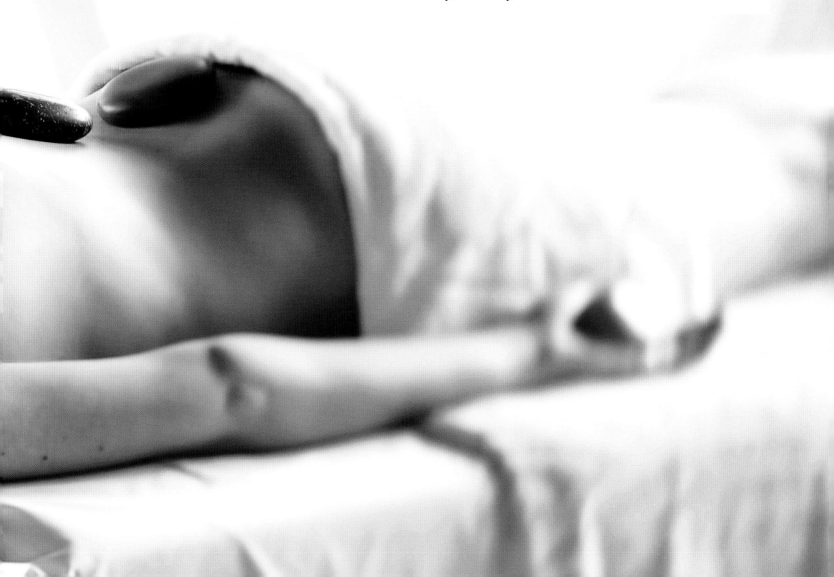

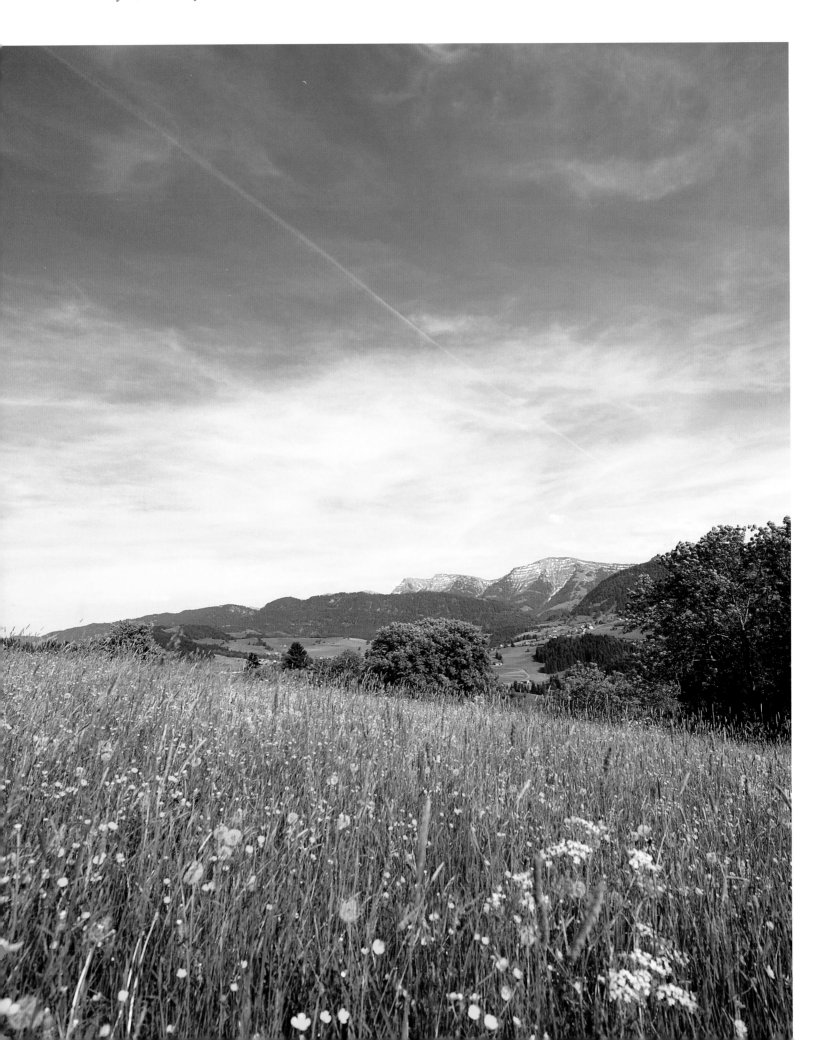

Oberstaufen, Germany

Intensive Health Programs in Heavenly Surroundings

Intensive Gesundheitsprogramme in traumhafter Umgebung

Allgäu Sonne

What is a Schroth cure? And what precisely does metabolic balance mean? Both nutrition programs are well balanced at the Allgäu Sonne alpine resort in Germany. The Schroth cure relieves all stress and detoxifies the body over a period of two to three weeks, while Metabolic Balance, a doctor-supervised metabolic program, helps patients achieve new vitality and reach their target weight for the long term. The hotel's unique health programs take place in a sunny location with enchanting panoramic vistas and revitalizing views of the Allgäu Alps. An innovative fitness area, professional therapists, and a medical practice help make the programs a success.

Was ist eine Schrothkur? Und was genau bedeutet Metabolic Balance? Die beiden Ernährungsprogramme sind in dem deutschen Alpenresort Allgäu Sonne bestens aufeinander abgestimmt. Während die Schrothkur den Körper in zwei bis drei Wochen gründlich entlastet und entgiftet, wird durch das ärztlich geleitete Stoffwechselprogramm Metabolic Balance neue Vitalität und ein dauerhaftes Wunschgewicht erlangt. Die einzigartigen Gesundheitsprogramme finden in zauberhafter Panorama-Sonnenlage statt, mit malerischem Blick auf die Allgäuer Alpen. Eine innovative Fitnesswelt, professionelle Therapeuten und eine Arztpraxis unterstützen den Erfolg.

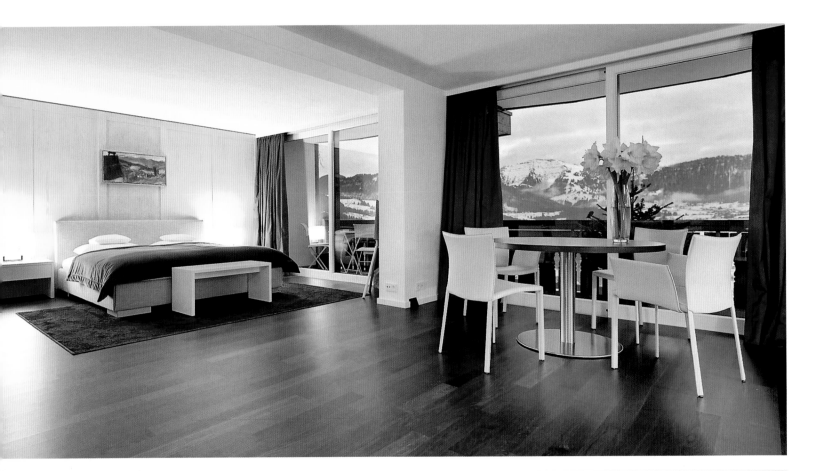

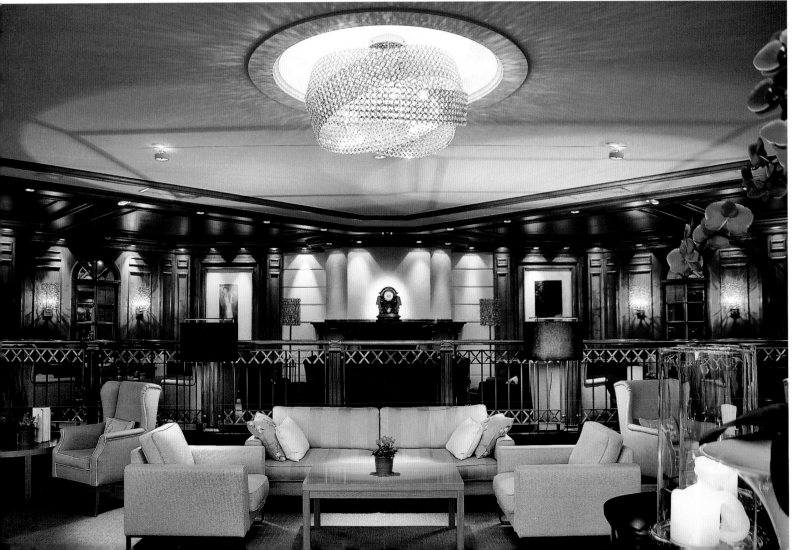

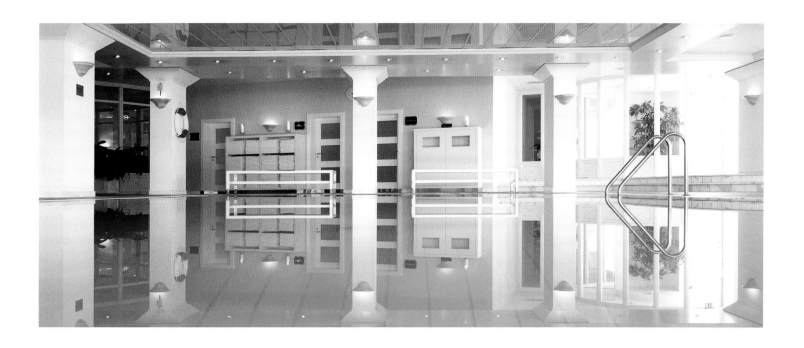

Spa, Health & Other Facilities
22,600 square feet (2,100 square meters) wellness oasis comprising 2 indoor pools, heated outdoor pool in summer, whirlpool, sauna, fitness area with Technogym exercise machines and personal coach, beauty farm. Half-board and à la carte restaurant, diet restaurant, shops, banquet facilities, conference room, elevator.

Treatments & Services
Baths, beauty treatments and classical cosmetics, dermatology, detox and weight loss programs, individual coaching, individual fitness schedules, informational lectures, massages, medical cosmetics (micro-dermabrasion, radiofrequency treatments, Swiss Cell Spa Experience), packages, physical prevention, physical therapy (lymphatic drainage, manual therapy, remedial gymnastics), Pilates, Qigong, rehabilitative postoperative care, Soft Aging, thalassotherapy treatments, wellness for men, yoga. Gourmet and vitality menu, Schrothkur and Metabolic Balance diet. 24-hour front desk, 24-hour room service available, airport transfer, babysitting/childcare, breakfast in the room, free public parking, free Wi-Fi, laundry service, private parking, turndown service, valet parking.

Activities
Airplane tours, Aqua fitness, fishing, fitness training, golf, guided hiking tours, gymnastics, group cycling, horseback riding, mountain bike tours, Nordic walking, parasailing; rafting, rowing, or canoeing; sailing, skiing, snowshoeing, swimming, tennis. Event programs including cocktail mixing classes, theme nights, and live music.

Rooms
141 rooms and 12 suites. Most rooms feature a balcony.

Located
10 minutes by foot to the town of Oberstaufen. 25 miles (40 kilometers) from Friedrichshafen Airport, 50 miles (80 kilometers) from Allgäu Airport Memmingen.

Stießberg 1
87534 Oberstaufen, Germany
www.allgaeu-sonne.de

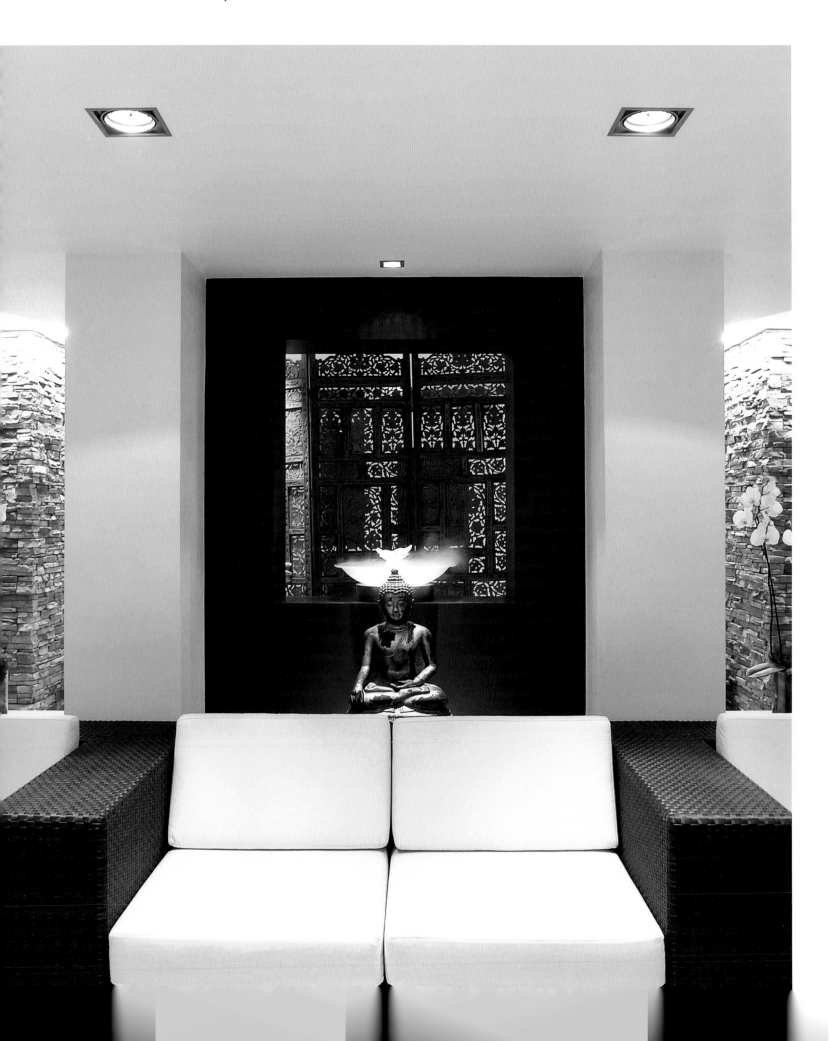

Ayurveda: A New Approach to Life

Ayurveda: eine neue Lebenseinsicht

Ayurveda Parkschlösschen Bad Wildstein

Ayurveda is the "knowledge of life," and one can immerse oneself in this ancient Indian healing art without booking a flight to India. This small castle surrounded by its own parkland is located in picturesque Bad Wildstein near the Moselle River. It has embodied medical and traditional Ayurveda cures in Europe for nearly 20 years. From medical diagnosis at the start of the cure to traditional oil massages, vegetarian meals, meditation, and yoga—everything is based on the principles of Ayurvedic healing developed thousands of years ago. Even the castle's interior design and the materials used were selected on the basis of Ayurvedic principles. The hotel's entire team, from the Ayurvedic physicians and therapists to the nutrition experts, operate according to holistic knowledge and thinking. All these aspects combine to form a complete, health-promoting whole. Everything centers around Panchakarma—a holistic method of detoxifying the body. It is the basis for restoring life energy and individual equilibrium.

Ayurveda ist das „Wissen vom Leben", und wer ganz tief in die uralte indische Heilkunst einsteigen möchte, braucht dafür nicht einmal nach Indien zu fliegen. Im romantischen Bad Wildstein nahe der Mosel steht das Ayurveda Parkschlösschen, das seit fast 20 Jahren der Inbegriff für medizinische und traditionelle Ayurvedakuren in Europa ist. Angefangen bei der medizinischen Diagnose bei Kurbeginn über die traditionellen Ölmassagen, die vegetarischen Mahlzeiten, Meditation und Yoga – alles basiert auf den jahrtausendealten Prinzipien der ayurvedischen Heilkunst. Sogar die Innenarchitektur und die dazu verwendeten Materialien sind nach den Erkenntnissen des Ayurveda ausgesucht. Das gesamte Team des Hotels, von den Ayurveda-Ärzten über die Ayurveda-Therapeuten bis zu den Ernährungsexperten, handelt nach dem ganzheitlichen Wissen und Denken. Dies alles verbindet sich zu einem großen heilsamen Ganzen. Im Mittelpunkt des Parkschlösschens steht die Panchakarma-Kur – die ganzheitliche Entgiftung des Körpers. Sie bildet die Grundlage zur Wiederherstellung der Lebensenergie und des ureigenen Gleichgewichts.

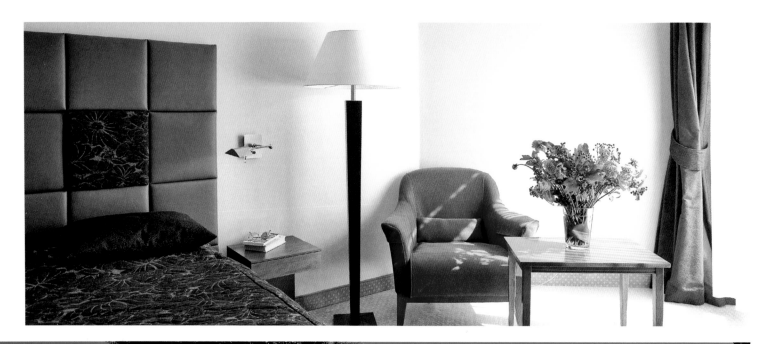

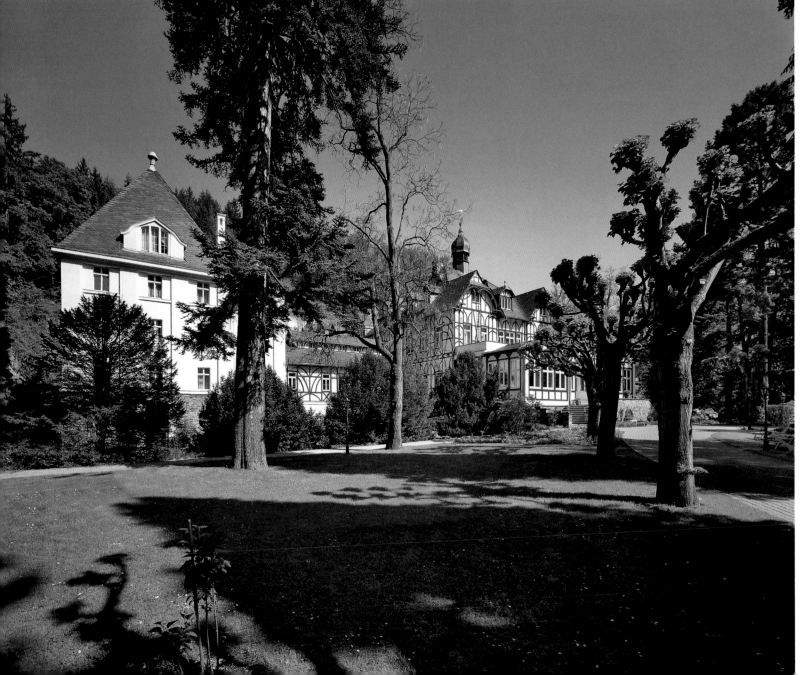

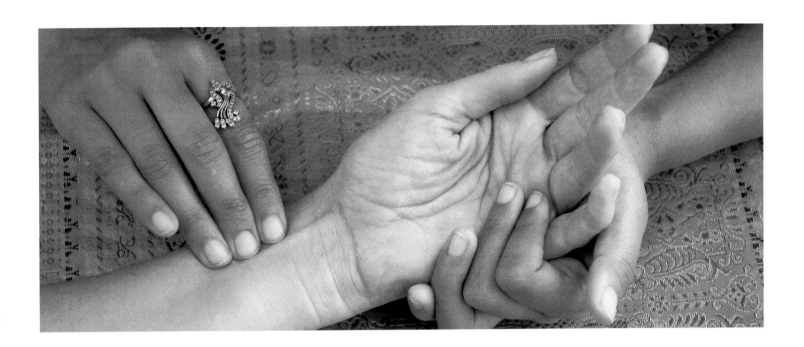

Spa, Health & Other Facilities
21,500 square feet (2,000 square meters) spa area with indoor thermal pool, 2 saunas, steam bath,
fitness center, yoga and gymnastics area, cosmetic studio. Ayurveda therapy area with 24 treatment
and relaxation rooms.

Treatments & Services
Medical team with Ayurvedic and orthodox medical education. Ayurvedic massages and treatments, daily
rotating fitness program, personal training, programs for prevention and regeneration, yoga classes twice
daily. Cooking workshops, daily lectures, free parking, vegetarian gourmet cuisine using organic ingredients.

Activities
Bicycling, golf, hiking, inline skating, tennis.

Rooms
60 comfortable rooms designed according to Ayurvedic principles:
15 junior suites, 30 double rooms, 15 single rooms.

Located
20 minutes from Frankfurt/Hahn Airport, 1.5 hours from Frankfurt Airport.
The next train station is Traben-Trarbach.

Wildbadstraße 201
56841 Traben-Trarbach, Germany
www.parkschloesschen.de

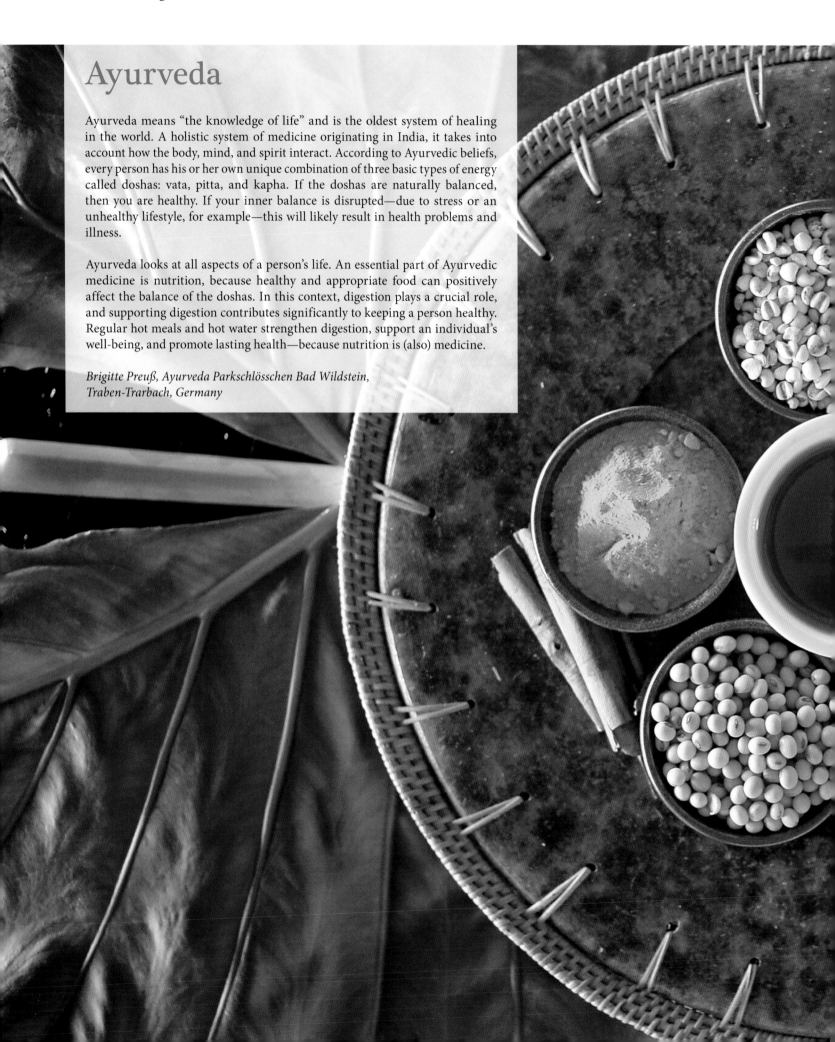

Ayurveda

Ayurveda means "the knowledge of life" and is the oldest system of healing in the world. A holistic system of medicine originating in India, it takes into account how the body, mind, and spirit interact. According to Ayurvedic beliefs, every person has his or her own unique combination of three basic types of energy called doshas: vata, pitta, and kapha. If the doshas are naturally balanced, then you are healthy. If your inner balance is disrupted—due to stress or an unhealthy lifestyle, for example—this will likely result in health problems and illness.

Ayurveda looks at all aspects of a person's life. An essential part of Ayurvedic medicine is nutrition, because healthy and appropriate food can positively affect the balance of the doshas. In this context, digestion plays a crucial role, and supporting digestion contributes significantly to keeping a person healthy. Regular hot meals and hot water strengthen digestion, support an individual's well-being, and promote lasting health—because nutrition is (also) medicine.

Brigitte Preuß, Ayurveda Parkschlösschen Bad Wildstein,
Traben-Trarbach, Germany

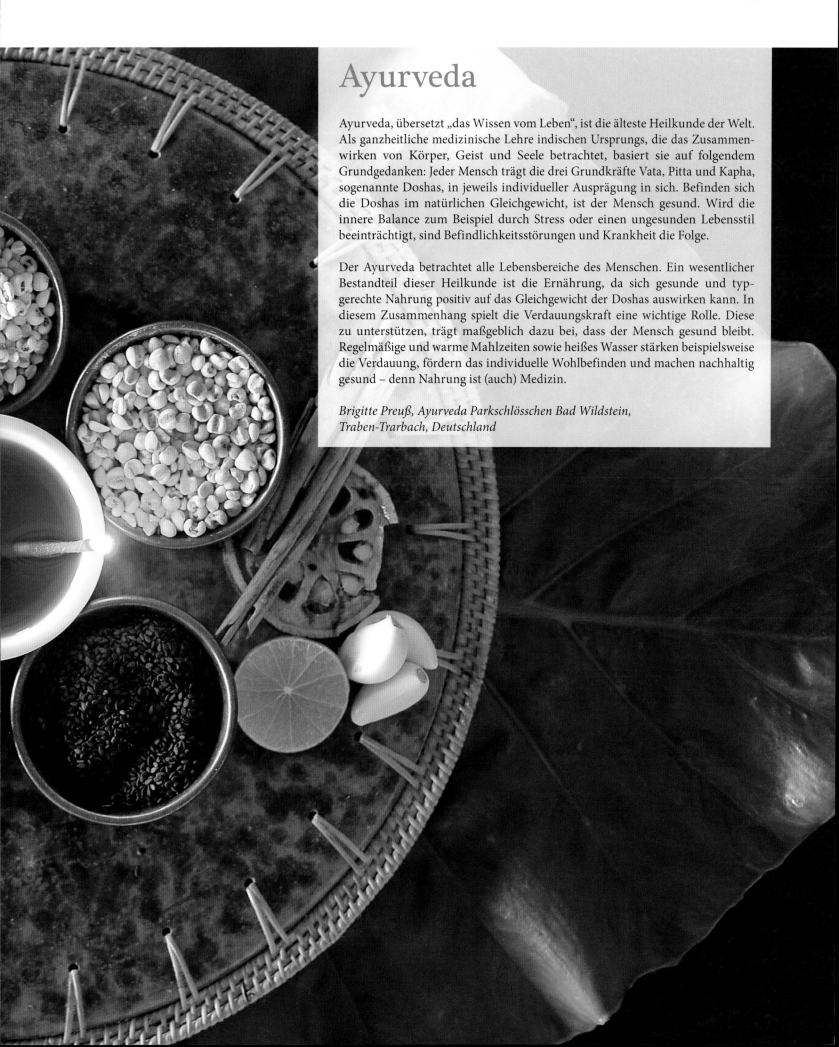

Ayurveda

Ayurveda, übersetzt „das Wissen vom Leben", ist die älteste Heilkunde der Welt. Als ganzheitliche medizinische Lehre indischen Ursprungs, die das Zusammenwirken von Körper, Geist und Seele betrachtet, basiert sie auf folgendem Grundgedanken: Jeder Mensch trägt die drei Grundkräfte Vata, Pitta und Kapha, sogenannte Doshas, in jeweils individueller Ausprägung in sich. Befinden sich die Doshas im natürlichen Gleichgewicht, ist der Mensch gesund. Wird die innere Balance zum Beispiel durch Stress oder einen ungesunden Lebensstil beeinträchtigt, sind Befindlichkeitsstörungen und Krankheit die Folge.

Der Ayurveda betrachtet alle Lebensbereiche des Menschen. Ein wesentlicher Bestandteil dieser Heilkunde ist die Ernährung, da sich gesunde und typgerechte Nahrung positiv auf das Gleichgewicht der Doshas auswirken kann. In diesem Zusammenhang spielt die Verdauungskraft eine wichtige Rolle. Diese zu unterstützen, trägt maßgeblich dazu bei, dass der Mensch gesund bleibt. Regelmäßige und warme Mahlzeiten sowie heißes Wasser stärken beispielsweise die Verdauung, fördern das individuelle Wohlbefinden und machen nachhaltig gesund – denn Nahrung ist (auch) Medizin.

Brigitte Preuß, Ayurveda Parkschlösschen Bad Wildstein,
Traben-Trarbach, Deutschland

Two Names Work Together for Beauty

Zwei Namen im Auftrag der Schönheit

Le Royal Monceau, Raffles Paris

This hotel offers an unusual yet relaxing blend: The magnificent 19th-century building in the heart of the City of Love combines with contemporary luxury by legendary designer Philippe Starck, which is in line with the Raffles' own philosophy. Throughout the hotel, guests can escape from the hectic pace of everyday life and leave behind all cares. On entering the lobby, a library invites you to relax. And the spa, one of the best in Paris, bears Starck's signature. Its white-on-white design offers a wall of silver-framed mirrors and the city's largest hotel pool. In the Spa My Blend by Clarins, another prominent name comes into play: Beauty expert Dr. Olivier Courtin-Clarins created a line of skin care products specifically for Raffles. From manicures and peelings to massages and whole-body care—after the spa treatments, you are ready for one of the world's most beautiful cities.

Eine ausgefallene und zugleich entspannende Mischung: Das prächtige Gebäude aus dem 19. Jahrhundert, mitten in der Stadt der Liebe, wurde im Sinne der Raffles-Philosophie mit zeitgemäßem Luxus der Design-Legende Philippe Starck ausgestattet. Im gesamten Haus ruht sich der Gast von der Alltagshektik aus und kann seine Seele baumeln lassen. Schon die Bibliothek in der Lobby lädt zum Entspannen ein. Auch das Spa, eines der besten in Paris, trägt Starcks Handschrift. Es ist weiß in weiß gestaltet mit einer Wand aus silbergerahmten Spiegeln und dem größten Hotelpool der Stadt. Hier im Spa My Blend by Clarins kommt noch ein weiterer Name ins Spiel: Schönheitsexperte Dr. Olivier Courtin-Clarins kreierte eigens für das Raffles eine Pflegeserie. Von Maniküre über Peelings, Massagen bis hin zu Ganzkörperbehandlungen – nach den Spa-Anwendungen ist man bereit für eine der schönsten Städte der Welt.

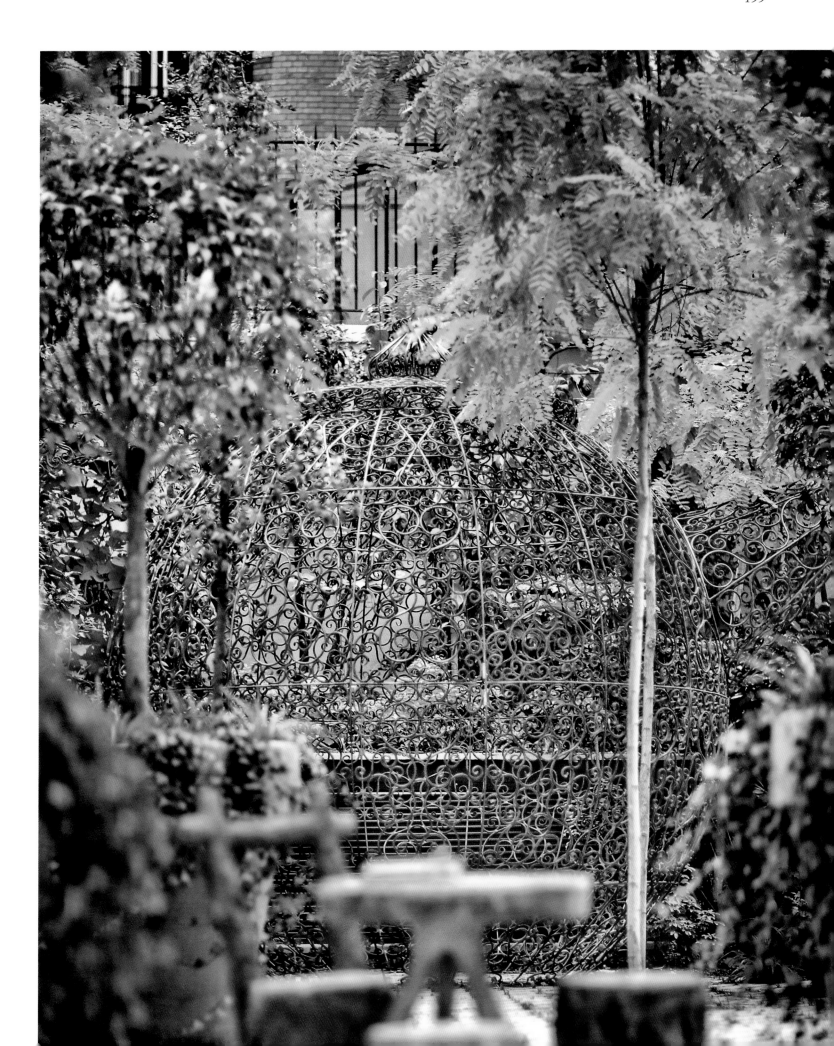

Spa, Health & Other Facilities
7 treatment rooms, couples treatment rooms, swimming pool, sauna, spa tub, hammam, steam room, ice bath and sauna, Watsu basin, fitness and cardio training room, 3 individual rooms for yoga, kinesis, and Pilates. 3 restaurants and bars, shops, meeting rooms.

Treatments & Services
Ayurvedic treatments, body treatments, color therapy, facials, hammam, hot stone, hydrotherapy, manicures, massages, pedicures, reflexology, shiatsu, Watsu, yoga. 24-hour front desk service, babysitting/childcare, business services, concierge, laundry service, multilingual staff.

Activities
Bicycling, golf, jogging, shopping, tennis.

Rooms
149 luxurious rooms and suites including 3 presidential suites. All rooms designed by Philippe Starck.

Located
5 minutes away from Arc de Triomphe and Champs-Élysées. 9 miles (15 kilometers) to Le Bourget Airport, 10 miles (16 kilometers) to Orly Airport, 15 miles (24 kilometers) to Charles de Gaulle Airport.

37 Avenue Hoche
75008 Paris, France
www.leroyalmonceau.com

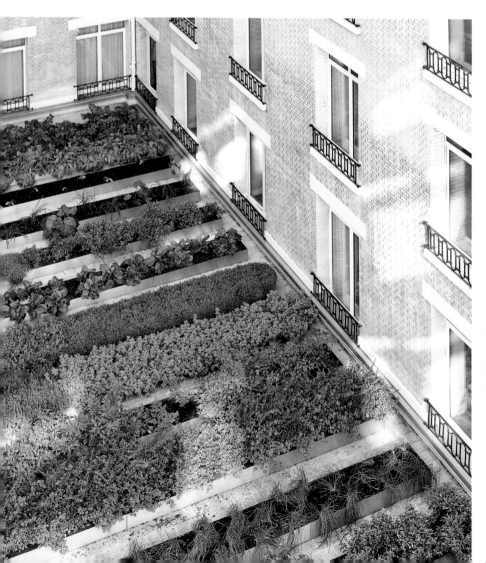
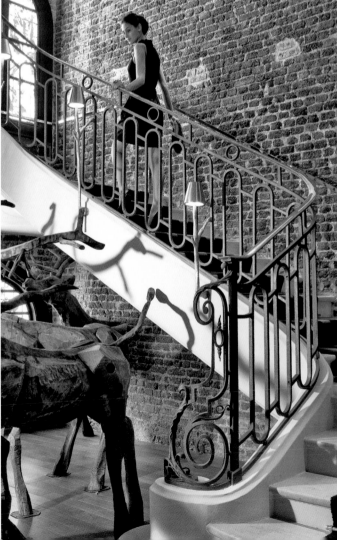

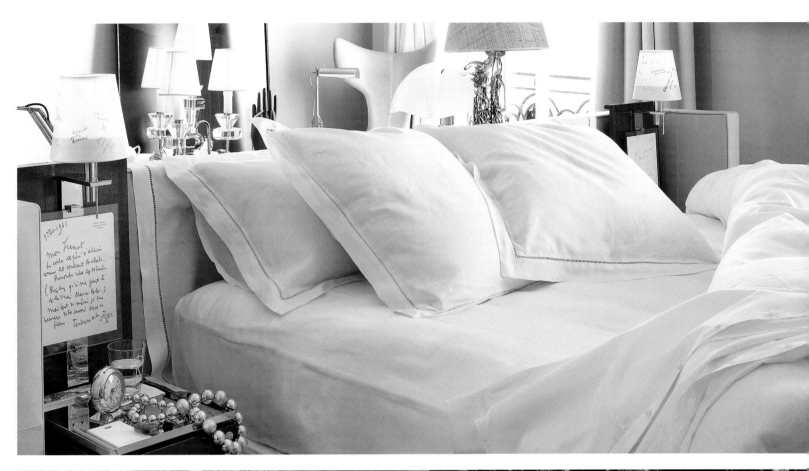

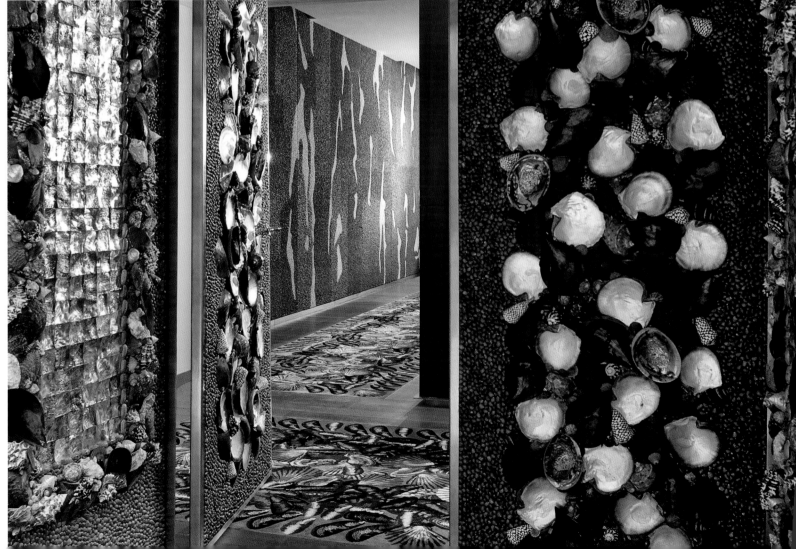

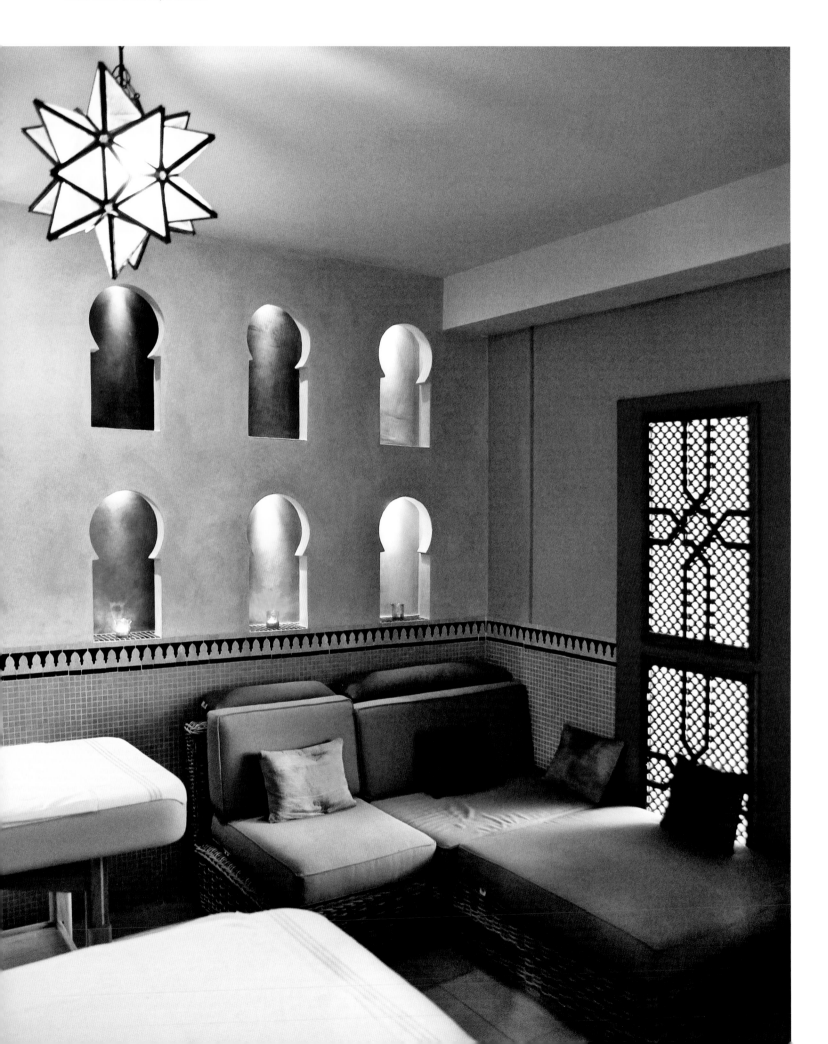

A Clearing in the Vosges Region's Nature Park

Lichtung im Naturpark der Vogesen

La Clairière Spa Hotel

Some people visit Alsace to recharge their batteries in pristine nature, while others come here for the gourmet cuisine. A third type of person wants both, plus a good portion of health and well-being—these are the guests of the La Clairière Spa Hotel. In the ancient, hilly woodlands of the Vosges region, they find a place of peace —a genuine "clearing in the forest." The health program, which focuses on the four elements of earth, fire, water, and air, is aimed at restoring and harmonizing life energy. The organic cuisine also helps. An entirely different form of grounding awaits guests in the hotel's own high ropes course, where psychological and emotional challenges reinforce positive self-esteem and generate vitality.

Während die einen ins Elsass fahren, um in ursprünglicher Natur aufzutanken, kommen andere der Gourmet-küche wegen. Eine dritte Spezies will beides und noch dazu ein riesiges Paket Wellbeing und Gesundheit – das sind die Gäste des La Clairière Spa Hotels. In den alten hügeligen Waldgebieten der Vogesen finden sie hier einen Ort des Friedens, eine wahre „Lichtung". Die Gesundheitsangebote rund um die vier Elemente Erde, Feuer, Wasser, Luft sind darauf ausgerichtet, die Lebensenergie wieder aufzubauen und zu harmonisieren. Dabei hilft auch die Bio-Küche. Einer ganz anderen Form der Erdung begegnen die Gäste im hoteleigenen Hochseilgarten. Dort stärken psychische und emotionale Herausforderungen ein positives Selbstbild und wecken die Lebendigkeit.

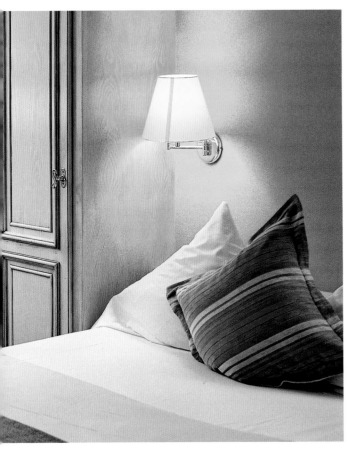

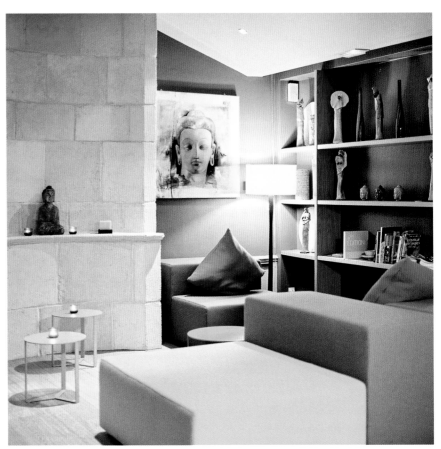

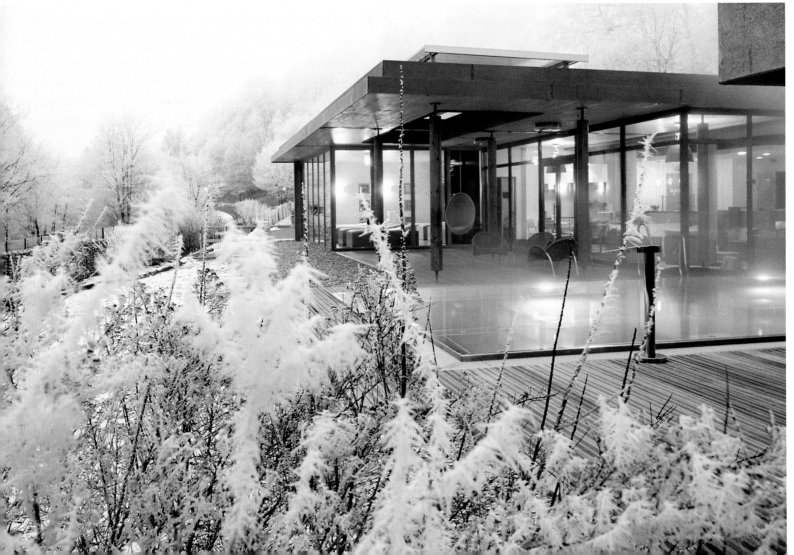

Spa, Health & Other Facilities
8 treatment rooms, Ayurveda center, wellness suites, indoor pool, heated outdoor pool, sauna, aroma and steam bath, relaxation rooms, fitness room. Restaurant with organic cuisine, 6 conference rooms, elevator.

Treatments & Services
Ayurvedic treatments and packages, body wrap in dry float, Dr. Hauschka facials, hot stone massage, Pantai Luar treatment, shiatsu, signature treatments with local products, YuNoHaNa. Free parking, laundry service.

Activities
Golf, hiking, mountain biking, team-building activities, walks in the surrounding forest.

Rooms
50 rooms – 4 categories: classique, comfort, supérieure, suite.

Located
50 minutes by car from Strasbourg and Karlsruhe, 105 minutes from Luxemburg Airport.

63 route d'Ingwiller
67290 La Petite-Pierre, France
www.la-clairiere.com

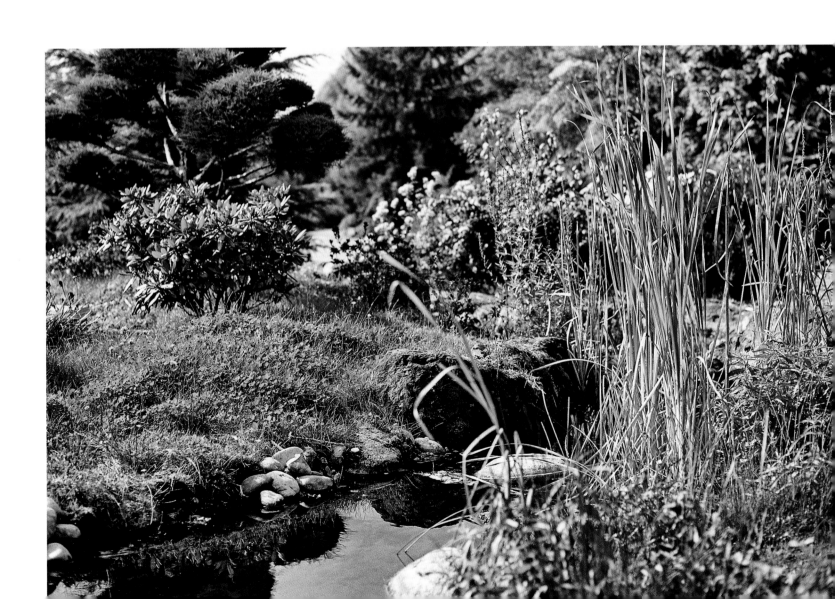

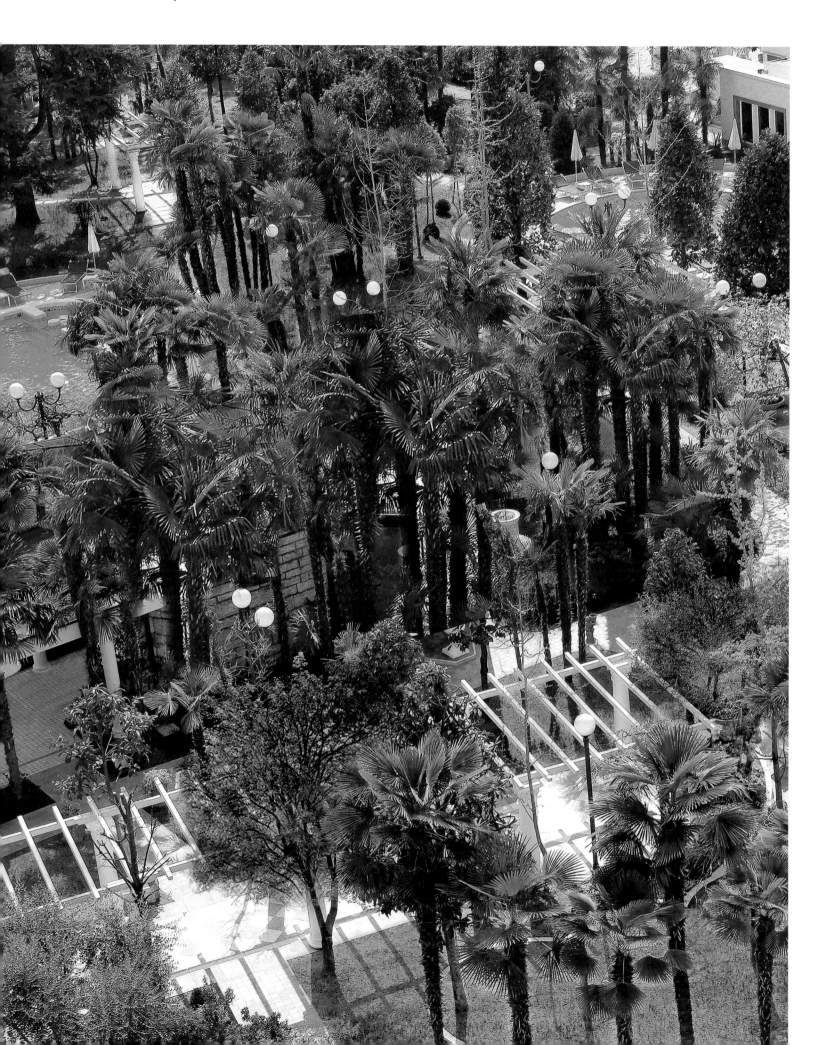

The 100-Year-Old Fountain of Youth

Der hundertjährige Jungbrunnen

Grand Hotel Terme Trieste & Victoria

In 1912, a young man from Padua had a dream, and not exactly a modest one. He wanted to build the world's grandest hotel—and that's where the story began. The "dream hotel" with its fin de siècle atmosphere soon began to attract Europe's rich and famous, who struck gold here on their quest for eternal youth. The secret flows right under the building and its seven-acre park: thermal springs with a health-giving blend of natural gases. The Borile family runs the house with the same inspiration it all started with 100 years ago. Today, the precious liquid and fango mud from the surrounding area still form the basis for the hotel's therapeutic success. A team of doctors uses the time-tested remedy for health, beauty, and fitness, based on the latest scientific findings. The Vital Thermal Spa offers a diversity of programs that help guests get back into top shape.

1912 hatte ein junger Mann aus Padua einen nicht gerade bescheidenen Traum: Er wollte das schönste aller Hotels schaffen – und so entstand es. Das „Traumhotel" mit Atmosphäre der Jahrhundertwende entwickelte sich bald zum Anziehungspunkt für die Schönen und Reichen Europas, die hier auf der Suche nach ewiger Jugend fündig wurden. Das Geheimnis fließt direkt unter dem Gebäude und seinem 30 000 Quadratmeter großen Park: heißes Thermalwasser mit einem heilsamen Naturgas-Gemisch. Heute führt Familie Borile das Haus mit der gleichen Inspiration, mit der vor 100 Jahren alles begann. Das kostbare Nass und Fango aus der Region bilden nach wie vor den Grundstein für den therapeutischen Erfolg des Hauses. Ein Ärzteteam wendet die bewährten Heilmittel nach neuesten wissenschaftlichen Erkenntnissen für Gesundheit, Schönheit und Fitness an. Das Vital Thermal Spa des Hotels bietet dazu diverse Programme, die den Gast wieder in Bestform bringen.

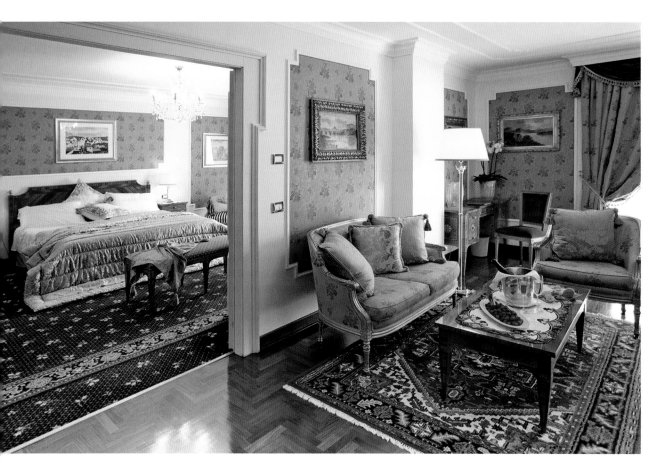

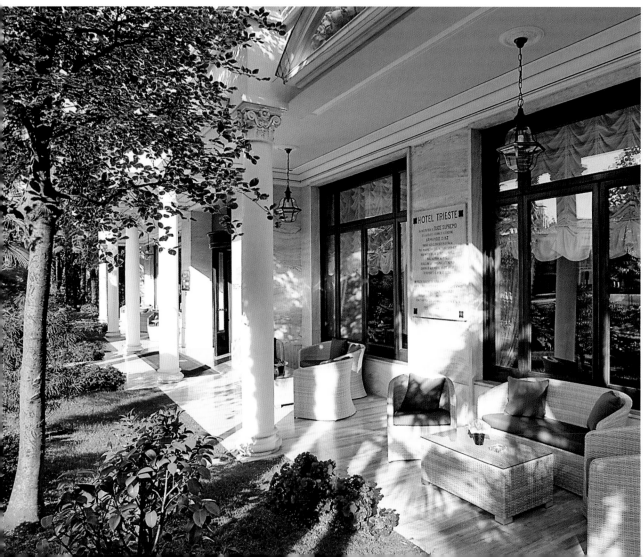

Spa, Health & Other Facilities
4 thermal pools set at different temperatures, whirlpool, oasis outdoor pool, resistance pool, cervical massage jets, waterfalls, water games, thermal steam bath, hydromassage beds, fitness facilities. Restaurant, summer restaurant, conference room.

Treatments & Services
Anti-stress, Ayurveda, bio thermal mud, body peelings, deep muscular body massage, detox programs, fango & forme, fango aesthetic treatments, fango plus, hot stone massage, hydrokinesitherapy, lymphatic drainage, personal trainer, physiokinesitherapy, physiotherapy, shiatsu. Healthy diet. 24-hour front desk, babysitting/childcare, concierge services, express check-in, free high-speed Internet, laundry service, luggage storage, room service, secretarial services.

Activities
Biking, fitness, golf, Nordic walking, horseback riding, shopping, sightseeing, tennis, wine tasting in the Eugean Hills.

Rooms
223 rooms in different categories in the Belle Epoque, Elegance, and Exclusive wings. Some rooms feature private spa cabins.

Located
In the historical center of Abano Terme's pedestrian zone.
1 hour by car from Venice, Treviso, Verona, and Bologna Airport.

Via Pietro d'Abano, 1
35031 Abano Terme, Italy
www.hoteltriestevictoria.com

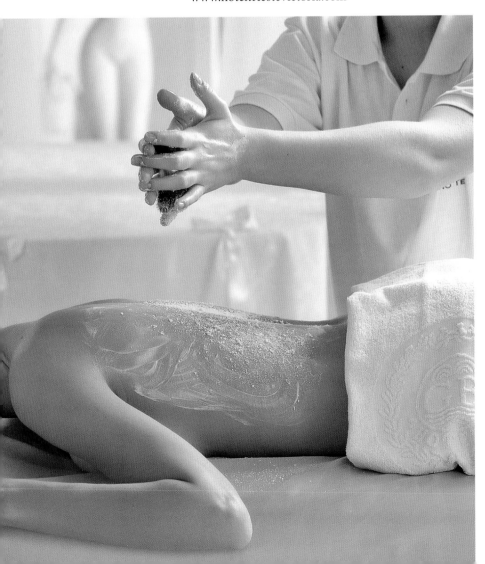

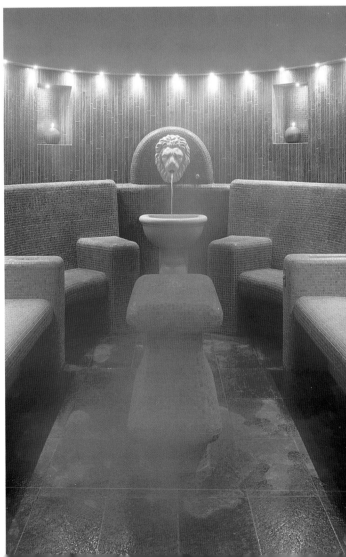

Health Secrets of Ancient Rome

Gesundheit wie die alten Römer sie pflegten

Abano Grand Hotel

Guests of the Abano Grand Hotel experience the glamour of days gone by while enjoying a range of health services based on modern research results. Whether you want to improve your health, enhance your appearance, or increase your athletic performance: The many different effects of thermal springs and fango mud have been the subject of scientific study, and their positive results can be applied through a variety of treatments. The high-end resort has large thermal pools located right in the middle of a beautiful garden. The Thermal Spa with its highly trained doctors offers unique anti-stress, remise en forme, fitness, and well-being programs. The spa specializes in anti-aging programs for men and women, which the team of doctors puts together according to the guest's individual needs. Delicious Italian and regional cuisines support the guests' health goals, while delivering true dining pleasure. Rejuvenated and refreshed, you can then tour the nearby city of Venice with renewed energy.

Im Abano Grand Hotel lebt man im Glanz vergangener Zeiten und kann gleichzeitig ein Gesundheitsangebot genießen, das auf modernen Forschungsergebnissen beruht. Ob man die Gesundheit verbessern, schöner sein oder seine sportlichen Leistungen steigern will: Die vielfache Wirkung von Thermalwasser und Fango ist wissenschaftlich untersucht, und ihre positiven Effekte können mittels verschiedener Behandlungen umgesetzt werden. Das edle Resort hat große Thermal-Schwimmbecken, die inmitten eines wunderschönen Gartens liegen. Das Thermal Spa mit hochqualifizierten Ärzten bietet einzigartige Programme in Sachen Anti-Stress, Remise en Forme, Fitness und Wellbeing. Den Schwerpunkt des Hauses bilden die Anti-Aging-Programme für Frauen und Männer, die das Ärzteteam individuell für den Gast zusammenstellt. Die köstliche italienische und regionale Küche unterstützt die Gesundheitsziele und verspricht gleichzeitig kulinarischen Genuss. Verjüngt und erfrischt sieht man dann das nahe gelegene Venedig mit neuen Augen.

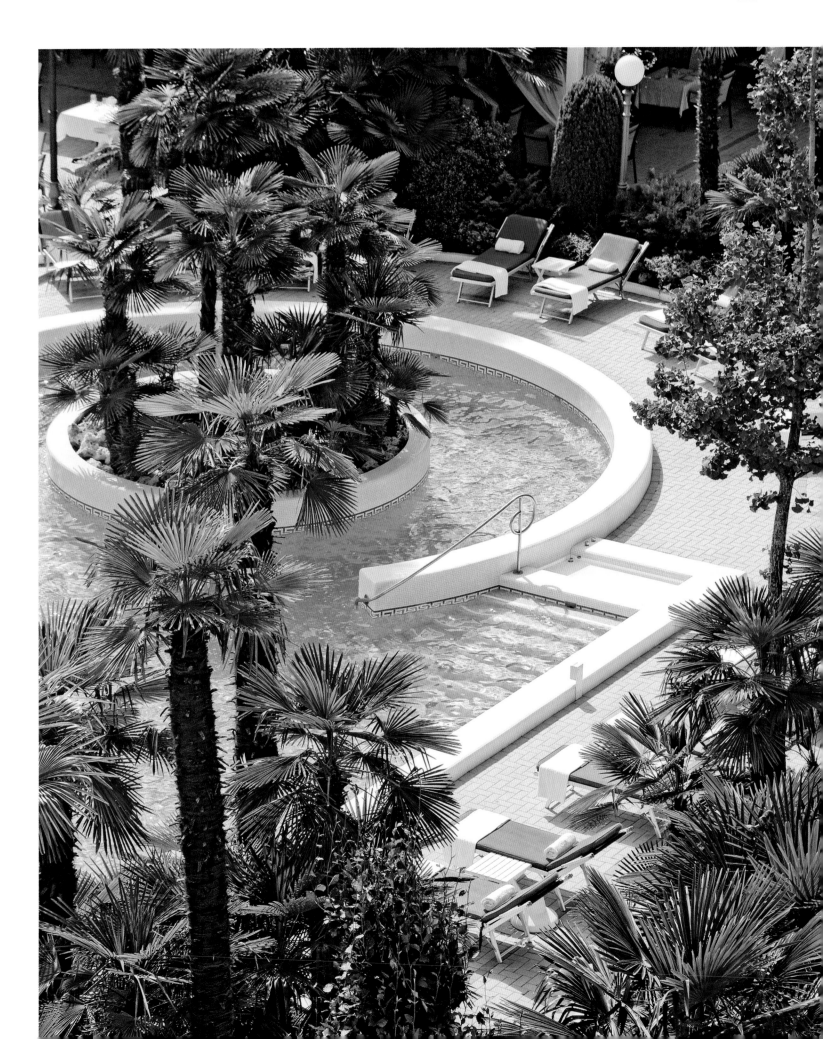

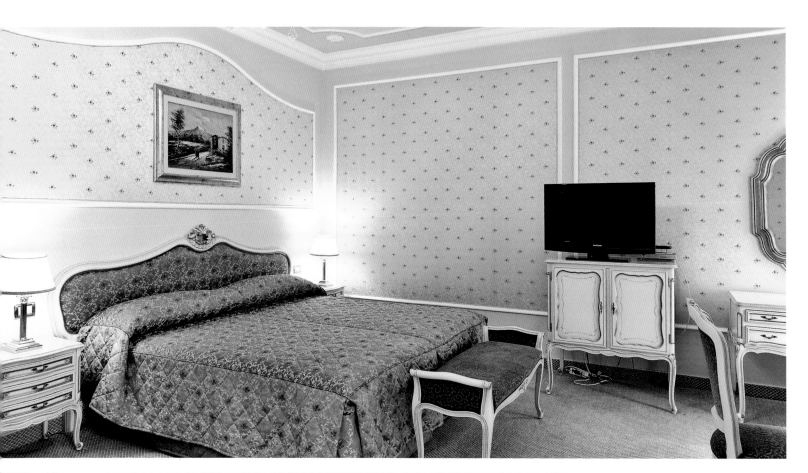

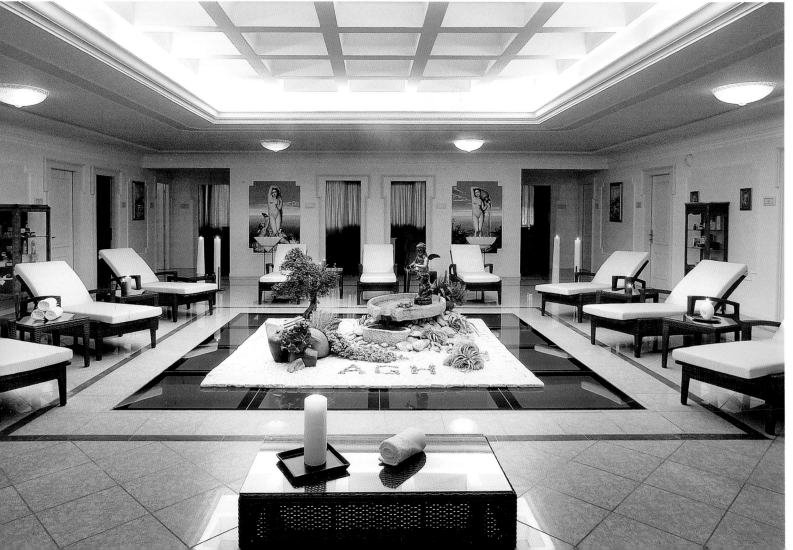

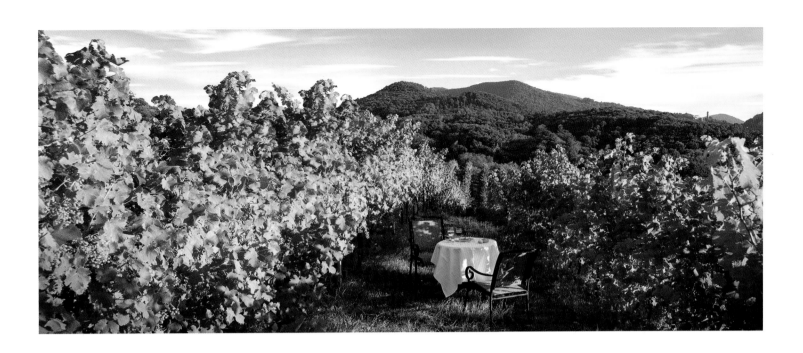

Spa, Health & Other Facilities
3 thermal pools (indoor and outdoor), relaxation area, Kneipp Path, fitness studio, thermal steam grotto.
Restaurant, poolside bar.

Treatments & Services
Antioxidant stress test, anti-stress, Ayurveda, Bacchus therapie, body peelings, deep muscular body massage,
fango, fango anti-aging, fango plus, healthy diet, hot stone massage, hydrokinesitherapy, lymphatic drainage,
physic therapy, physiokinesitherapy, personal trainer, Pilates, shiatsu, thermal bath. 24-hour front desk,
babysitting/childcare, free parking.

Activities
Aerobics, biking, golf, horseback riding, Nordic walking, shopping,
sightseeing, tennis, wine tasting in the Eugean Hills.

Rooms
189 rooms, soundproofed – 5 categories: Deluxe, Deluxe Panorama, Junior Suite, Imperial Suite,
Presidential Suite. Each with a balcony and a minimum space of 452 square feet (42 square meters).

Located
In Abano Terme, 7 miles (11 kilometers) from Padua.
1 hour by car from Venice, Treviso, Verona, and Bologna Airport.

Via Valerio Flacco, 1
35031 Abano Terme, Italy
www.abanograndhotel.com

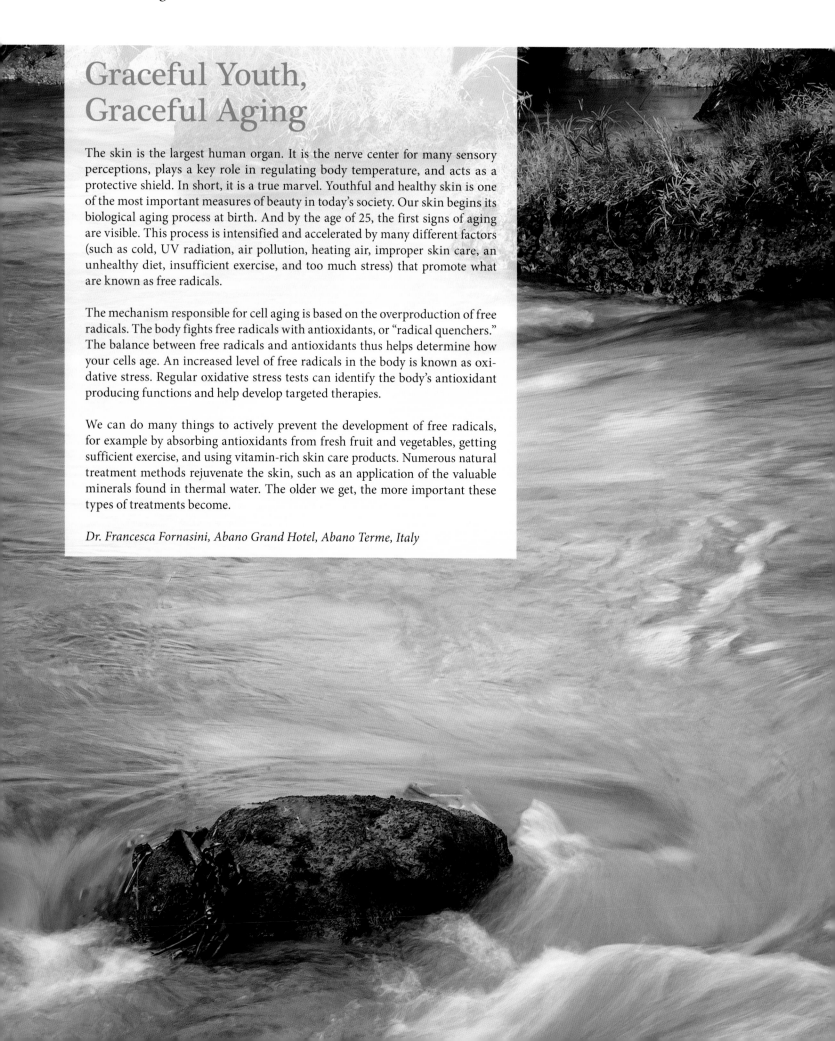

Graceful Youth, Graceful Aging

The skin is the largest human organ. It is the nerve center for many sensory perceptions, plays a key role in regulating body temperature, and acts as a protective shield. In short, it is a true marvel. Youthful and healthy skin is one of the most important measures of beauty in today's society. Our skin begins its biological aging process at birth. And by the age of 25, the first signs of aging are visible. This process is intensified and accelerated by many different factors (such as cold, UV radiation, air pollution, heating air, improper skin care, an unhealthy diet, insufficient exercise, and too much stress) that promote what are known as free radicals.

The mechanism responsible for cell aging is based on the overproduction of free radicals. The body fights free radicals with antioxidants, or "radical quenchers." The balance between free radicals and antioxidants thus helps determine how your cells age. An increased level of free radicals in the body is known as oxidative stress. Regular oxidative stress tests can identify the body's antioxidant producing functions and help develop targeted therapies.

We can do many things to actively prevent the development of free radicals, for example by absorbing antioxidants from fresh fruit and vegetables, getting sufficient exercise, and using vitamin-rich skin care products. Numerous natural treatment methods rejuvenate the skin, such as an application of the valuable minerals found in thermal water. The older we get, the more important these types of treatments become.

Dr. Francesca Fornasini, Abano Grand Hotel, Abano Terme, Italy

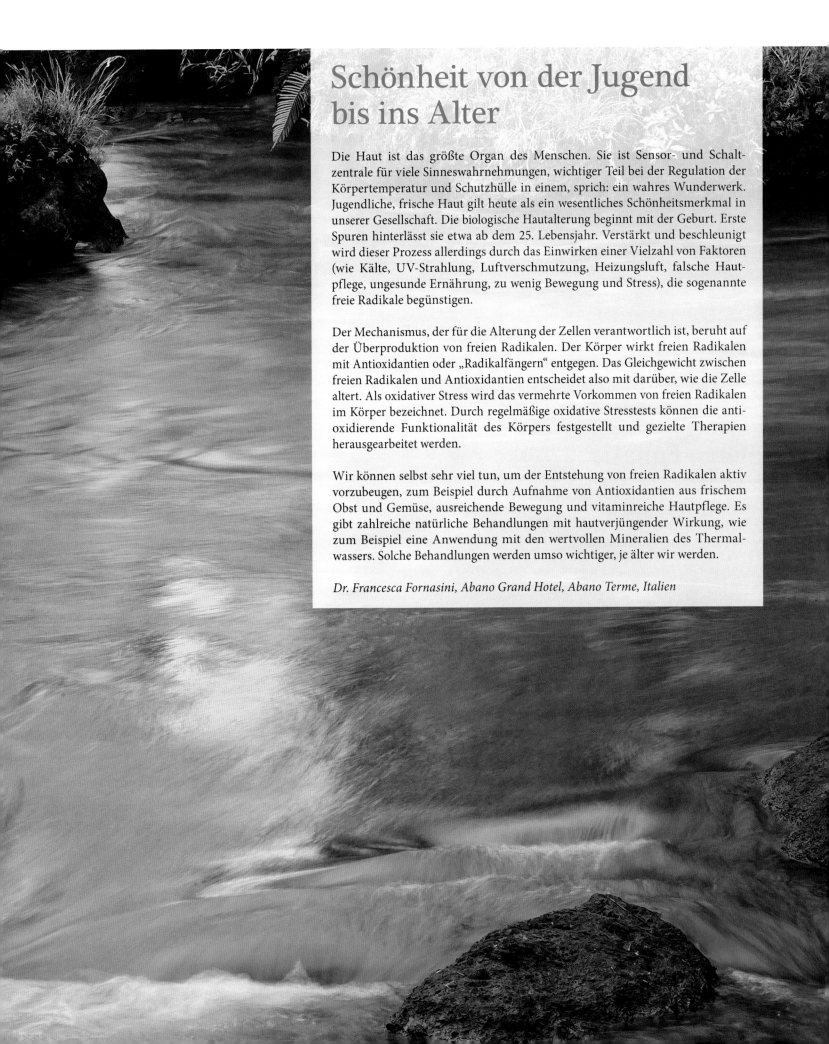

Schönheit von der Jugend bis ins Alter

Die Haut ist das größte Organ des Menschen. Sie ist Sensor- und Schaltzentrale für viele Sinneswahrnehmungen, wichtiger Teil bei der Regulation der Körpertemperatur und Schutzhülle in einem, sprich: ein wahres Wunderwerk. Jugendliche, frische Haut gilt heute als ein wesentliches Schönheitsmerkmal in unserer Gesellschaft. Die biologische Hautalterung beginnt mit der Geburt. Erste Spuren hinterlässt sie etwa ab dem 25. Lebensjahr. Verstärkt und beschleunigt wird dieser Prozess allerdings durch das Einwirken einer Vielzahl von Faktoren (wie Kälte, UV-Strahlung, Luftverschmutzung, Heizungsluft, falsche Hautpflege, ungesunde Ernährung, zu wenig Bewegung und Stress), die sogenannte freie Radikale begünstigen.

Der Mechanismus, der für die Alterung der Zellen verantwortlich ist, beruht auf der Überproduktion von freien Radikalen. Der Körper wirkt freien Radikalen mit Antioxidantien oder „Radikalfängern" entgegen. Das Gleichgewicht zwischen freien Radikalen und Antioxidantien entscheidet also mit darüber, wie die Zelle altert. Als oxidativer Stress wird das vermehrte Vorkommen von freien Radikalen im Körper bezeichnet. Durch regelmäßige oxidative Stresstests können die antioxidierende Funktionalität des Körpers festgestellt und gezielte Therapien herausgearbeitet werden.

Wir können selbst sehr viel tun, um der Entstehung von freien Radikalen aktiv vorzubeugen, zum Beispiel durch Aufnahme von Antioxidantien aus frischem Obst und Gemüse, ausreichende Bewegung und vitaminreiche Hautpflege. Es gibt zahlreiche natürliche Behandlungen mit hautverjüngender Wirkung, wie zum Beispiel eine Anwendung mit den wertvollen Mineralien des Thermalwassers. Solche Behandlungen werden umso wichtiger, je älter wir werden.

Dr. Francesca Fornasini, Abano Grand Hotel, Abano Terme, Italien

"Authentic" Beauty

„Echte" Schönheit

Borgo Egnazia

The history of Borgo Egnazia is the story of a passion—the passion to build a health resort in the style of an Apulian village, with colors and stones from the surrounding area and elements reminiscent of Roman times. Surrounded by lemon and olive trees, this oasis of beauty is situated a short distance from a picturesque fishing port and the deep blue Adriatic Sea. The magic word here is "vair" (which means "authentic" in the local dialect). It stands for a treatment method based on Apulian traditions, ancient natural remedies, and the region's vital spirit. For example, cleansing massages with Apulian sea salt and oil are "vair," as are body wraps using volcanic minerals and even a session that goes beyond verbal communication with the music therapist, Dr. Rotondo. Of course, the spa's cucina italiana also helps to create a sense of well-being. The kitchen serves traditional Mediterranean dishes, and the region's practice of cultivating olives and grapes has left its own culinary mark.

Die Geschichte des Borgo Egnazia ist die Geschichte einer Leidenschaft – der Leidenschaft, einen Erholungsort im Stil eines apulischen Dorfes zu bauen, mit den Farben und den Steinen der Umgebung sowie Reminiszenzen an die Römerzeit. Umgeben von Zitronen- und Olivenbäumen, nicht weit von einem malerischen Fischerhafen und der tiefblauen Adria, liegt diese Oase der Schönheit. „Vair" (was im einheimischen Dialekt „echt" bedeutet) heißt hier das Zauberwort. Es steht für eine Behandlungsmethode auf der Grundlage apulischer Traditionen, alter Naturheilmittel und des lebendigen Geistes der Region. „Vair" sind zum Beispiel reinigende Massagen mit apulischem Meersalz und Öl, Körperwickel mit vulkanischen Mineralien aber auch eine Reise jenseits der verbalen Kommunikation mit Musiktherapeut Dr. Rotondo. Natürlich trägt auch die Cucina Italiana zum Wohlbefinden bei: Die Küche serviert traditionelle mediterrane Gerichte, und die regionale Anbaukultur von Oliven und Trauben hinterlässt ihre kulinarischen Spuren.

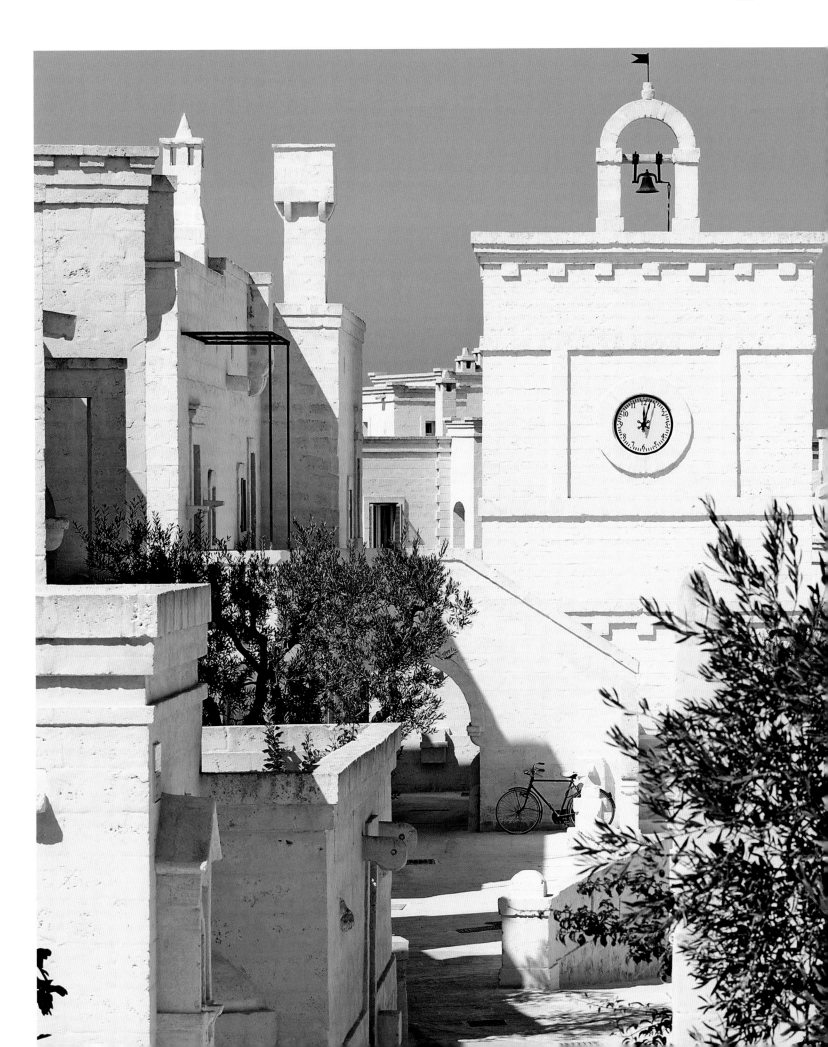

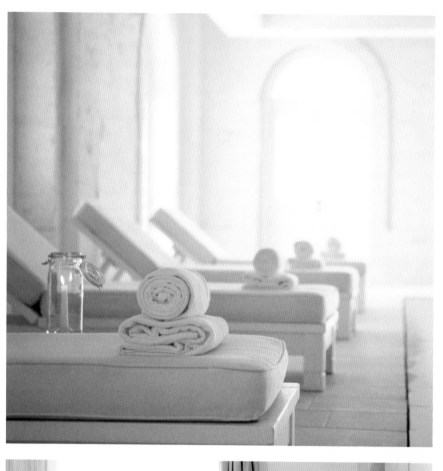

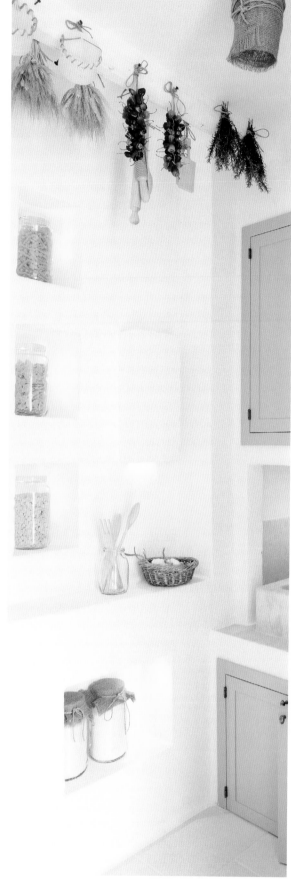

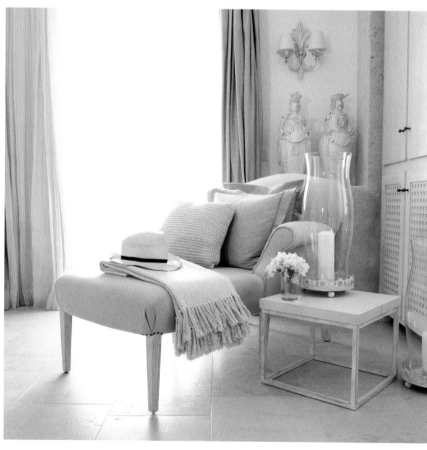

Spa, Health & Other Facilities
13 treatment rooms, indoor pool, gym, sauna, tepidarium, frigidarium, caldarium, spa cinema, relaxation area, Roman bath area with scrub rooms and flotation room, fitness and yoga studio. 4 restaurants, 4 bars, terrace, 18-hole golf course, bicycle rental, banquet facilities, conference room, children's club, hair studio, social room for hands and feet, makeup area, elevator.

Treatments & Services
Ancient beauty rituals, aromatherapy, color therapy, manicure, massages, medical consultant, pedicure. 24-hour front desk, babysitting/childcare, billiards, event catering, free parking, infant beds available, laundry service, valet parking.

Activities
Beach club, biking, cooking lessons, fishing, golf, horseback riding, rowing/canoeing, sailing, scuba diving, snorkeling, swimming, tennis, windsurfing.

Rooms
183 rooms.

Located
34 miles (55 kilometers) from Bari Airport, 31 miles (50 kilometers) from Brindisi Airport.

72010 Savelletri di Fasano, Italy
www.borgoegnazia.com/en

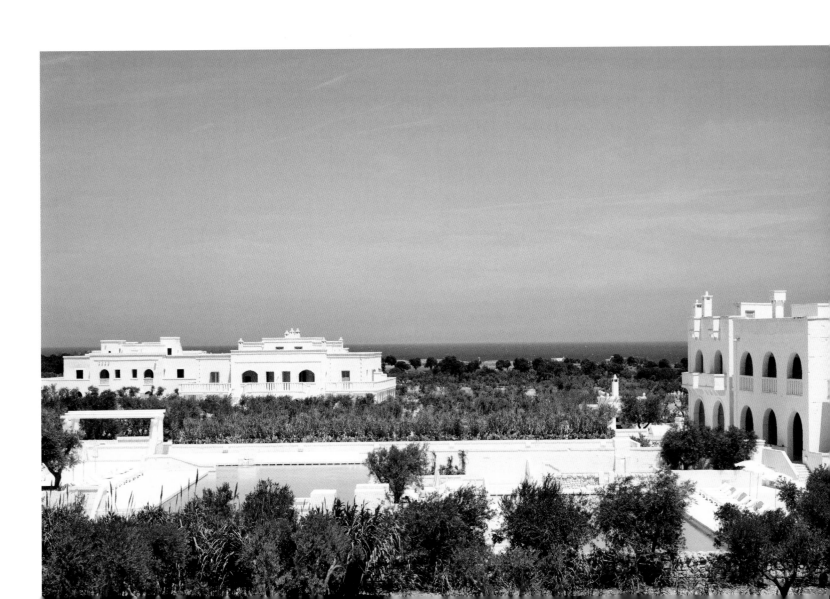

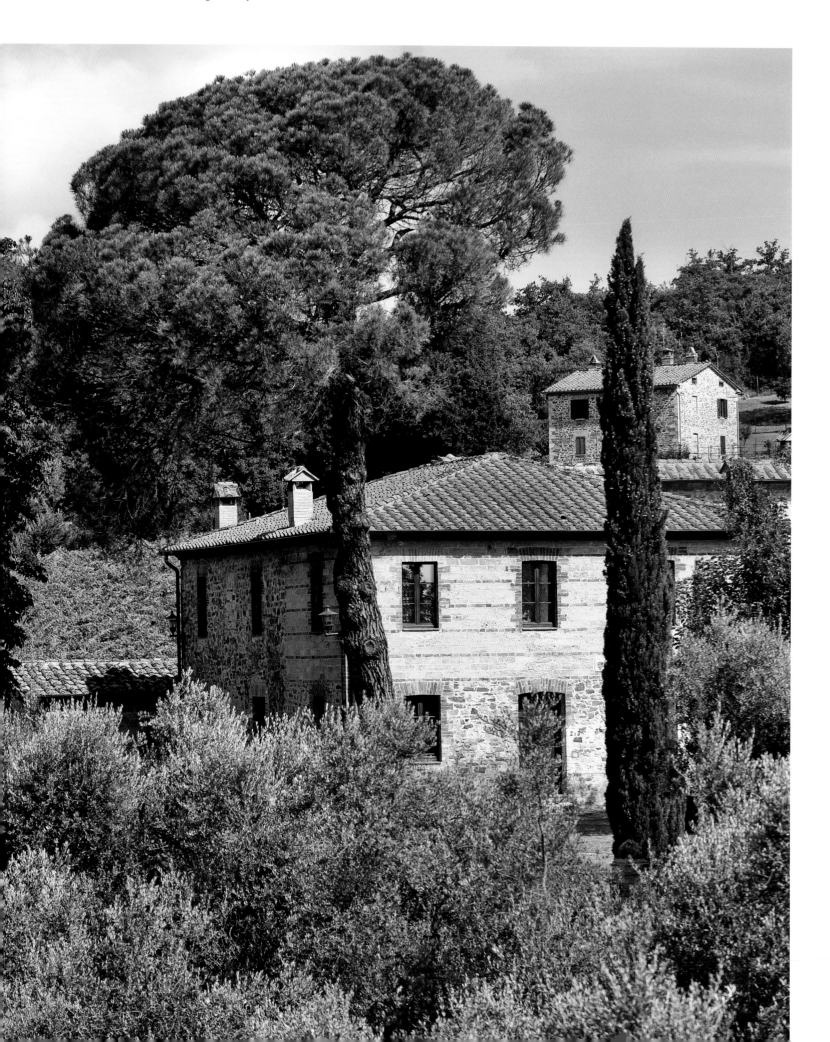

Tuscany's Energy Castle

Die Energie-Burg in der Toskana

Castel Monastero

Castel Monastero, a meticulously restored medieval village and monastery, is situated in a typical Tuscan landscape. Here, a team of doctors trained in holistic medicine offers special health programs aimed at restoring the balance between body and soul. The programs, which were designed by Dr. Mosaraf Ali, director of the Integrated Medical Centre in London and a leading expert in the field of integrative medicine, are tailored to individual needs. The choices include detox, weight loss, and revitalization, supported by a prescription for a healthy diet and exercise. Herbal teas from the castle garden, massages, and yoga classes where you learn correct breathing techniques and how to relax are also part of the program. On your way to your morning yoga class, you cross the small plaza and pass the tiny chapel—following the same route that monks used to take back in the 12th century. Guests immerse themselves in the spa's saunas, hammam, and salt water pool and emerge again, feeling like a new person. Gordon Ramsay had a hand in planning the imaginative nutrition plans, which are based on a low-sugar, low-fat diet. The castle's beautiful courtyard provides the right ambiance for enjoying delicious meals featuring natural foods.

In typisch toskanischer Landschaft liegt Castel Monastero, ein sorgsam restauriertes mittelalterliches Dorf und Kloster. Hier bringt heute ein ganzheitlich geschultes Ärzteteam mit speziellen Gesundheitsprogrammen Körper und Seele wieder ins Gleichgewicht. Die individuell abgestimmten Programme stammen von Dr. Mosaraf Ali, Direktor des Integrated Medical Centre in London und führender Experte auf dem Gebiet der Integrativen Medizin. Zur Auswahl stehen etwa Detox, Gewichtsreduzierung und Revitalisierung. Unterstützend werden eine gesunde Diät und Bewegung verschrieben. Kräutertees aus dem Burggarten, Massagen und Yogastunden, in denen die richtige Atemtechnik und die Fähigkeit zur Entspannung unterrichtet werden, gehören ebenfalls dazu. Der Weg zur morgendlichen Yogaklasse führt über die kleine Plaza und vorbei an der winzigen Kapelle – das ist der Weg, den schon die Mönche im 12. Jahrhundert beschritten. Im Spa-Bereich mit seinen Saunen, Hamam und dem Salzwasserpool taucht der Gast ab und wie neugeboren wieder auf. Die einfallsreichen Ernährungspläne wurden in Zusammenarbeit mit Gordon Ramsay erstellt und basieren auf einer zuckerarmen, fettreduzierten Ernährung. Der wunderschöne Hof bietet das richtige Ambiente für genussvolle, natürliche Mahlzeiten.

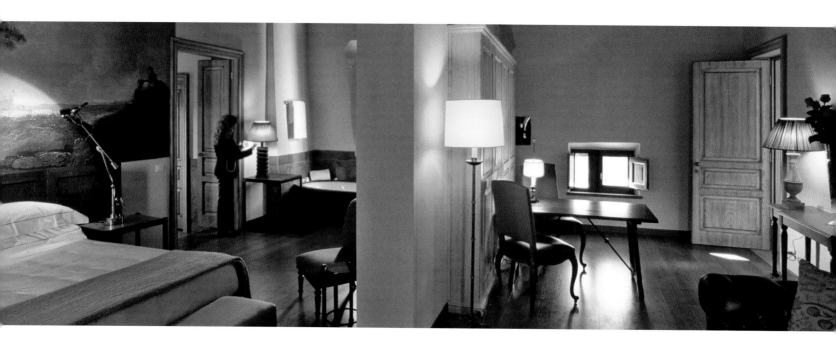

Spa, Health & Other Facilities
10,800 square feet (1,000 square meters) spa treatment area comprising 8 treatment rooms, 3 outdoor pools surrounded by gardens, 2 indoor pools, Finnish sauna, bio sauna, steam room, experience showers, Kneipp and phlebologic circuit, fitness room. Audio-visual equipment, banquet facilities, health club, conference room.

Treatments & Services
Exclusive wellness programs by the international expert in integrated medicine, Dr. Mosaraf Ali: detox, revitalizing programs, therapeutic yoga, weight-loss. 24-hour front desk, babysitting/childcare, doorman, free breakfast, free parking, infant beds available, laundry service, luggage storage, town car service available, valet parking, wedding service.

Activities
Excursions to Siena and its wineries, horseback riding, tennis.

Rooms
74 rooms and suites plus 1 villa.

Located
In the Chianti countryside, 14 miles (23 kilometers) from Siena, 56 miles (90 kilometers) from Florence.

Loc. Monastero d'Ombrone, 19
53019 Castelnuovo Berardenga, Italy
www.castelmonastero.com/it

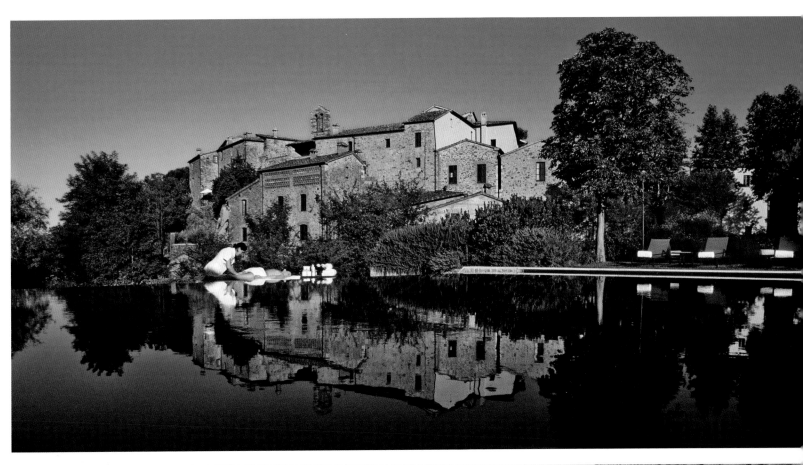

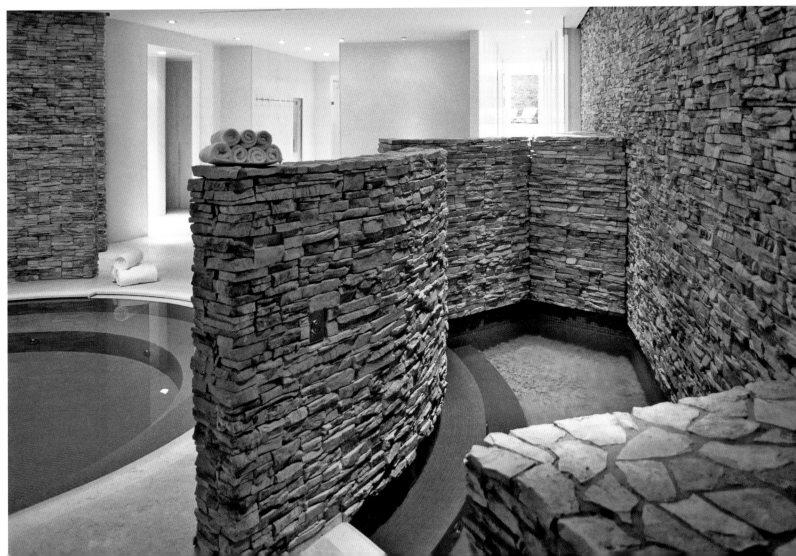

Integrated Medicine

Conventional medicine treats the disease, often ignoring the individuality of the patient, and even the cause, in the blind rush to recreate normality. Integrated medicine treats the patient as an individual and as a cooperative partner to restore health and therefore fight off the disease. You may sometimes need that packet of pills but 80 percent of the healing will still come from you, mostly through nutritional care, with exercise and therapeutic massage as well.

Conventional medicine is called allopathic, from allo (other), patho (agent of disease). In other words, conventional medicine introduces other pathogens, usually toxins (in the case of drugs or chemotherapy) to counter the original pathogen (the disease). Integrated medicine adjusts the lifestyle of the patient to restore the defensive network and the balance of the systems to their healthy state. Conventional medicine therefore requires least effort from the patient, who simply remains passive. Integrated medicine demands full mental and physical cooperation and effort to build up defences, but with a far higher ultimate reward—good health.

Dr. Mosaraf Ali, Integrated Medical Centre in London and Castel Monastero, Italy

Integrative Medizin

In der Schulmedizin werden Krankheiten oftmals behandelt, ohne den individu-ellen Patienten oder gar die Ursache genauer zu betrachten, um auf schnellstem Wege den Normalzustand wiederherzustellen. In der Integrativen Medizin wird der Patient im Kampf gegen die Krankheit als Individuum und kooperativer Partner behandelt. Tabletten sind zwar hin und wieder notwendig, jedoch hängen 80 Prozent der Heilung vom Patienten selbst ab, der mit gesunder Ernährung, körperlicher Bewegung und therapeutischen Massagen am Genesungsprozess teilnimmt.

Die Schulmedizin wird als allopathisch bezeichnet, wobei sich allo von „anders" und patho von „Krankheitserreger" ableitet. Das heißt mit anderen Worten, die Schulmedizin nutzt andere Krankheitserreger – üblicherweise Giftstoffe (Medikamente oder Chemotherapie) –, um die ursprünglichen Krankheitserreger (die Krankheit) zu bekämpfen. Die Integrative Medizin stellt die Lebensweise des Patienten so um, dass das Abwehrsystem wiederhergestellt und das Gleich-gewicht der Systeme wieder zu seinem gesunden Zustand zurückgeführt wird. Die Schulmedizin fordert nur sehr geringe Bemühungen seitens des Patienten, der sich passiv verhält. Die Integrative Medizin verlangt dagegen umfassende mentale und körperliche Zusammenarbeit und Anstrengung, um Abwehrkräfte aufzubauen. Dafür erhält der Patient die größte aller Belohnungen: Gesundheit.

Dr. Mosaraf Ali, Integrated Medical Centre in London und Castel Monastero, Italien

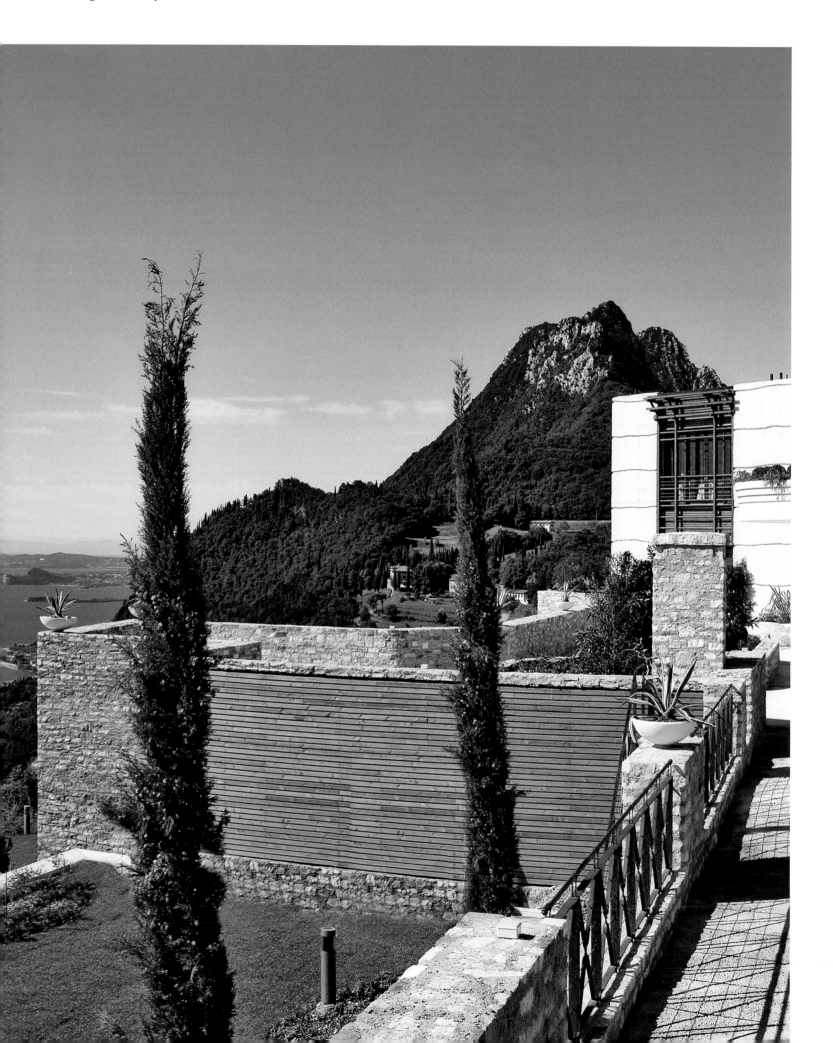

Awareness of People and the Environment

Bewusstsein für Mensch und Umwelt

Lefay Resort & Spa Lago di Garda

Situated between gently rolling hills and olive groves, the Lefay Resort stands high above Lake Garda in northern Italy. Everything here is based on the principle that luxury is whatever is good for the body and the environment. The spa, a temple to well-being, is where you renew body and spirit by getting back in touch with genuine feelings. This goal is achieved through oriental rituals, thalassotherapies, cosmetic treatments, and the special Lefay SPA Method, which combines the thousand-year-old principles of Classical Chinese Medicine with those of research based on Western science. Various types of massage, cures, gymnastics, energy work, and healing teas help restore your individual energy flow. The concept of holistic health and personal wellness consistently incorporates the natural surroundings. Even the rooms, which are built entirely from recyclable materials, demonstrate that ecological principles played an important role when the resort was constructed. A beautiful garden, dedicated to energy therapy and intended to symbolize the different stages of life, is one of the resort's main highlights. A small wood, which beckons guests with its mystical atmosphere, lies right behind the complex.

Eingebettet zwischen sanften Hügeln und Olivenhainen, hoch über dem Gardasee in Norditalien, liegt das Lefay Resort. Hier lautet das Motto: Luxus ist, was Mensch und Umwelt gut tut. Im Spa, einem Tempel des Wohlbefindens, sollen sich Geist und Körper durch die Wiederentdeckung authentischer Gefühle selbst regenerieren. Dafür sorgen orientalische Rituale, Thalasso-Therapien, kosmetische Behandlungen und die spezielle Lefay SPA Method. Sie vereint die jahrtausendealten Prinzipien der Klassischen Chinesischen Medizin mit denen der wissenschaftlichen Forschung der westlichen Welt. Mit unterschiedlichen Massagen, Kuren, Gymnastiken, Energie-Arbeiten und Heiltees wird dabei der individuelle Energiefluss wiederhergestellt. Konsequent bezieht das Konzept der Ganzheitlichkeit und persönlichen Wellness auch die umgebende Natur ein. An den Zimmern, die zu 100 Prozent aus recycelbarem Material bestehen, lässt sich erkennen, dass ökologische Prinzipien beim Bau des Resorts maßgeblich waren. Besonderes Highlight der Anlage ist der wunderschöne energetisch-therapeutische Garten, der an den Lauf des Lebens erinnern soll. Gleich hinter dem Resort liegt ein kleines Waldstück, das mit seiner mystischen Stimmung zum Verweilen einlädt.

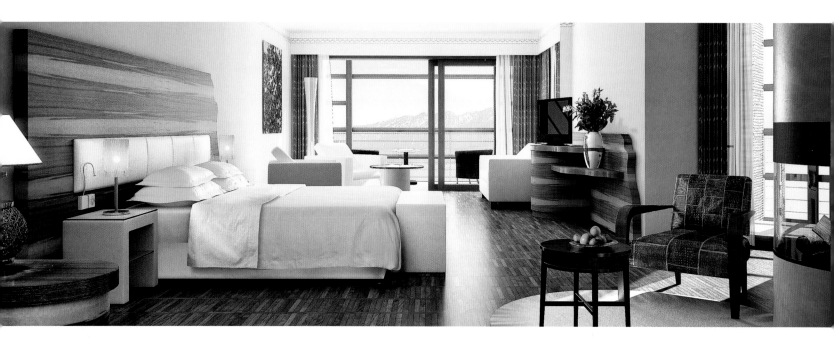

Spa, Health & Other Facilities
Wellness spa, whirlpool, steam bath, sauna, fitness studio, outdoor wellness paths, energetic-therapeutic gardens. Restaurant, trattoria, bar, pool bar, hair salon.

Treatments & Services
Acupuncture, anti-stress, body massages from the oriental as well as the western tradition, detox, energy therapy, hydrotherapy, lifestyle coaching, lymphatic drainage, medical, meditation, naturopathy, nutritional consultancy, oriental rituals for body and face, osteopathy, physiotherapy, phytotherapy, Pilates, reflexology, shiatsu, Talgo thalassotherapy, thermal water, weight loss, yoga. 24-hour front desk, 24-hour room service, activities for children, airport transfer, babysitting/childcare, free parking, laundry service, town car rental, valet parking.

Activities
Biking, bungee jumping, fishing, golf, motorcycling, rafting, sailing, surfing, tennis, trekking, volleyball, walking, windsurfing.

Rooms
90 rooms and suites – 4 categories: Lefay prestige junior suites, deluxe junior suites, exclusive suites, family suites. Each room features a terrace or balcony with lake view.

Located
In an 11 hectares natural park. 55 miles (88 kilometers) from Verona Airport, 4 miles (6 kilometers) from Gargnano.

Via Angelo Feltrinelli, 118
25084 Gargnano, Italy
www.lefayresorts.com

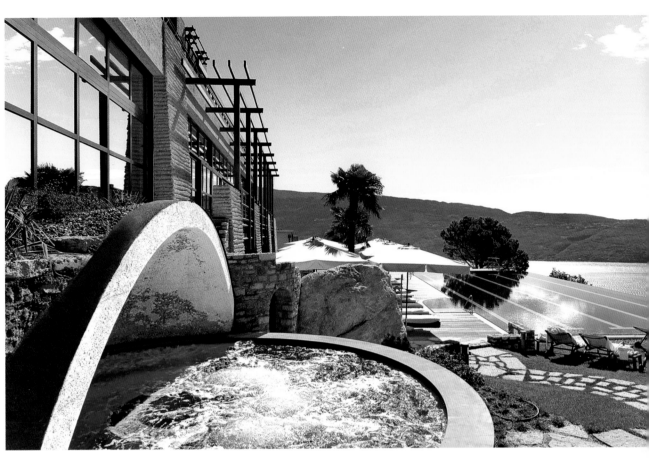

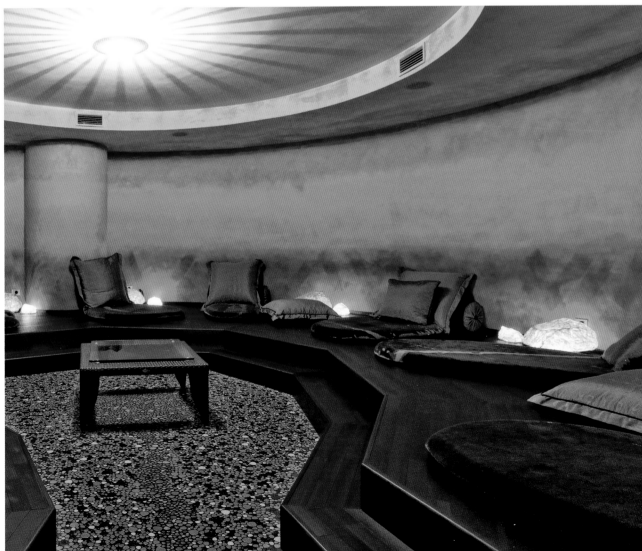

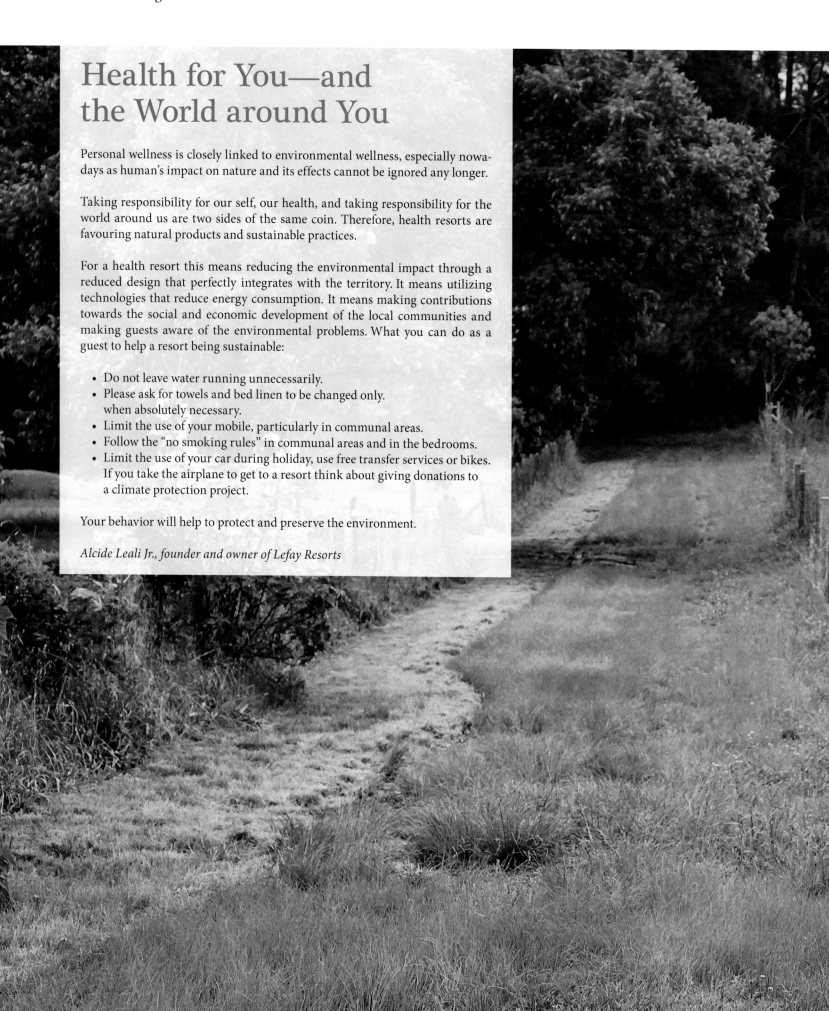

Health for You—and the World around You

Personal wellness is closely linked to environmental wellness, especially nowadays as human's impact on nature and its effects cannot be ignored any longer.

Taking responsibility for our self, our health, and taking responsibility for the world around us are two sides of the same coin. Therefore, health resorts are favouring natural products and sustainable practices.

For a health resort this means reducing the environmental impact through a reduced design that perfectly integrates with the territory. It means utilizing technologies that reduce energy consumption. It means making contributions towards the social and economic development of the local communities and making guests aware of the environmental problems. What you can do as a guest to help a resort being sustainable:

- Do not leave water running unnecessarily.
- Please ask for towels and bed linen to be changed only. when absolutely necessary.
- Limit the use of your mobile, particularly in communal areas.
- Follow the "no smoking rules" in communal areas and in the bedrooms.
- Limit the use of your car during holiday, use free transfer services or bikes. If you take the airplane to get to a resort think about giving donations to a climate protection project.

Your behavior will help to protect and preserve the environment.

Alcide Leali Jr., founder and owner of Lefay Resorts

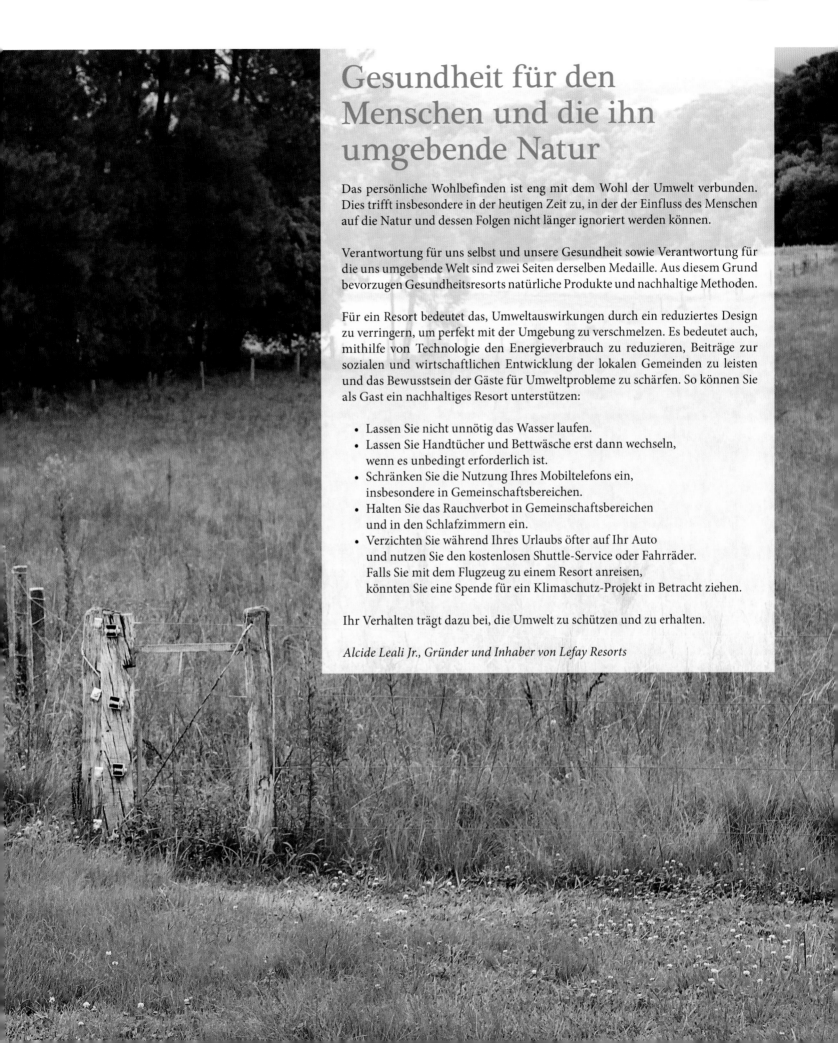

Gesundheit für den Menschen und die ihn umgebende Natur

Das persönliche Wohlbefinden ist eng mit dem Wohl der Umwelt verbunden. Dies trifft insbesondere in der heutigen Zeit zu, in der der Einfluss des Menschen auf die Natur und dessen Folgen nicht länger ignoriert werden können.

Verantwortung für uns selbst und unsere Gesundheit sowie Verantwortung für die uns umgebende Welt sind zwei Seiten derselben Medaille. Aus diesem Grund bevorzugen Gesundheitsresorts natürliche Produkte und nachhaltige Methoden.

Für ein Resort bedeutet das, Umweltauswirkungen durch ein reduziertes Design zu verringern, um perfekt mit der Umgebung zu verschmelzen. Es bedeutet auch, mithilfe von Technologie den Energieverbrauch zu reduzieren, Beiträge zur sozialen und wirtschaftlichen Entwicklung der lokalen Gemeinden zu leisten und das Bewusstsein der Gäste für Umweltprobleme zu schärfen. So können Sie als Gast ein nachhaltiges Resort unterstützen:

- Lassen Sie nicht unnötig das Wasser laufen.
- Lassen Sie Handtücher und Bettwäsche erst dann wechseln, wenn es unbedingt erforderlich ist.
- Schränken Sie die Nutzung Ihres Mobiltelefons ein, insbesondere in Gemeinschaftsbereichen.
- Halten Sie das Rauchverbot in Gemeinschaftsbereichen und in den Schlafzimmern ein.
- Verzichten Sie während Ihres Urlaubs öfter auf Ihr Auto und nutzen Sie den kostenlosen Shuttle-Service oder Fahrräder. Falls Sie mit dem Flugzeug zu einem Resort anreisen, könnten Sie eine Spende für ein Klimaschutz-Projekt in Betracht ziehen.

Ihr Verhalten trägt dazu bei, die Umwelt zu schützen und zu erhalten.

Alcide Leali Jr., Gründer und Inhaber von Lefay Resorts

One Step Closer to Heaven

Dem Himmel ein Stück näher

Alpina Dolomites – Gardena Health Lodge & Spa

The world is far away—it literally lies somewhere in the valley below, and it's not important at the moment. The view from your breakfast table—the Dolomite peaks and gently rolling alpine meadows on Europe's largest high-altitude plateau—is much more interesting. At an elevation of 5,900 feet, the air alone is a health elixir. "Experience nature" lies at the very heart of the philosophy of the Alpina Dolomites resort. The spa uses products with natural ingredients for cosmetic applications; in the wellness oasis, you will find hay and herbal bath treatments based on deep-rooted South Tyrolean traditions. The meals served in the dining room are based on the use of regional and local foods. The lodge's architecture was inspired by the surrounding landscape, and the building was constructed according to environmentally friendly standards. Whether you come to the Alpina Dolomites in search of relaxation, fitness, or a way to prevent burnout, the Seiser Alm brings you closer to heaven than anywhere else.

Die Welt ist weit weg – sie liegt buchstäblich irgendwo unten im Tal und ist gerade nicht wichtig. Viel interessanter ist der Blick vom Frühstückstisch auf die Gipfel der Dolomiten und die sanften Almwiesen der größten Hochalm Europas. Auf 1 800 Metern Höhe ist allein die Luft schon ein Gesundheitselixier. „Natur erleben" – das ist im Alpina Dolomites zentral. So werden für Kosmetikanwendungen Produkte mit natürlichen Inhaltsstoffen benutzt; in der Wellness-Oase gibt es Heu- und Kräuterbadbehandlungen nach alter Südtiroler Tradition. Auf den Tisch kommen Speisen aus regionalen Zutaten. Die Architektur der Lodge ist von den Formen der umgebenden Landschaft inspiriert, das Gebäude nach umweltfreundlichen Standards erbaut. Egal ob man zur Entspannung, Fitness oder zur Burn-Out-Prävention ins Alpina Dolomites kommt: Auf der Seiser Alm ist man dem Himmel immer ein Stückchen näher als anderswo.

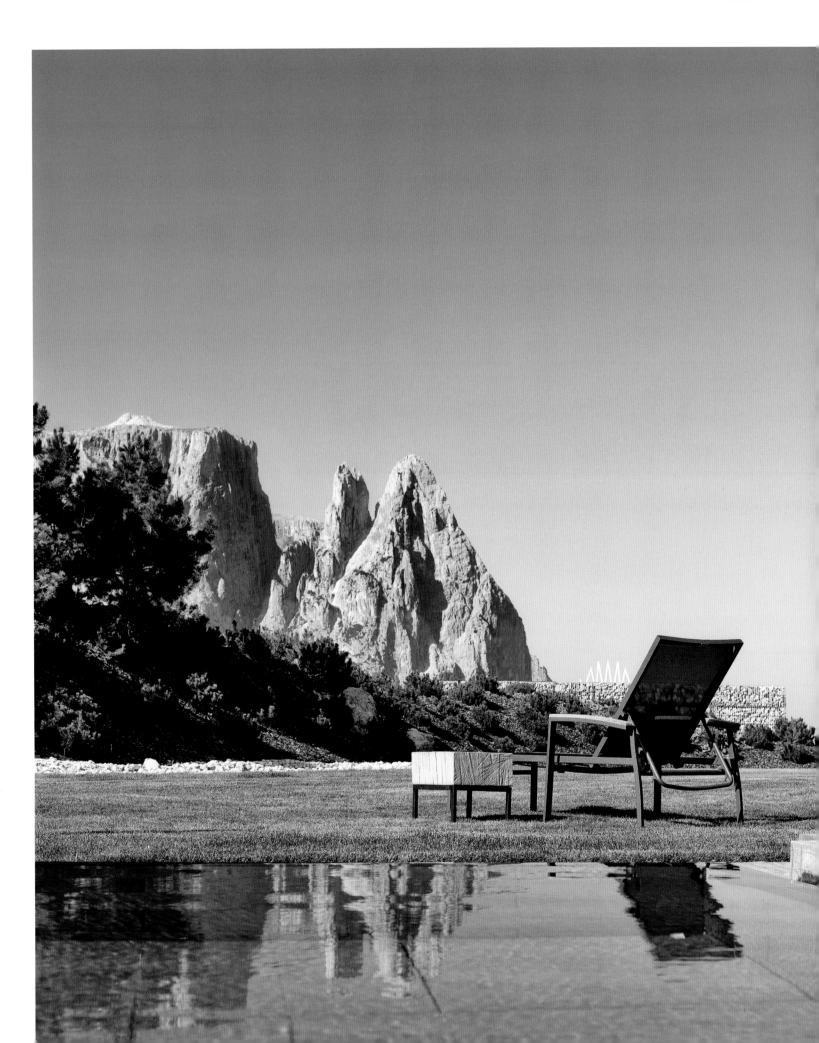

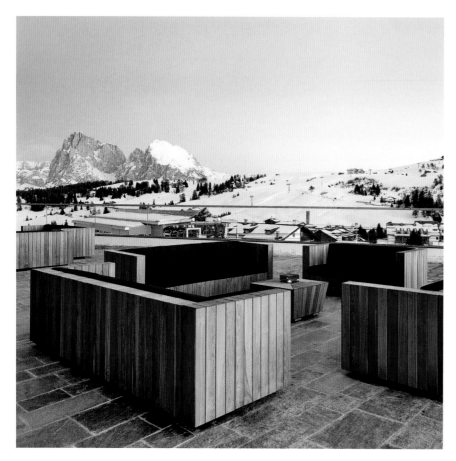

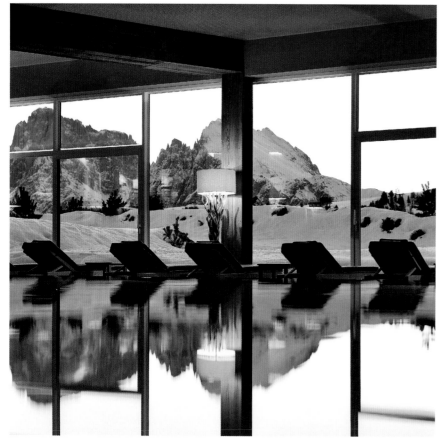

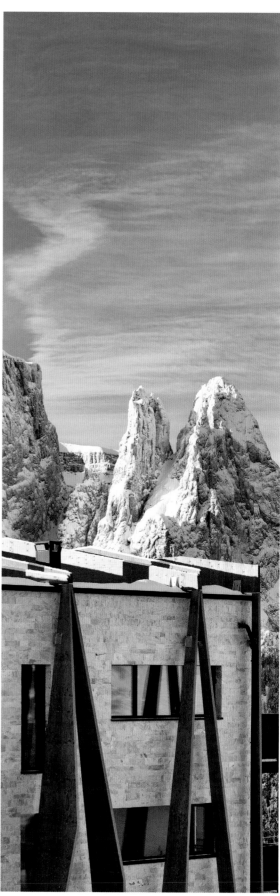

Spa, Health & Other Facilities

Indoor and outdoor panoramic swimming pool with massage loungers and massaging jet sprays, aquagym, sauna, bio-sauna, steam bath, relaxation areas with water beds, fitness area with modern equipment. Mountain Restaurant & Stuben, Mountain Lounge & Bar with view of the Dolomites, Cigar Lounge, library, indoor golf simulator, hair salon.

Treatments & Services

Alpine treatments, aromatherapy, Ayurveda, baths, beauty care treatments, body art, Californian massage, fitball, gentle gymnastics, La Stone massage, Lomi Lomi, lymphatic drainage, massages, Pantai Luar, Pilates, reflexology, Thai massage, Tibetan massage, yoga. Mountain bike rental, ski rental.

Activities

Biking, climbing, cross-country skiing, golf, hiking, horseback riding, jogging, mountain biking, Nordic walking, skiing, snowshoeing, space curling, swimming.

Rooms

56 elegant rooms and suites, all furnished with natural materials, various categories: superior room, exclusive room, molignon suite. Each room and suite feature a balcony or terrace.

Located

On the Seiser Alm/Alpe di Siusi, Europe's largest high-altitude plateau.
25 miles (40 kilometers) from Bolzano, 112 miles (180 kilometers) from Verona.

Compatsch, 62/3
39040 Seiser Alm/Alpe di Siusi
Südtirol/South Tyrol – Dolomites – Italy
www.alpinadolomites.it

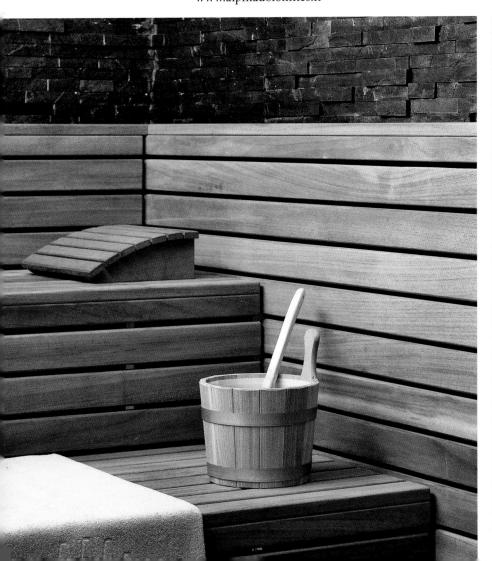

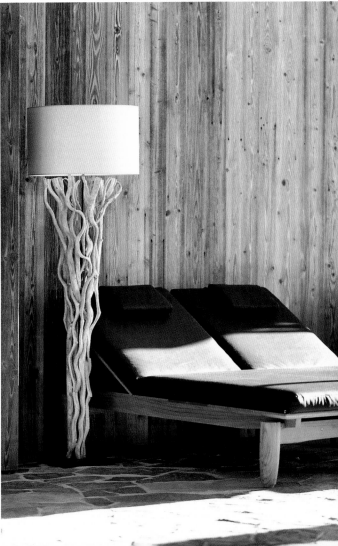

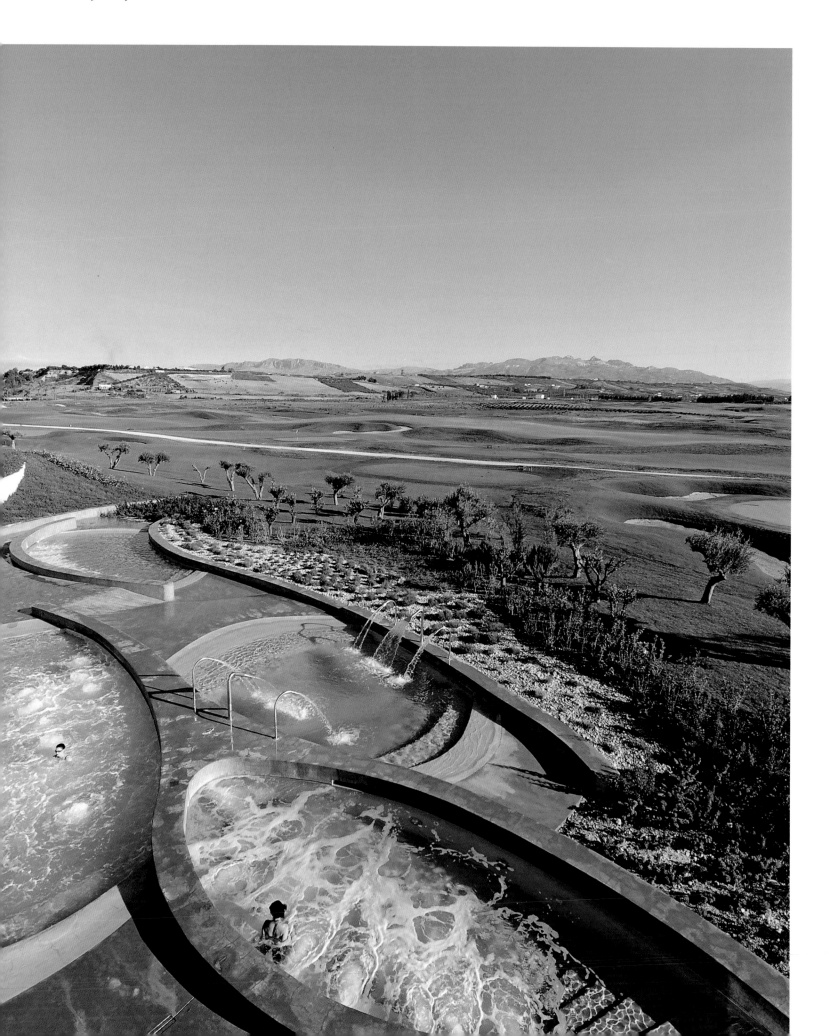

Golfing and Thermal Springs

Golf und Therme

Verdura Golf & Spa Resort

A light breeze carries the scent of olive groves and colorful flowers across green lawns. Time seems to stand still. Now and then, a gentle clicking sound blends with the soft lapping of waves against the shore—it's the sound of a tee shot. Music to any golfer's ears! When Sir Rocco Forte planned the resort, he had two main things in mind that he wanted to bring to his native land: golfing and thermal springs. Situated in one of Italy's prettiest valleys around the Verdura River, the Verdura Golf & Spa Resort stretches along the southern coast of Sicily. The location is a gift from Mother Earth and an ideal place to revitalize body and spirit. With a prominent doctor of integrative medicine and a nutrition expert at the helm, the Vita Health Centre in the Verdura Valley offers programs that focus on detox, weight loss, stress relief, and better aging. While enjoying the spa treatments, you can also experience the effects of cold-pressed vegetable oils and natural plant extracts native to the Mediterranean island. The resort's eight restaurants serve healthy delicacies that are part of traditional Sicilian cuisine. In fact, Germany's national soccer team came here to recuperate in preparation for the 2012 World Cup games—with success, as it turned out. Incidentally, the resort's breathtaking interior design is by Olga Polizzi.

Eine leichte Brise trägt den Duft von Olivenhainen und farbenprächtigen Blumen über grüne Rasenflächen. Die Zeit scheint still zu stehen. Nur ab und zu mischt sich ein leises Klicken in das Rauschen der Meeres- brandung – das Geräusch von Abschlägen. Musik in den Ohren eines jeden Golfers! Als Sir Rocco Forte das Resort plante, waren es vor allem zwei Dinge, die er in seiner Heimat verwirklicht sehen wollte: Golf und Thermalgewässer. In einer der schönsten Talebenen Italiens, um den Fluss Verdura, erstreckt sich das Verdura Golf & Spa Resort entlang der Südküste Siziliens. Die Lage ist ein Geschenk von Mutter Erde und bestens geeignet, Seele und Körper neu zu beleben. Geleitet von einem renommierten Arzt für Integrative Medizin und einer Ernährungsexpertin, bietet das Vita Health Centre im Verdura Programme in den Bereichen Entgiftung, Gewichtsverlust, Anti-Stress und Better Aging. Während der Spa-Anwendungen kann man auch die Wirkung der kaltgepressten Pflanzenöle und natürlichen Pflanzenextrakte der Mittelmeerinsel erfahren. Die acht Restaurants der Anlage bieten gesunde Köstlichkeiten der traditionellen sizilianischen Küche. Vor der Fußball-WM 2012 erholte sich hier die deutsche Nationalmannschaft – mit Erfolg, wie sich zeigte. Das atemberaubende Design der Innenräume stammt übrigens von Olga Polizzi.

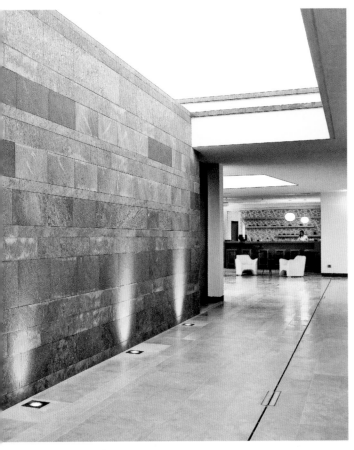

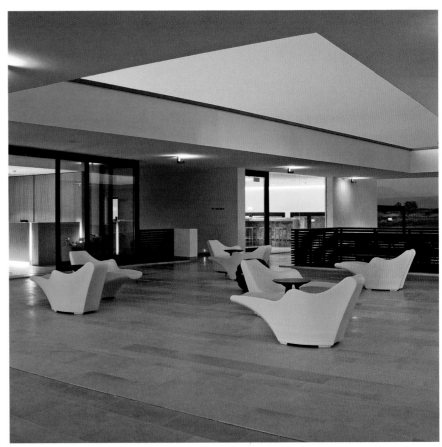

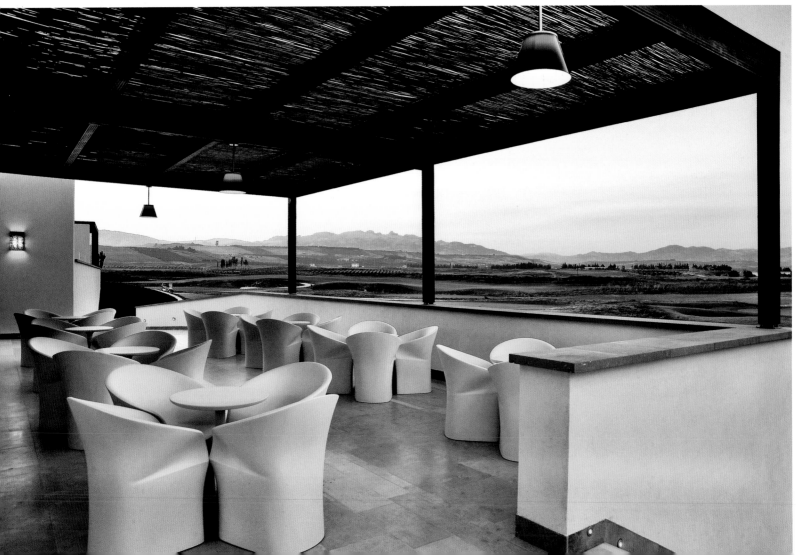

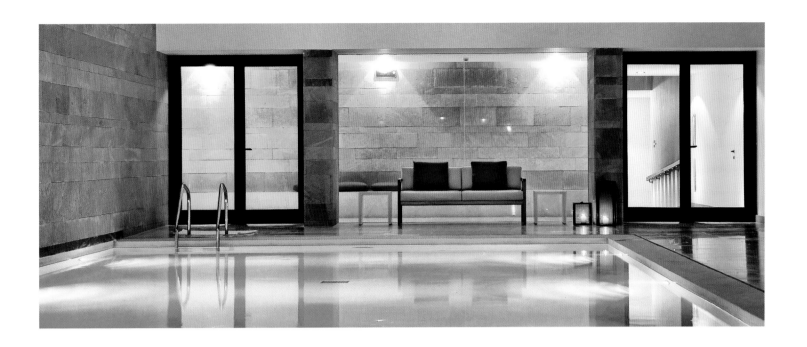

Spa, Health & Other Facilities
43,000 square feet (4,000 square meters) spa comprising 11 treatment rooms, swimming pools,
4 thalassotherapy pools, whirlpools, relaxation rooms, saunas, yoga room, hammam, gym.
Health bar and restaurant bars, 10 meeting rooms (fully equipped), ballroom, beauty and hair salon,
golf courses, tennis courts. Amphitheater.

Treatments & Services
Better Aging, detoxification, spa treatment menus, stress management, Vita Health program, weight loss, yoga.
24-hour business center, latest audiovisual equipment, secretarial and translation services, video conferencing,
Wi-Fi in meeting rooms, worldwide courier services.

Activities
Excursions to local wineries, golf, jogging, sailing, stand-up paddling, tennis, water sports, windsurfing.

Rooms
156 rooms and 47 suites with view across the Mediterranean Sea from a private terrace.

Located
On the south-west coast of Sicily, 15 minutes from the attractive seaside town of Sciacca.
80 minutes from Palermo Airport, 2.5 hours from Catania Airport.

S.S. 115 Km 131
92019 Sciacca, Sicily, Italy
www.verduraresort.com

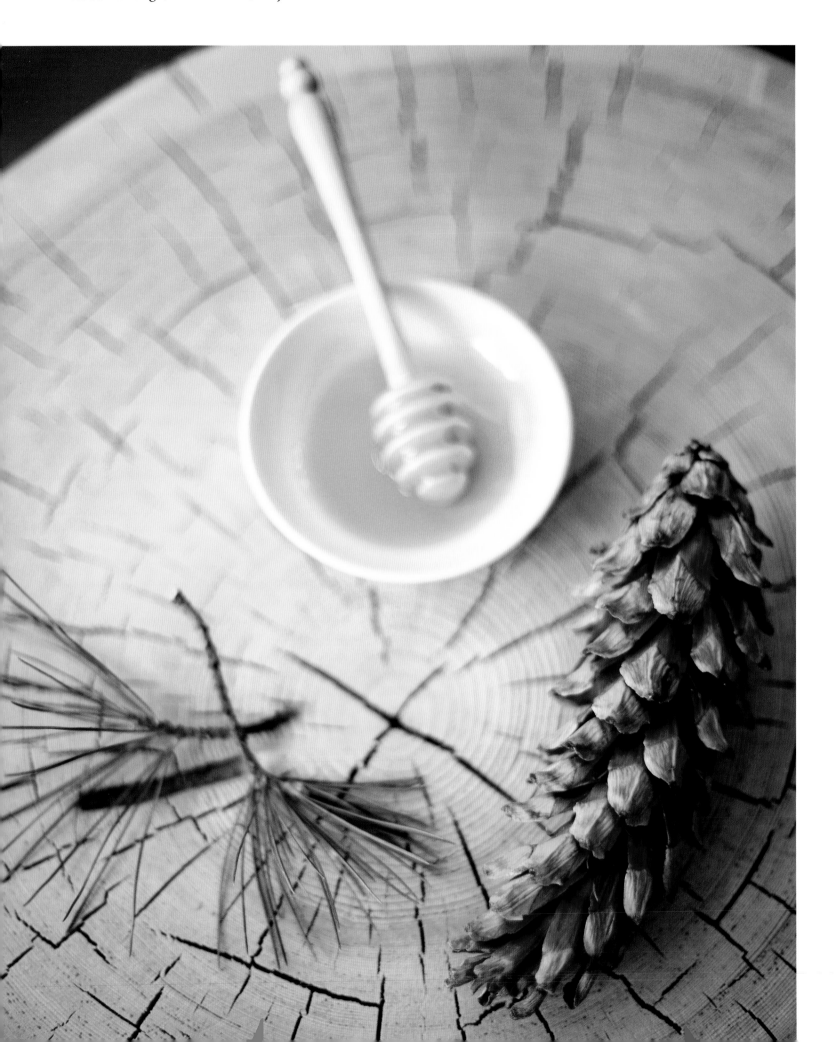

Ancient Healing Methods in Modern Surroundings

Heilen wie in alten Zeiten in moderner Umgebung

AROSEA Life Balance Hotel

Tim, Tom, and Anne—the team at the heart of AROSEA—are joined by an herbalist and a natural health practitioner who doubles as the chef and leads tours through the healing mountain landscape of South Tyrol. Pleasantly comfortable beds, the scent of fresh mountain air and pine, as well as health-promoting sheep's wool—all these things await guests who stay at the AROSEA Life Balance Hotel near Merano. Locally grown organic food is a real treat for the senses, while spa healing takes place on a very deep, natural level. The water in the indoor pool is energized, as is the food. How does that work? Wolfgang, the natural health practitioner, will explain it to you. The hotel with its ultramodern design is equally enticing due to its wonderfully quiet location. Summer or winter, the Val d'Ultimo, with its 8,200-foot mountain range and impressive, ancient larches, invites you to embark on a journey of discovery.

Tim, Tom, Anne – das ist das Team, die Seele von AROSEA. Dazu kommen eine Kräuterhexe und ein Heilpraktiker, der auch kocht und Wanderungen durch die heilende Bergwelt Südtirols leitet. Wohlig-kuschelige Betten, der Duft von frischer Bergluft und Pinienholz, gesundheitsfördernde Schafwolle – all das erwartet die Gäste beim Aufenthalt im AROSEA Life Balance Hotel bei Meran. Das biologische Essen aus der Region ist ein wahrer Sinnesgenuss, das Spa-Healing geschieht auf einer sehr tiefen, natürlichen Ebene. Das Wasser im Indoor-Pool ist energetisiert, ebenso das Essen. Wie das geht? Das erklärt Wolfgang, der Heilpraktiker. Das Hotel im topmodernen Design besticht außerdem durch seine wundervoll ruhige Lage. Im Sommer wie im Winter lädt das Ultental mit seinen 2 500 Meter hohen Bergketten und seinen eindrucksvollen Urlärchen zu Entdeckungsreisen ein.

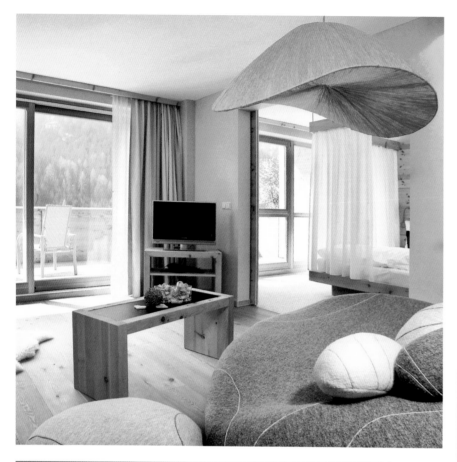

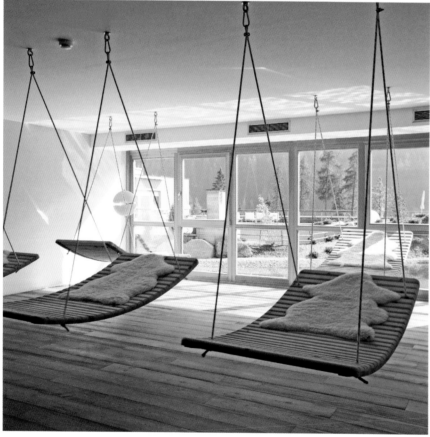

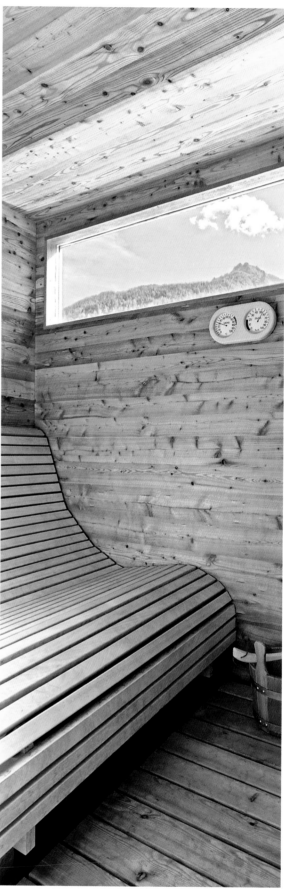

Spa, Health & Other Facilities
Indoor and outdoor pool, 7,500 square feet (700 square meters) biological swimming pond, pine wood
bio sauna, herbs-stone sauna, Finnish panoramic outdoor sauna, steam snail with light therapy, ice trough,
sensory shower experience, sound stumping tunnel, quiet rooms, fitness room, gym.

Treatments & Services
Body treatments, relaxation and wellness treatments, use of exclusive,
natural wellness products by Farfalla. Enriched water, healthy cuisine.

Activities
Biking, climbing, scuba diving, fishing, golf, horseback riding, ice skating,
Nordic walking, paragliding, running, sledging, snowshoe hiking.

Rooms
63 rooms: 51 double rooms, 7 family suites, 4 Life Balance Suites, 1 Deluxe Life Balance Suite.

Located
In the Ultimo Valley, 30 minutes from the spa town of Merano. 1 hour by car to Bozen Airport,
2.5 hours to Verona Airport, and 2 hours to Innsbruck Airport.

Kuppelwies am See 355
39016 St. Walburg/Ultental bei Meran, Italy
www.arosea.it/en

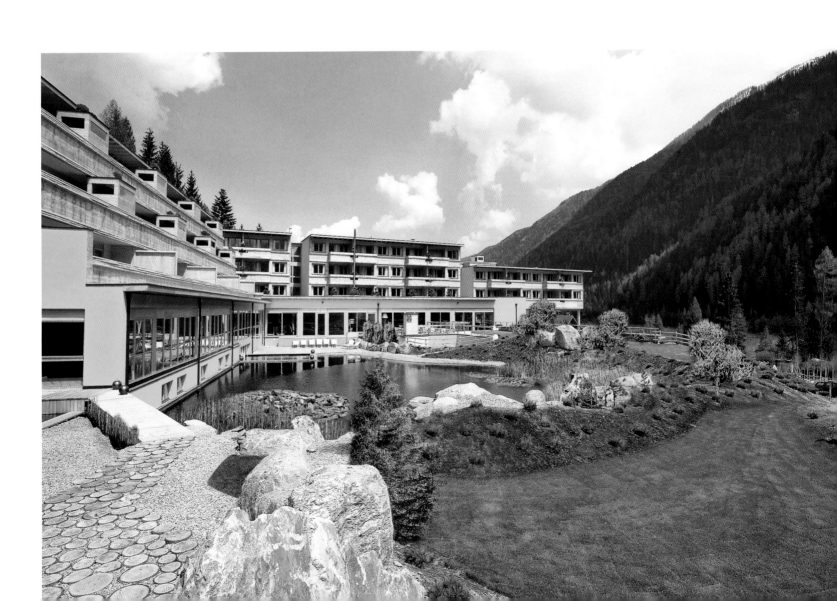

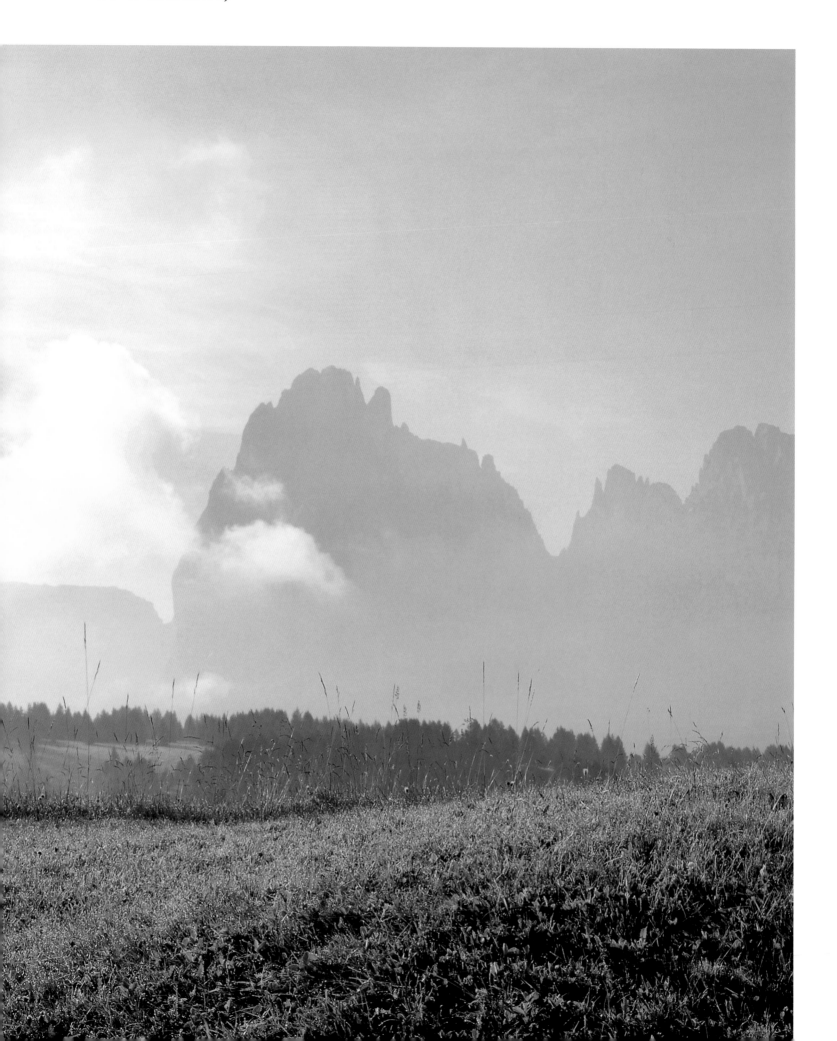

Ortisei, Val Gardena, Italy

Happiness Hormones at Lofty Heights

Glückshormone in luftigen Höhen

Adler Balance

Like an island, the Adler Balance Spa & Health Resort lies right in the middle of the South Tyrolean Dolomites, with a view of Ortisei. To be happy, all you need to do is sit in front of the mountain scenery and take a deep breath. After all, scientists have proven that the body releases endorphins ("happiness hormones") when exposed to alpine air at high elevations. And yet, it is hard to sit still given that each new season offers a different set of opportunities: hiking, biking, tobogganing, skiing—exercise that helps you slow down. At the same time, you can enjoy nearly every conceivable kind of beauty and relaxation treatment. From the sauna and swimming pool, you can experience a special highlight: the breathtaking panoramic views of the massive mountains. Where detox, anti-aging treatments, revitalization, and weight loss are concerned, a team of doctors and experts specializing in traditional medicine and alternative healing methods will design an efficient health program tailored to your specific preferences. When it's time to descend the mountain again, you will feel several years younger.

Wie eine Insel liegt das Adler Balance Spa & Health Resort inmitten der Südtiroler Dolomiten mit Blick auf Sankt Ulrich. Um glücklich zu werden, genügt es eigentlich, sich hier vor die Bergkulisse zu setzen und tief einzuatmen. Wissenschaftler haben nämlich nachgewiesen, dass der Körper in alpiner Höhenluft Glückshormone freisetzt. Doch hier ruhig sitzen zu bleiben, fällt schwer. Allein der Wechsel der Jahreszeiten bringt immer wieder neue Möglichkeiten mit sich: Wandern, Biken, Rodeln, Skifahren – Bewegung, die entschleunigt. Daneben kann man nahezu alle denkbaren Anwendungen für Schönheit und Entspannung genießen. Besonderes Highlight beim Saunen und Schwimmen: der überwältigende Blick auf das massive Bergpanorama. In Sachen Detox, Anti-Aging, Revitalisierung und Gewichtsabnahme entwirft ein Ärzte- und Expertenteam mit Spezialisierung auf traditionelle Medizin und alternative Heilverfahren ein individuelles und effizientes Gesundheitsprogramm. Wer von diesem Berg wieder heruntersteigt, fühlt sich um mehrere Jahre verjüngt.

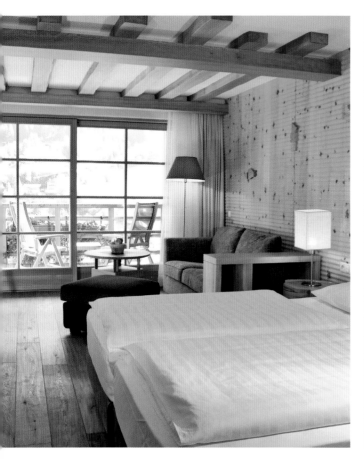
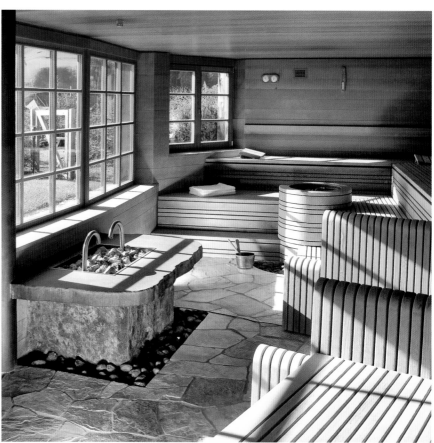
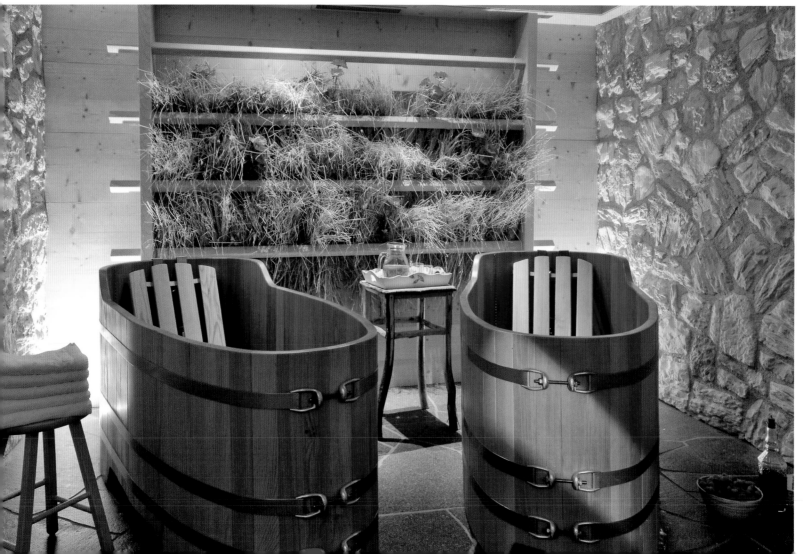

Spa, Health & Other Facilities

Spa and water world, indoor swimming with crystal pool, open-air pool, open-air brine pool, panorama brine pool, hot whirlpool, Finnish panorama sauna, organic hay sauna, blossom steam bath, lady's sauna with rose bath, mountain lake with whirlpool features, rhassoul bath (extra charge), subterranean salt lake and rock salt grotto, panorama relaxation areas with water beds, salt grottos (extra charge). 96,900 square feet (9,000 square meters) park, health center, Balance Restaurant offering healthy nutrition, elevator.

Treatments & Services

Aesthetic medicine, Ayurveda and oriental applications, baths, beauty services, body styling, facial treatments, hair spa, man spa, medical checkups, medical diagnostics, medical treatments and therapies, packs, personal coaching, skin care rituals, special items for mums with babies, spiritual treatments, thalasso, therapeutic treatments, treatments for twosomes. Classes of aquagym, body tonic, breathing & relaxing, Dyna-Band gym, leg-abdominals-hips, Pilates, Staby-Bar gym, Thera-Ball gym, yoga, Zen stretching.

Activities

Climbing, golf, hiking, horseback riding, jogging, mountain biking,
Nordic walking, paragliding, skiing, snowshoeing, swimming.

Rooms

29 junior suites.

Located

25 miles (40 kilometers) from Bolzano, 75 miles (120 kilometers) from Innsbruck,
115 miles (185 kilometers) from Verona.

39046 Ortisei – Val Gardena/Gröden – Italy
www.adler-balance.com

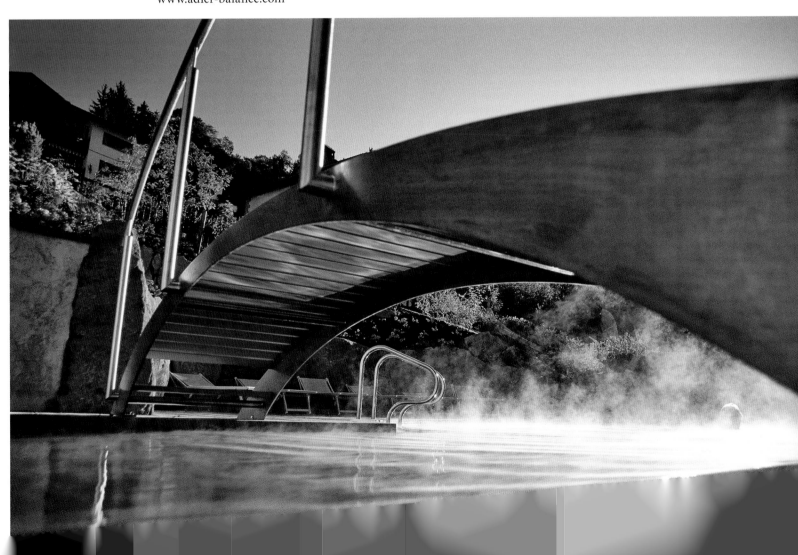

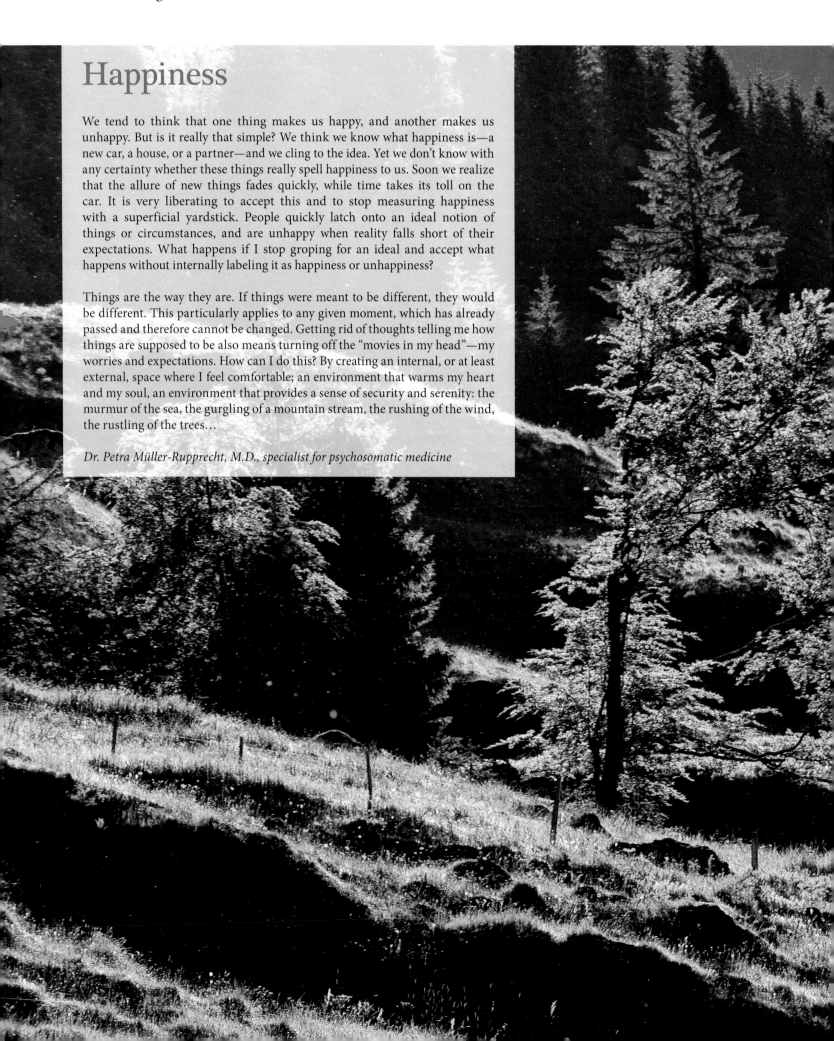

Happiness

We tend to think that one thing makes us happy, and another makes us unhappy. But is it really that simple? We think we know what happiness is—a new car, a house, or a partner—and we cling to the idea. Yet we don't know with any certainty whether these things really spell happiness to us. Soon we realize that the allure of new things fades quickly, while time takes its toll on the car. It is very liberating to accept this and to stop measuring happiness with a superficial yardstick. People quickly latch onto an ideal notion of things or circumstances, and are unhappy when reality falls short of their expectations. What happens if I stop groping for an ideal and accept what happens without internally labeling it as happiness or unhappiness?

Things are the way they are. If things were meant to be different, they would be different. This particularly applies to any given moment, which has already passed and therefore cannot be changed. Getting rid of thoughts telling me how things are supposed to be also means turning off the "movies in my head"—my worries and expectations. How can I do this? By creating an internal, or at least external, space where I feel comfortable; an environment that warms my heart and my soul, an environment that provides a sense of security and serenity: the murmur of the sea, the gurgling of a mountain stream, the rushing of the wind, the rustling of the trees…

Dr. Petra Müller-Rupprecht, M.D., specialist for psychosomatic medicine

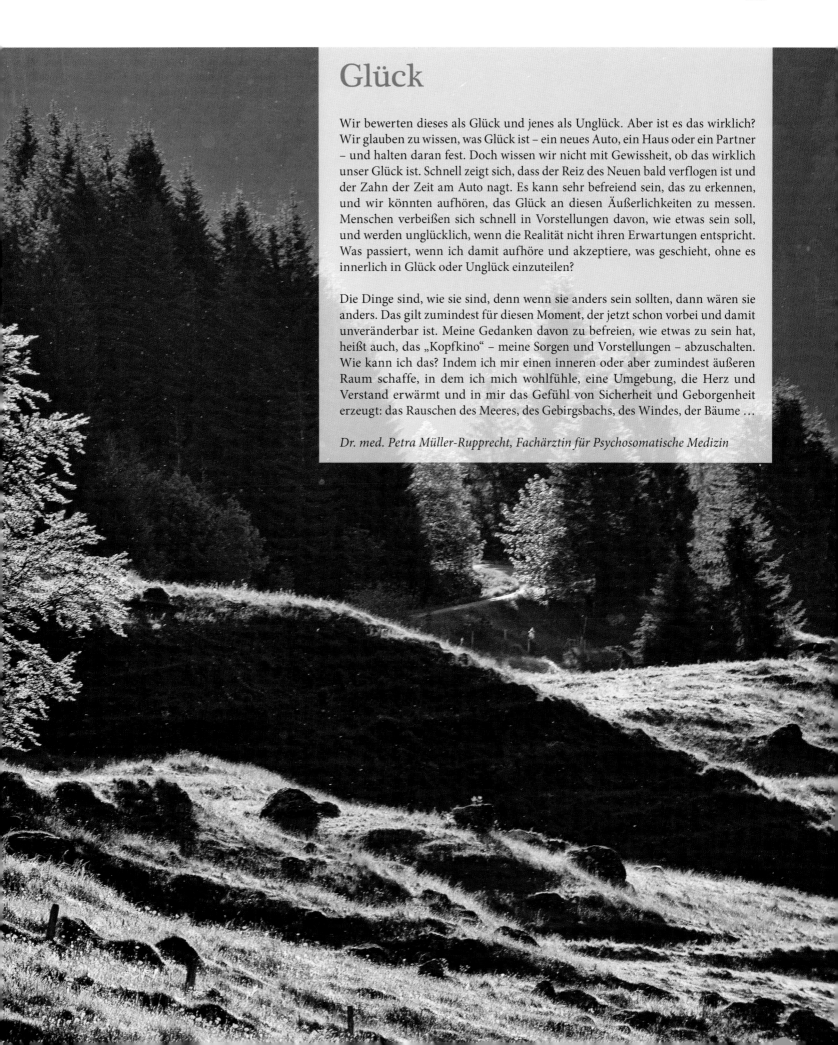

Glück

Wir bewerten dieses als Glück und jenes als Unglück. Aber ist es das wirklich? Wir glauben zu wissen, was Glück ist – ein neues Auto, ein Haus oder ein Partner – und halten daran fest. Doch wissen wir nicht mit Gewissheit, ob das wirklich unser Glück ist. Schnell zeigt sich, dass der Reiz des Neuen bald verflogen ist und der Zahn der Zeit am Auto nagt. Es kann sehr befreiend sein, das zu erkennen, und wir könnten aufhören, das Glück an diesen Äußerlichkeiten zu messen. Menschen verbeißen sich schnell in Vorstellungen davon, wie etwas sein soll, und werden unglücklich, wenn die Realität nicht ihren Erwartungen entspricht. Was passiert, wenn ich damit aufhöre und akzeptiere, was geschieht, ohne es innerlich in Glück oder Unglück einzuteilen?

Die Dinge sind, wie sie sind, denn wenn sie anders sein sollten, dann wären sie anders. Das gilt zumindest für diesen Moment, der jetzt schon vorbei und damit unveränderbar ist. Meine Gedanken davon zu befreien, wie etwas zu sein hat, heißt auch, das „Kopfkino" – meine Sorgen und Vorstellungen – abzuschalten. Wie kann ich das? Indem ich mir einen inneren oder aber zumindest äußeren Raum schaffe, in dem ich mich wohlfühle, eine Umgebung, die Herz und Verstand erwärmt und in mir das Gefühl von Sicherheit und Geborgenheit erzeugt: das Rauschen des Meeres, des Gebirgsbachs, des Windes, der Bäume …

Dr. med. Petra Müller-Rupprecht, Fachärztin für Psychosomatische Medizin

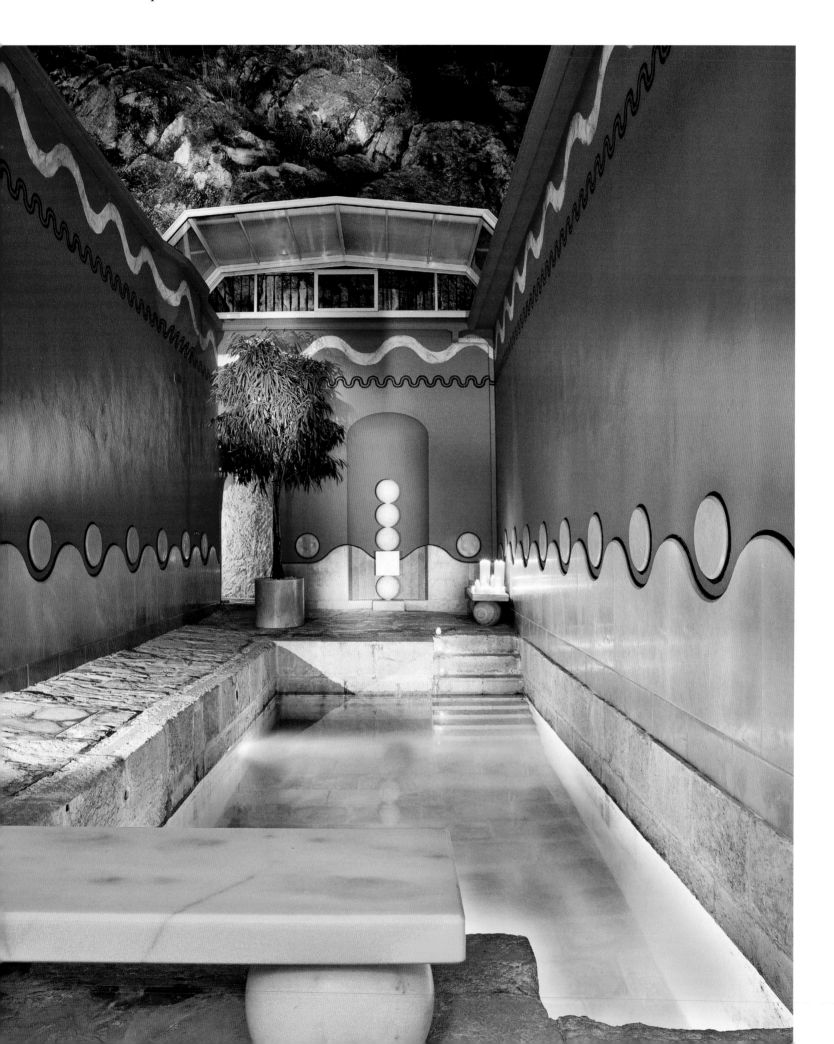

Spanish Dreams and Fountains of Health

Spanische Träume und Gesundbrunnen

Villa Padierna Thermas de Carratraca

At the Villa Padierna Thermas Hotel, you immerse yourself in the world of a traditional Spanish village. High up in the idyllic village of Carratraca, you will find a mineral spring that was once sought out by such historic luminaries as the wife of Napoleon III and Lord Byron. All of the hotel's programs are based on the healing effects of this spring, whose water contains a unique combination of sulfates, calcium, and magnesium and has antioxidant properties—ideal for facial, body, and beauty treatments that are combined in order to provide a real rejuvenation cure. The resort's overall concept is a blend of relaxation, balance, and detoxification. In the serene mountain atmosphere of Andalusia's Serranía de Ronda, with the scent of lemon and orange trees filling your senses, it is not difficult to leave all your cares behind.

Im Villa Padierna Thermas Hotel taucht man in die traditionelle dörfliche Welt Spaniens ein. Hoch oben im idyllisch gelegenen Dörfchen Carratraca befindet sich eine Heilquelle, in der bereits historische Größen wie die Gattin von Napoleon III. und Lord Byron badeten. Alle vom Hotel angebotenen Programme basieren auf der heilenden Wirkung dieses Wassers, das aus einer einzigartigen Kombination aus Sulfaten, Kalzium und Magnesium besteht und antioxidante Eigenschaften hat – ideal für Gesichts-, Körper- und Schönheitsbehandlungen, die zu wahren Verjüngungskuren zusammengeführt werden. Entspannung, Balance und Entgiftung bilden das Gesamtkonzept des Resorts. In der friedlichen Atmosphäre der Berge der andalusischen Serranía de Ronda, mit dem Duft von Zitronen- und Orangenbäumen in der Nase, fällt es nicht schwer, sich völlig fallen zu lassen.

Spa, Health & Other Facilities
21 treatment rooms, 5 Roman thermal pools, outdoor swimming pool, sauna, steam room, hammam, gymnasium. Restaurant, rooftop terrace, library, elevator.

Treatments & Services
Body, facial, and massage treatments, hydrotherapy. 24-hour front desk, airport transfer, healthy gourmet cuisine, luggage storage, unique spring water.

Activities
Canoeing, excursions to Málaga city, golf, horseback riding, rappelling.

Rooms
43 guest rooms and suites – 4 categories: classic, deluxe room, junior suite, suite.

Located
In Valle del Guadalhorce, a typical white village in Andalusia. 28 miles (45 kilometers) from Málaga Airport.

Avenida Antonio Rioboo 11
29551 Carratraca, Spain
www.hotelvillapadierna.com/Blog/de

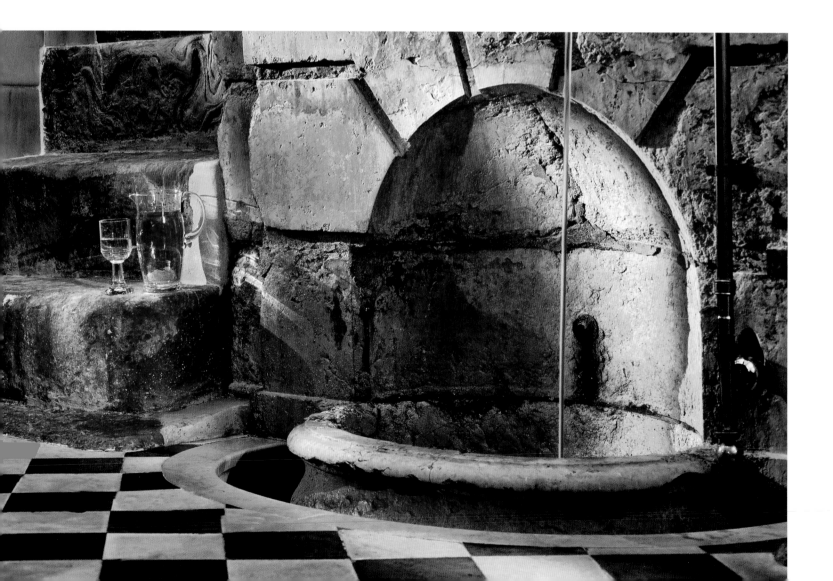

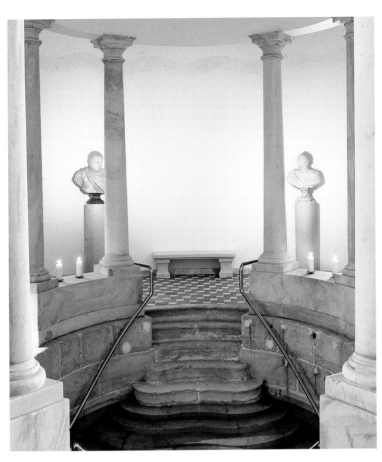

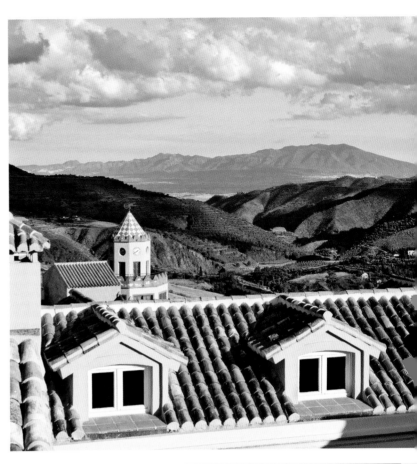

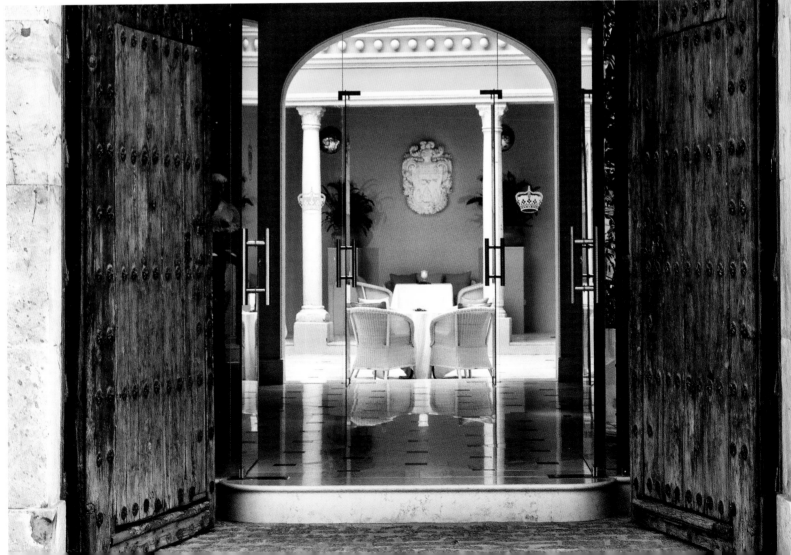

"Long Life" and Japanese Brightness

„Langes Leben" und die japanische Helligkeit

SHA Wellness Clinic

SHA Wellness Clinic came about through a man's personal journey back to health. After an alarming diagnosis and years of unsuccessful treatment, resort founder Alfredo Bataller Parietti recovered completely by changing his diet and undergoing natural therapies. He wanted to share his wealth of knowledge with others—and so he built SHA (Japanese for brightness and radiance). The naturopath who taught Bataller about the special diet known as macrobiotics is now as much a part of the team as are family members. Bataller has a personal connection to SHA's location in the Sierra Helada in an unspoilt coastal area, since his family often spent their vacations here. In building SHA, the owners created an unparalleled, stylish place of rest and recovery. After all, macrobiotics literally means "long life." And that's what SHA is all about: preventing illness and healing disease in a marvelous atmosphere, bringing body, mind, and spirit back into equilibrium.

Grundstein für die SHA Wellness Clinic war die persönliche Erfahrung einer Genesung. Nach einer beängstigenden Diagnose und Jahren erfolgloser Behandlung wurde Alfredo Bataller Parietti, Gründer des Resorts, durch eine Ernährungsumstellung und natürliche Therapien wieder vollständig gesund. Seinen Wissensschatz wollte er mit anderen teilen – so entstand das SHA (japanisch für Helligkeit und Glanz). Der Naturheilkundler, der Bataller seinerzeit in der speziellen Diät der Makrobiotik anwies, gehört heute ebenso zum Team wie Familienangehörige. Auch der Standort des SHA, in der Sierra Helada in einem naturbelassenen Küstengebiet, hat einen persönlichen Bezug, da die Familie Bataller hier oft ihre Ferien verbracht hatte. Mit dem SHA haben die Eigentümer einen stilvollen, unvergleichlichen Ort der Ruhe und Genesung geschaffen. Makrobiotik bedeutet schließlich nichts Geringeres als „langes Leben". Und eben darum geht es im SHA: Krankheiten vorzubeugen und in wundervollem Ambiente zu heilen, sodass Körper, Geist und Seele wieder im Gleichgewicht stehen.

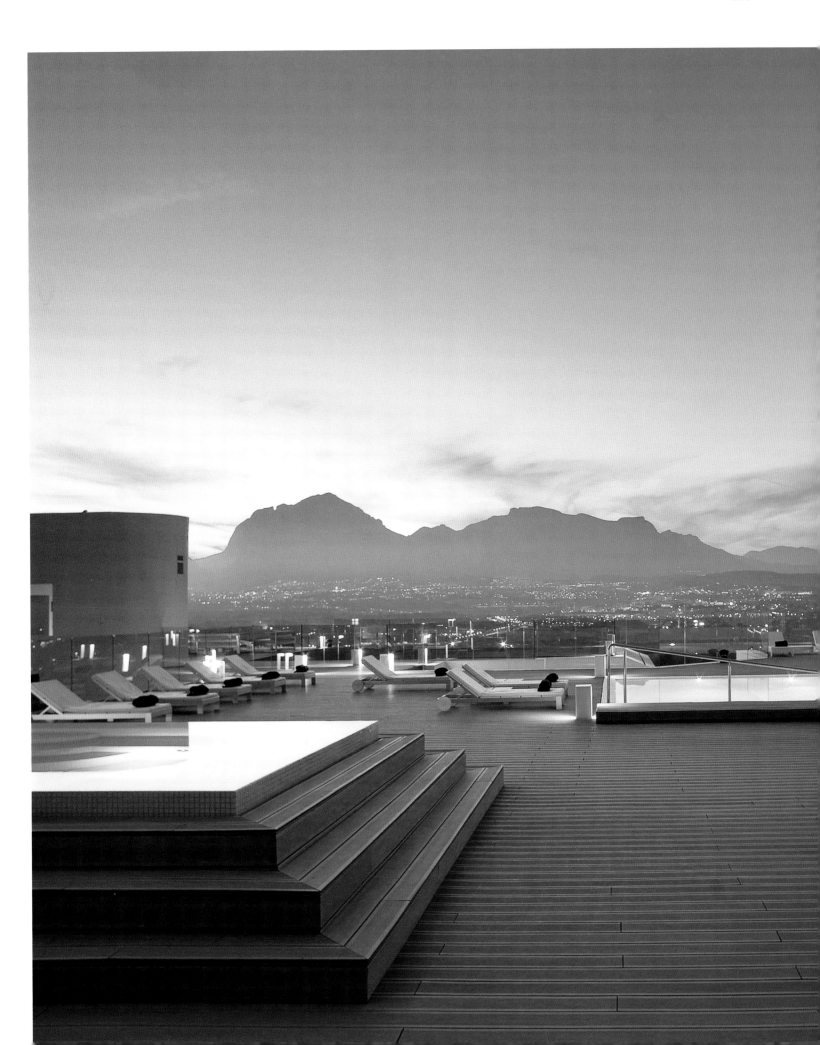

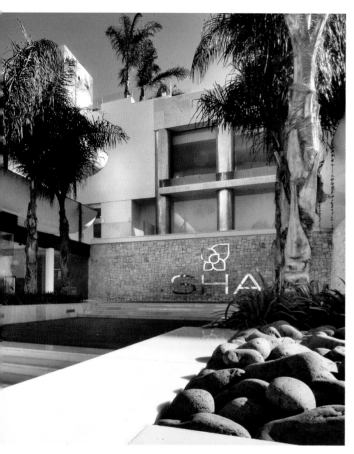
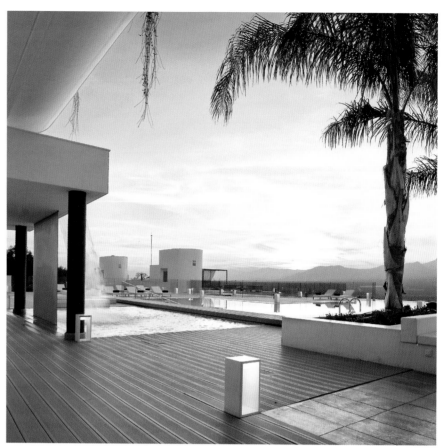
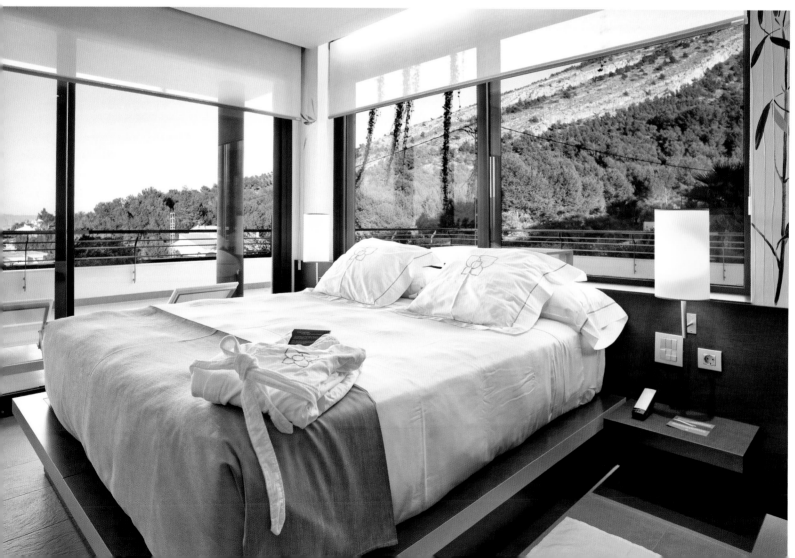

Spa, Health & Other Facilities
22,000 square feet (2,000 square meters) wellness area, hydrotherapy area with therapeutic pools, physiotherapy and hydro-massage beds, invigorating pool, pebbles path, tepidarium, sauna, caldarium, feelings shower and several areas of relax, Zen garden.

Treatments & Services
Aesthetic medicine, anti-smoking unit, anti-stress, aromatherapy, Ayurveda, beauty treatments, bioenergy test, burn out, chromotherapy, craniosacral, crystal massage, dermatology, detox, detox massage, diabetes, emotional balance, energy therapy, genetics, health consultancy, healthy aging medicine, holistic lifestyle coaching, hot stone massage, hydrotherapy, laboratory tests, lymphatic drainage, meditation, music therapy, naturopathy, nutritional consultancy, osteopathy, personal coaching, physiotherapy, Pilates, reflexology, Reiki, shiatsu, sleeping orders unit, spiritual lectures, therapeutic and relaxing massages, water therapies, yoga.

Activities
Daily SHA Life Learning Program: healthy cooking lessons, Nordic walking, swimming, talks, walks, etc. Other activities: biking, bird-watching, canoeing, climbing, scuba diving, fishing, golf, horseback riding, jogging, kayaking, sailing, snorkeling, tennis, windsurfing.

Rooms
93 spacious suites, all with terraces and nice views to the sea or mountains. Optional Jacuzzi.

Located
2 hours from Valencia and 45 minutes from Alicante International Airport.

Calle de Verderol 5
03581 El Albir, Spain
www.shawellnessclinic.com

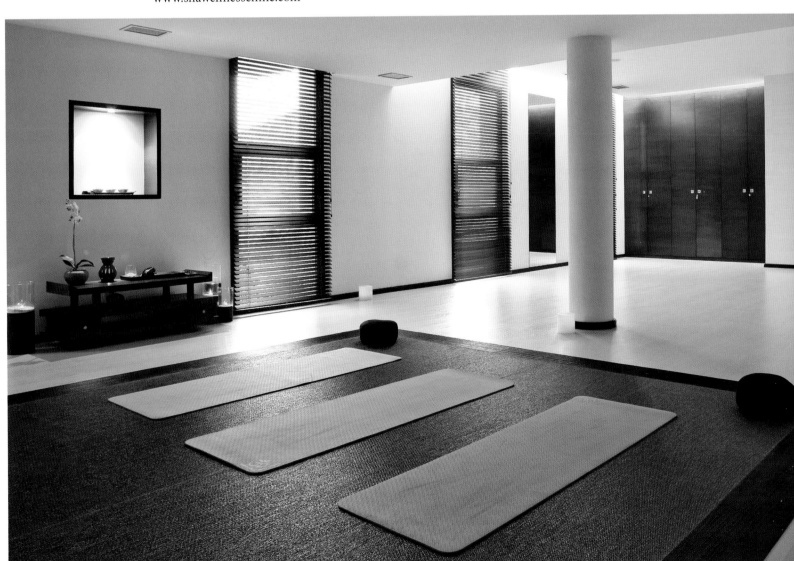

The Power of Food

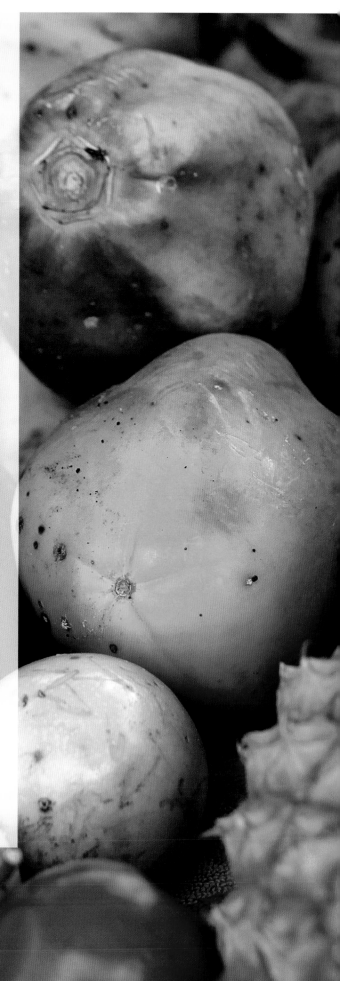

A vital formula for dealing with ill-health and promoting and maintaining wellness is eating an abundance of fresh, organic, whole foods. The fewer preserved, processed, and fragmented foods consumed, the more the body will flourish.

In the Western world, we have become accustomed to consuming preservative-rich produce that we have forgotten the taste of real food. Modern science, fuelled by economic pressure, has made fruit and vegetables available throughout the year. However, nature has intended us to eat seasonally. Combine this with a preference for highly refined carbohydrates, battery hens, and nutritionally unsustainable supermarket convenience foods, and the cause of our poor state of health becomes blatantly obvious.

There is an undoubted link between industrial processing of food and degenerative diseases. In countries where there is less industrialization and the staple diet predominantly consists of mainly whole foods: nuts, seeds, legumes, fresh fruit, and vegetables, research indicates that there is a lower risk of refined diet-related illnesses, which include Diabetes mellitus II and cancer. The cancer-preventative-and-ameliorating role of vegetables has proven consistent, especially one rich in dark green leafy and cruciferous vegetables.

All structures of the body—organs, glands, bones, circulatory system, etc., although specialized in function, are designed to work in concert. When one begins to deteriorate a note of disharmony is sounded, not only to the brain, but also to all other parts of the body via changes in the blood, alterations in glandular secretions, and nerve conduction. As the metabolism shifts in response to an organ malfunction, every cell in the body is alerted to this.

Maintaining homeostasis, or balance, underlies the principle objectives of many ancient and traditional cultures. The foundations of the Chinese principles of Yin and Yang, and the Ayurvedic practices of the Indian subcontinent, rest in the solid wisdom of the power of food as a healing, nurturing, and life-enhancing medicine. They believe that without this balance, the vital force known by the Chinese as "qi" (pronounced "chi") or "prana" (the Sanskrit word) will be blocked, thus causing imbalance within the body.

The Western world has been slow in embracing the fact that such a vital energy force does exist in the human body and in the foods it needs to live healthily, but, as we become more interconnected globally, the wisdom of the East may marry that of the West. Our conventional medical equivalent is homeostasis—a state when the body exists in an ideal chemical balance.

No longer can the individual afford to be ignorant about, or ignore, the harmful effects of processed, preserved foodstuffs and unhealthy cooking techniques—let alone the myriad of other food facts which need to be understood if people are to prevent unnecessary illness and live healthy, happy, fulfilling lives.

Samantha Gowing, award-winning clinical nutritionist,
founder of the global wellness company Gowings Food Health Wealth

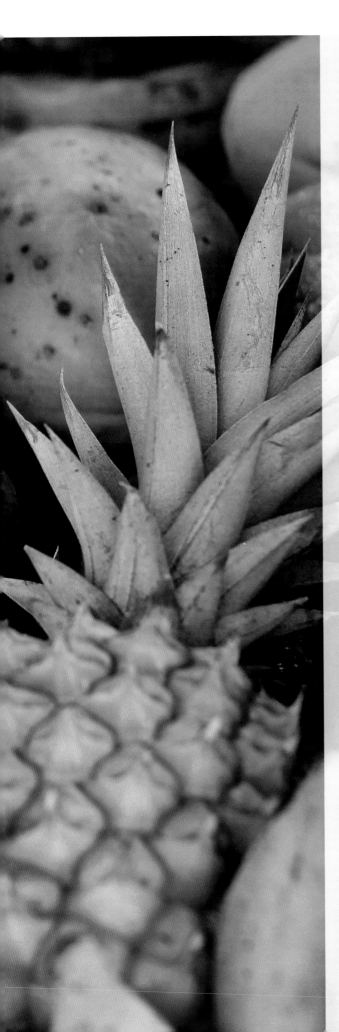

Die Kraft der Nahrungsmittel

Ein grundlegendes Rezept zur Heilung von Krankheiten und für dauerhaftes Wohlbefinden ist der Verzehr einer Vielfalt frischer, organischer und unverarbeiteter Lebensmittel. Je weniger konservierte, verarbeitete und raffinierte Nahrung wir zu uns nehmen, desto gesünder entwickelt sich der Körper.

In der westlichen Welt haben wir uns daran gewöhnt, Erzeugnisse mit einem großen Anteil von Konservierungsmitteln zu uns zu nehmen, sodass wir den Geschmack echter Nahrungsmittel vergessen haben. Angetrieben von wirtschaftlichem Druck hat die moderne Wissenschaft dafür gesorgt, dass Obst und Gemüse nahezu überall ganzjährig erhältlich sind. Die Natur sieht jedoch für den Menschen vor, sich den Jahreszeiten entsprechend zu ernähren. Nimmt man noch unsere Vorliebe für hoch raffinierte Kohlenhydrate hinzu, für Legebatteriehaltung und Fertiggerichte aus dem Supermarkt, die Ernährungsmängel verursachen, ist die Ursache für unseren schlechten Gesundheitszustand ganz offensichtlich.

Zweifellos besteht ein Zusammenhang zwischen industriell verarbeiteten Nahrungsmitteln und degenerativen Krankheiten. Untersuchungen deuten darauf hin, dass in weniger industrialisierten Ländern, wo hauptsächlich unverarbeitete Lebensmittel verzehrt werden (Nüsse, Samen, Hülsenfrüchte, frisches Obst und Gemüse), ein geringeres Risiko für Krankheiten wie etwa Diabetes mellitus II und Krebs besteht. Diese entstehen durch die Ernährung mit raffinierten Lebensmitteln. Die krebsvorbeugende und -heilende Rolle von Gemüsesorten, insbesondere von dunkelgrünem Blatt- und Kreuzblütlergemüse, hat sich ja bereits bewährt.

Alle Körperstrukturen – Organe, Drüsen, Knochen, Kreislaufsystem etc. – erfüllen zwar jeweils eine ganz eigene Aufgabe, sind jedoch zum Zusammenspiel vorgesehen. Wenn eine dieser Funktionen sich verschlechtert, werden nicht nur dem Gehirn, sondern auch allen anderen Körperteilen über Veränderungen des Bluts, der Drüsensekrete und Nervenleitungen Warnsignale gemeldet. Während sich der Stoffwechsel als Reaktion auf eine Organfehlfunktion verändert, ist jede einzelne Körperzelle darüber informiert.

Die Aufrechterhaltung der Homöostase (Gleichgewicht) ist Leitgedanke vieler alter und traditioneller Kulturen. Die Fundamente der chinesischen Prinzipien von Yin und Yang und die ayurvedischen Methoden des indischen Subkontinents beruhen auf der unumstößlichen Weisheit über die Kraft der Nahrungsmittel als heilende, nährende und lebensverbessernde Medizin. Beide Philosophien sind überzeugt, dass die lebenswichtige Kraft, die die Chinesen als „Qi" (gesprochen: „Chi") oder „Prana" (Wort aus dem Sanskrit) bezeichnen, ohne dieses Gleichgewicht blockiert wird und folglich im Körper ein Ungleichgewicht ensteht.

Die westliche Welt hat lange gebraucht, um die Tatsache zu akzeptieren, dass solch lebenswichtige Energie im menschlichen Körper existiert und in den Nahrungsmitteln für ein gesundes Leben vorhanden ist. Doch mit wachsender globaler Vernetzung werden die Weisheit des Ostens und die des Westens einander näher kommen. Das Äquivalent unserer Schulmedizin ist die Homöostase – ein Zustand, in dem sich der Körper in idealem chemischen Gleichgewicht befindet. Der Mensch kann es sich nicht länger erlauben, den schädlichen Auswirkungen verarbeiteter, konservierter Nahrungsmittel und ungesunder Zubereitungsformen mit Unwissenheit oder Ignoranz zu begegnen – ganz zu schweigen von den unzähligen anderen Fakten über Lebensmittel, die der Mensch begreifen muss, um unnötigen Krankheiten vorzubeugen und ein gesundes, glückliches und erfülltes Leben zu führen.

Samantha Gowing, preisgekrönte Ernährungswissenschaftlerin, Gründerin des globalen Wellness-Unternehmens Gowings Food Health Wealth

Golfing, the Ocean, and a Roman Bath in the Spanish Sun

Golf, Meer und ein römisches Bad unter spanischer Sonne

Villa Padierna Palace

Anyone who has undergone the treatments in this enchanting spa has emerged feeling like a new person. The backdrop to this relaxing stay is an elegant former manor house with a panoramic view of the mountains in the countryside near Marbella, Spain. From here, your gaze wanders across the vast expanse of the surrounding golf course to the nearby ocean. Feeling balanced by this vastness, you enter the peace and quiet of the spa. Built in the style of a Roman bath, the spa features eight different saunas and steam baths as well as a fitness center and an ice grotto. Here, a caldarium and massage therapies replace stress and daily routines. If you want your vacation to include more than just relaxation, a professional team of doctors in the Medical Wellness Institute will assist you with your goals—from healthy weight loss to thoroughly recharging your batteries.

Wer die Behandlungen in dem traumhaften Spa durchlaufen hat, fühlt sich wie neu geboren. Die Kulisse für diesen erholsamen Aufenthalt bildet ein elegantes ehemaliges Herrenhaus mit Panorama auf die Bergketten im Hinterland von Marbella. Von hier wandert der Blick über die Weite des umgebenden Golfplatzes auf das nahe gelegene Meer. Ausgeglichen von dieser Weite taucht man in die Ruhe und den Frieden des Spa-Bereichs ein. Er ist im Stil römischer Bäder gestaltet und bietet acht unterschiedliche Saunen und Dampfbäder sowie Fitnesscenter und eine Eisgrotte. Hier heißt es: Caldarium und Massagen statt Stress und Routine. Wer sich neben der Entspannung noch weitere Ziele für den Urlaub setzt, findet im Medical Wellness Institute passende Unterstützung durch ein professionelles Ärzteteam, zum Beispiel beim gesunden Abnehmen oder gründlichen Regenerieren.

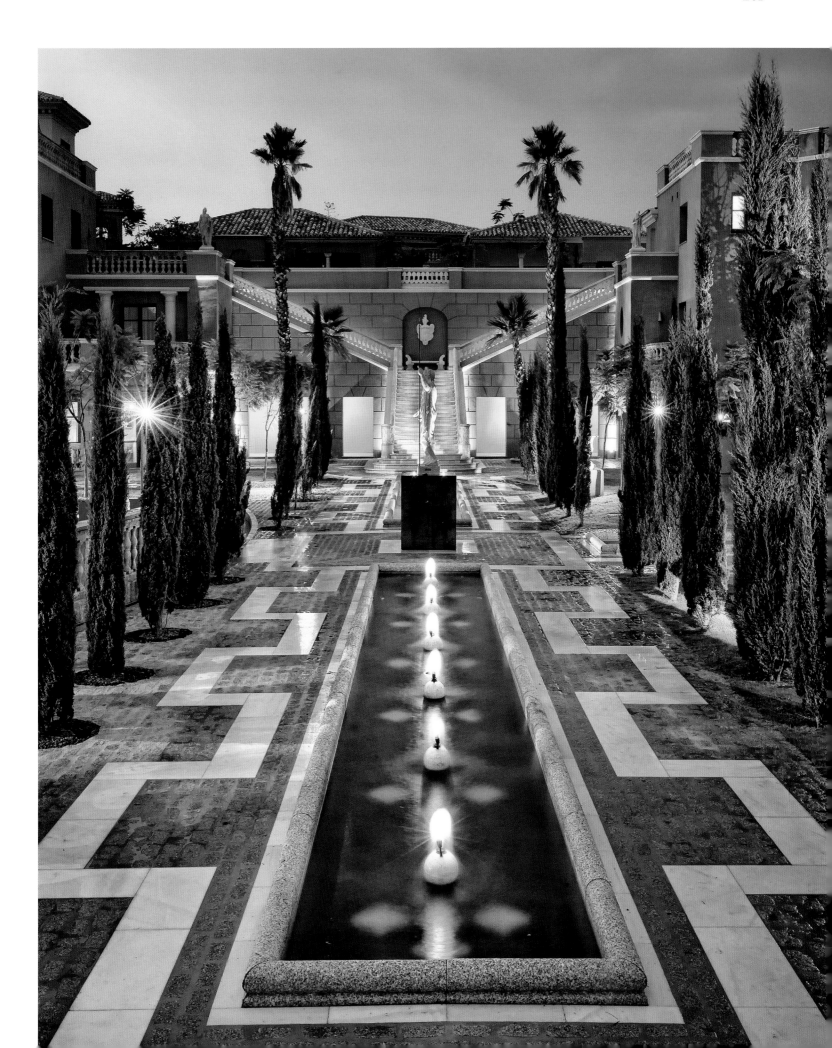

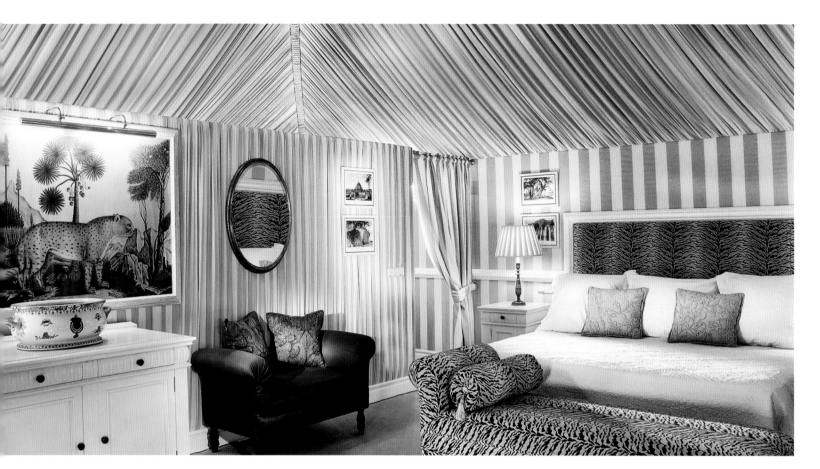

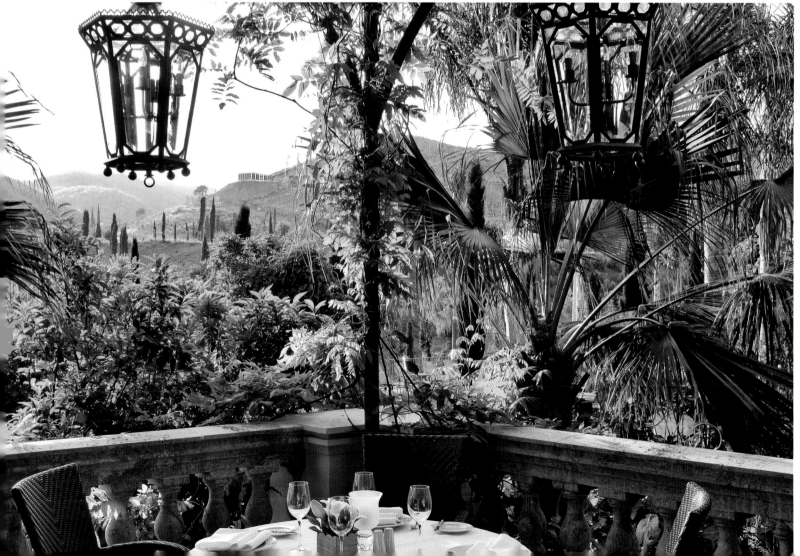

Spa, Health & Other Facilities
21,500 square feet (2,000 square meters) Thermae Spa comprising 12 treatment rooms for specialized treatments, dynamic indoor swimming pool with massage jets, plunge pool, showers with orange and lemon essences, ice fountain, aromatherapy steam rooms, Bali Steam, Indian Steam, Finnish sauna, hammam, laconium, relaxation room. Space for meetings, conferences, celebrations, or product launches, with 8 meeting rooms and 5 terraces, children's club, health club, Roman amphitheater for up to 400 people.

Treatments & Services
Medical, wellness, and beauty treatments. Make-up service, babysitting/childcare, turndown service.

Activities
Aerobics, basketball, bicycling, fishing, golf, horseback riding, hunting, mountain biking, racquetball, sailing, scooter/moped, surfing.

Rooms
132 rooms and suites.

Located
Located in Marbella at the Costa del Sol. 31 miles (50 kilometers) to Málaga Airport, 1 mile (2 kilometers) to the beach.

Ctra. de Cádiz Km 166
29679 Marbella, Spain
www.hotelvillapadierna.com

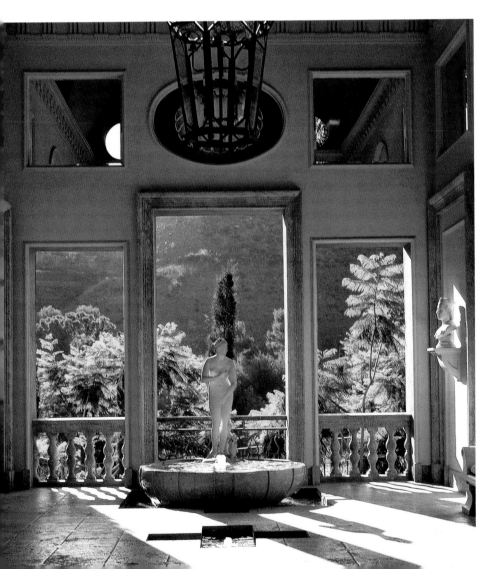

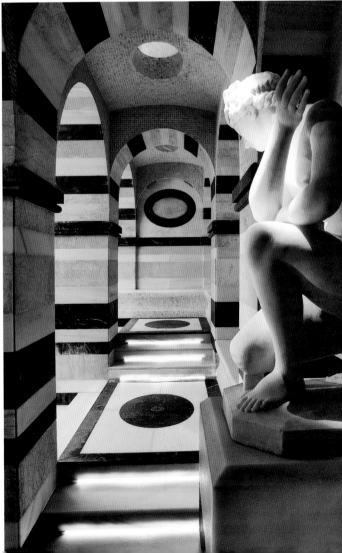

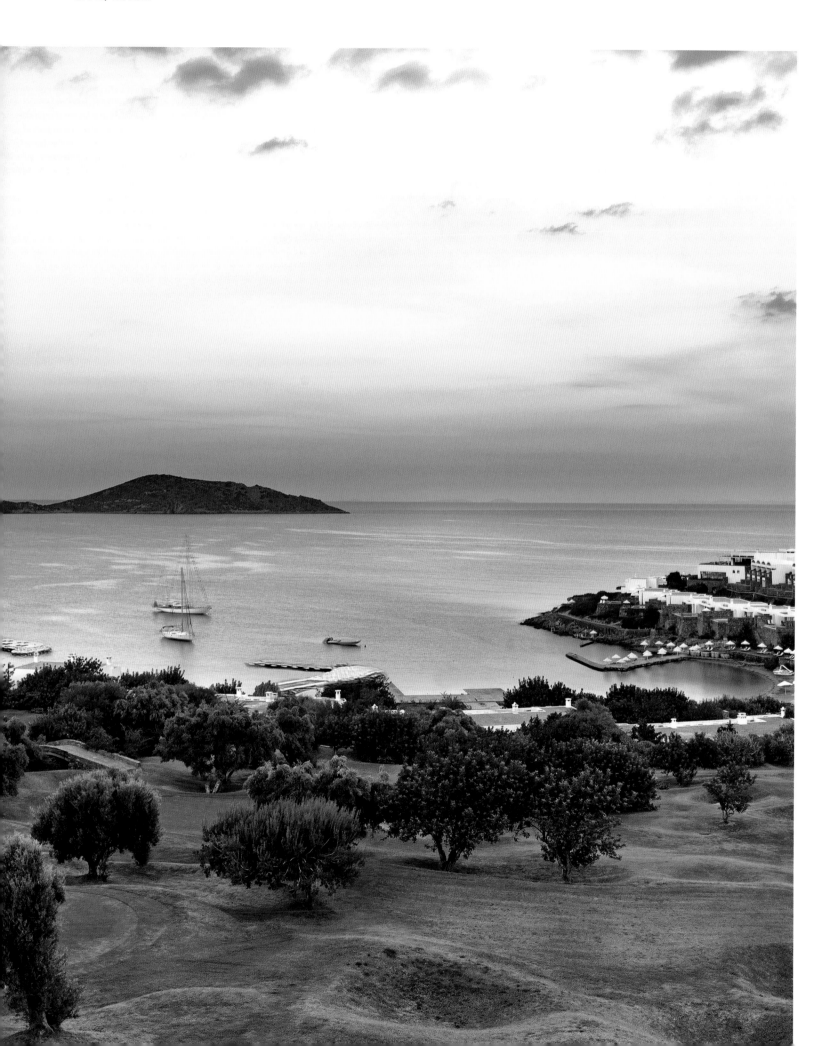

Crete, Greece

Crete's Endless Blue

Kretas wunderbares Blau

Porto Elounda Golf & Spa Resort

Green hills with golf courses surrounded by pleasant stillness. It is the perfect place to play a quiet round of golf and experience new heights of well-being with the help of holistic medical experts. The Six Senses Spa, which has won multiple awards, offers bathing rituals and effective body and energy work that ranges from Thai massage to Reiki, SLOW LIFE programs, Asian therapies, and an organic tomato-olive facial mask— the selection is enormous. And what's the best part? Whether enjoying a relaxing massage, leaning back in the tepidarium, or swimming laps in the infinity pool, guests can always enjoy views of the enchanting Gulf of Mirabello and Crete's azure coast. Anyone who comes here should make the sea a permanent part of the recuperation plan and dive into Greece's endless blue waters.

Grüne Hügel mit Golfplatz in angenehmer Stille. Der perfekte Ort, um eine ruhige Kugel zu schieben und mithilfe von Experten der ganzheitlichen Medizin neue Höhen des Wohlbefindens zu erfahren. Das mehrfach ausgezeichnete Six Senses Spa bietet Baderituale, effektive Körper- und Energiearbeit von Thai-Massage bis Reiki, SLOW-LIFE-Programme, asiatische Therapien oder eine Bio-Tomaten-Oliven-Maske – die Auswahl ist groß. Das Beste daran: Ob bei entspannenden Massagen, zurückgelehnt im Tepidarium oder während man im Infinity-Pool Bahnen zieht, stets schweift der Blick in die Weite über die bezaubernde Bucht von Mirabello und Kretas azurblaue Küste. Wer hierher kommt, sollte auch dem Meer in seinem Erholungsplan einen festen Platz geben: Dort taucht man ab, hinein ins Blau Griechenlands.

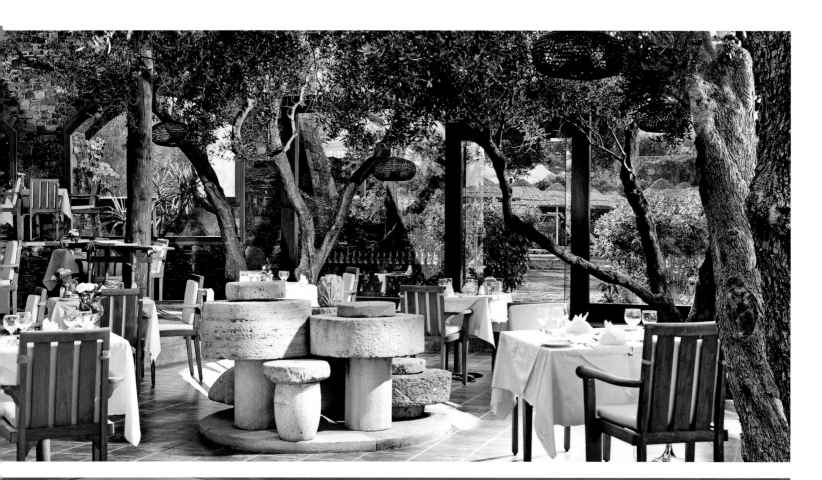

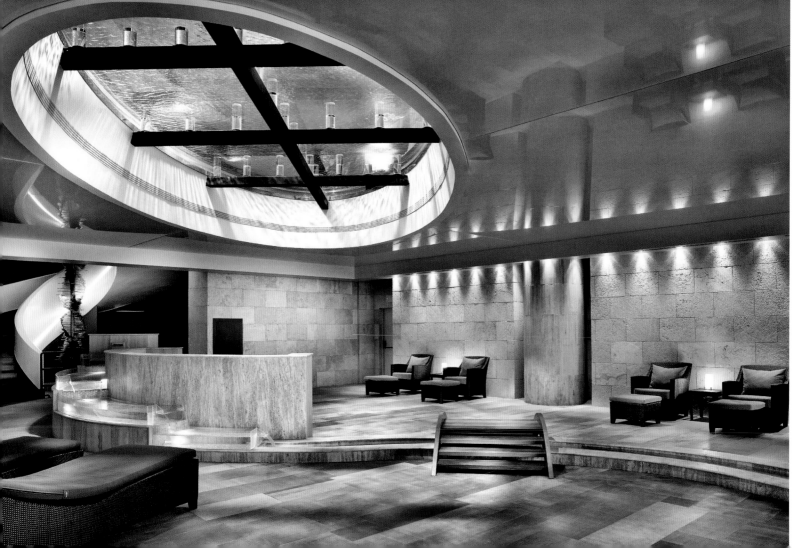

Spa, Health & Other Facilities
21 treatment rooms, rooms for couples, seawater swimming pool, children's paddling pool, sauna, steam bath, gymnasium, outdoor yoga area. Buffet restaurant, business center, conference rooms, roofterrace, sunloungers and sunshades.

Treatments & Services
Acupuncture, anti-stress, aromatherapy, Ayurveda, crystal massage, detox, emotional balance, energy therapy, fitness, graceful aging, Hawaiian massage, holistic health consultancy, hot stone massage, hydrotherapy, indigenous therapies, learning sessions, lifestyle coaching, lymphatic drainage, medical doctor, meditation, physiotherapy, Pilates, Qigong, reflexology, Reiki, shiatsu, spiritual lectures, Swedish massage, Tai Chi, Thai massage, thalassotherapy, Watsu, weight loss, yoga. 24-hour front desk, free parking, free Wi-Fi.

Activities
Biking, canoeing, fishing, golf, scuba diving, shopping, snorkeling, tennis, watersports, yachting.

Rooms
133 rooms and suites.

Located
In the picturesque fishing village Elounda, 43 miles (70 kilometers) from Heraklion International Airport.

72053 Elounda, Greece
www.portoelounda.com

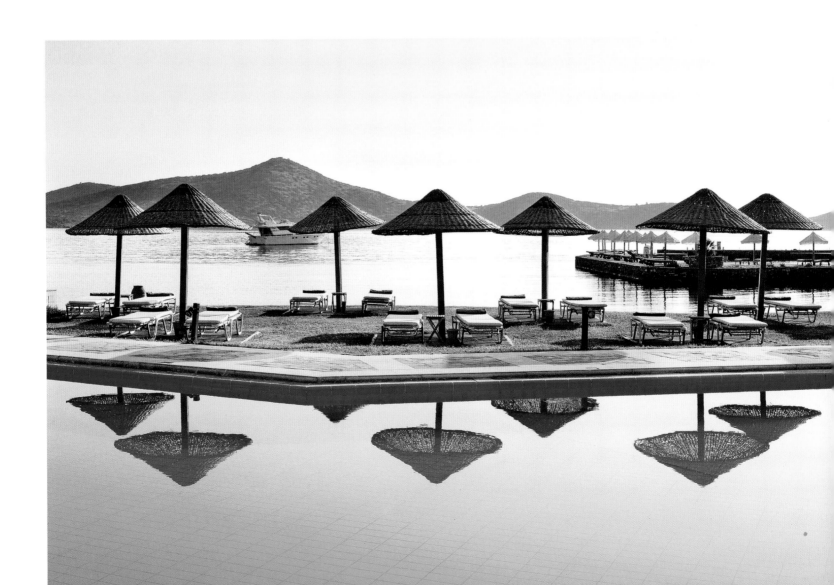

Biographies
Biografien

Dr. Mosaraf Ali (Castel Monastero, p. 224)

Dr. Mosaraf Ali is a pioneer of Integrated Medicine. Having studied medicine and taken courses in acupuncture, homeopathy, hypnosis, iridology, and Ayurveda, he runs the Integrated Medical Centre in London, attended by many high-profile clients such as Richard Branson, Michael Douglas, Claudia Schiffer, and Samuel L. Jackson. He is exclusively collaborating with Castel Monastero, Italy, designing and developing scientifically cutting-edge treatment programs in the field of preventative medicine. (See www.castelmonastero.com for more information.)

Dr. Mosaraf Ali ist ein Vorreiter im Bereich Integrative Medizin. Er studierte Medizin und besuchte verschiedene Kurse in Akupunktur, Homöopathie, Hypnose, Iridologie und Ayurveda. Er ist Leiter des Integrated Medical Centre in London, zu dessen Kunden zahlreiche weltbekannte Personen wie Richard Branson, Michael Douglas, Claudia Schiffer und Samuel L. Jackson gehören. Dr. Mosaraf Ali arbeitet exklusiv mit dem Castel Monastero in Italien zusammen und erarbeitet und entwickelt aus wissenschaftlicher Sicht zukunftsweisende Behandlungsprogramme im Bereich der Präventivmedizin (für nähere Informationen siehe: www.castelmonastero.com).

Dr. med. h. c. Günther W. Amann-Jennson (p. 116)

Dr. Günther W. Amann-Jennson, sleep psychologist, entrepreneur, book author, and director of the Institute for Sleep Research and Bioenergetics in Austria, has been a renowned expert in the field of healthy sleep for over 20 years. The internationally successful SAMINA Bioenergetic Healthy Sleep Concept is based on his many years of experience as a psychologist and psychotherapist.
(See www.samina.com for more information.)

Dr. Günther W. Amann-Jennson, Schlafpsychologe, Unternehmer, Buchautor und Leiter des Instituts für Schlafforschung und Bioenergetik in Österreich, ist seit über 20 Jahren ein angesehener Experte auf dem Gebiet des gesunden Schlafs. Aus seiner langjährigen Tätigkeit als Psychologe- und Psychotherapeut ging das heute international erfolgreiche Bioenergetische Schlaf-Gesund-Konzept SAMINA hervor (für nähere Informationen siehe: www.samina.com).

Sonia Bach (p. 52)

Sonia Bach owns the yogaloft, a yoga studio in Cologne, Germany. She has practiced yoga intensively for the past 14 years, inspired by a number of training courses and yoga workshops with pioneers such as David Swenson, Shiva Rea, Seane Corn, Richard Freeman, and many others. (See www.theyogaloft.de for more information.)

Sonia Bach ist Inhaberin des Yogastudios the yogaloft in Köln. Sie lebt seit 14 Jahren intensiv Yoga und ließ sich von mehreren Lehrertrainings und Yoga-Workshops mit Yogapionieren wie David Swenson, Shiva Rea, Seane Corn, und Richard Freeman und vielen anderen inspirieren (für nähere Informationen siehe: www.theyogaloft.de).

Prof. Dr. med. Dietrich Baumgart (p. 186)

Prof. Dr. Dietrich Baumgart is a cardiologist and internist who specializes in preventive medicine. A senior physician with the West German Heart Center in Essen for many years, he was appointed to the European Society of Cardiology as a member and belongs to the scientific advisory board of the Internationale Gesellschaft für Prävention e.V. (International Society for Preventive Medicine). He is the author of the guide book "Mut zur Gesundheit" (Courage to Be Healthy), published by Fackelträger Verlag.

Prof. Dr. Dietrich Baumgart ist Kardiologe, Internist und Präventivmediziner. Er war jahrelang Oberarzt des Westdeutschen Herzzentrums Essen, wurde als Mitglied der Europäischen Gesellschaft für Kardiologie berufen und ist Teil des wissenschaftlichen Beirats der Internationalen Gesellschaft für Prävention e.V. Er ist Autor des Ratgebers „Mut zur Gesundheit", erschienen im Fackelträger Verlag.

Ewald Eisen (p. 170)

Ewald Eisen was a mechanical engineer, teacher, and financial consultant before founding VitaJuwel in 2007. VitaJuwel produces gemstone vials to improve water quality. Eisen holds several patents in the field of holistic health and has authored several books. (See www.vitajuwel.com for more information.)

Ewald Eisen war Maschinenbauer, Lehrer und Finanzberater, bevor er 2007 das Unternehmen VitaJuwel gründete, das Edelstein-Phiolen zur Verbesserung der Wasserqualität herstellt. Er besitzt mehrere Patente im Bereich ganzheitlicher Gesundheit und ist auch Buchautor (für nähere Informationen siehe: www.vitajuwel.com).

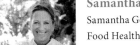

Dr. Francesca Fornasini (Abano Grand Hotel; Grand Hotel Terme Trieste & Victoria, p. 214)

Dr. Francesca Fornasini specializes in hydrology and aesthetic medicine and works as an internist, sports physician, and medical spa director of Levico Terme. Since 2010, she had headed the Anti-Aging Department of the GB Thermæ Hotel Group in Abano, which includes the Abano Grand Hotel and the Grand Hotel Terme Trieste & Victoria.

Dr. Francesca Fornasini ist spezialisiert auf Hydrologie und ästhetische Medizin und arbeitete als Internistin, Sportmedizinerin und leitende Kurärztin in der Levico Terme. Seit 2010 leitet sie den Fachbereich Anti-Aging für die GB Thermæ Hotelgruppe in Abano, zu der das Abano Grand Hotel und das Grand Hotel Terme Trieste & Victoria gehören.

Samantha Gowing (p. 258)

Samantha Gowing is a therapeutic chef, an award-winning clinical nutritionist, and a renowned teacher of Food as Medicine. She founded Gowings Food Health Wealth twelve years ago—a business service that celebrates organic produce and encompasses her teachings, complemented by her previous incarnation as a highly successful restaurateur and hotelier of the historic Grace Darling Hotel in Collingwood, Victoria. During this time, she has written extensively about food, fitness, travel, and nutrition.

Samantha Gowing ist therapeutische Köchin, preisgekrönte Ernährungswissenschaftlerin und angesehene Lehrerin im Bereich Nahrungsmittel als Medizin. Vor zwölf Jahren gründete sie Gowings Food Health Wealth, eine unternehmerische Dienstleistung, die Bioprodukte fördert und ihre Lehren umfasst. Sie ergänzt diesen Service durch ihre frühere selbstverwirklichende Tätigkeit als erfolgreiche Gastronomin und Besitzerin des historischen Grace Darling Hotels in Collingwood, Victoria. Während dieser Zeit schrieb sie ausführlich über Nahrungsmittel, Fitness, Reisen und Ernährung.

Dr. med. Roland G. Heber (p. 62)

Dr. Roland G. Heber heads the Indeo Healing and Teaching Institute in Lans, Austria. He holds a doctoral degree in Western medicine, and is a Master of Chinese Medicine. Collaborating with RMIT University in Melbourne in 2004, he developed and implemented a teaching program for energy medicine. At the Indeo Institute, Dr. Roland G. Heber teaches his approach to therapy and healing as well as related healing modalities and techniques for physicians, alternative medical specialists, and therapists. (See www.indeoinstitute.com for more information.)

Dr. Roland G. Heber leitet das Indeo Heil- und Lehrinstitut in Lans, Tirol. Er ist Doktor der Medizin und Master der Chinesischen Medizin. In Zusammenarbeit mit der RMIT Universität Melbourne entwickelte er 2004 ein Lehrprogramm für einen Kurs in Energiemedizin. Am Indeo Institut lehrt Dr. Roland G. Heber seine Praxis der Therapie und des Heilens sowie die entsprechenden Heilmodalitäten und Techniken für Ärzte, Heilpraktiker und Therapeuten (für nähere Informationen siehe www.indeoinstitute.com).

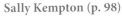

Ursula Karven (p. 144)

Ursula Karven was born in Ulm, Germany, and currently lives in Berlin. The multi-talented actress has appeared in many national and international productions. Since 1999, she has practiced yoga intensively and made it part of her life's philosophy. She completed her teacher training in Los Angeles, with a focus on Vinyasa Flow Yoga, and has headed a yoga school on Majorca for several years. The best-selling author has published a number of books and DVDs on the subject.

Ursula Karven wurde in Ulm geboren und lebt heute in Berlin. Die vielseitig talentierte Schauspielerin war in vielen nationalen und internationalen Produktionen zu sehen. Seit 1999 beschäftigt sie sich intensiv mit Yoga, das Teil ihrer Lebensphilosophie wurde. Sie absolvierte in Los Angeles eine Ausbildung zur Lehrerin mit Schwerpunkt Vinyasa-Flow-Yoga und leitete mehrere Jahre eine Yogaschule auf Mallorca. Die Bestseller-Autorin hat zu diesem Thema diverse Bücher und DVDs veröffentlicht.

Sally Kempton (p. 98)

Sally Kempton gives worldwide meditation workshops and writes a popular column, "Wisdom", for Yoga Journal. She teaches regular teleclasses on meditation and has published several CDs, including "Awakened Heart" and "Beginning Meditation", which are available on the internet. Her most recent book is "Meditation for the Love of It." (See www.sallykempton.com for more information.)

Sally Kempton veranstaltet Meditations-Workshops auf der ganzen Welt und schreibt die beliebte Kolumne „Wisdom" für das Magazin Yoga Journal. Sie bietet regelmäßig Fernlehrgänge in Meditation an und hat verschiedene CDs veröffentlicht, darunter „Awakened Heart" und „Beginning Meditation", die im Internet erhältlich sind. Ihr neuestes Buch heißt „Meditation – Das Tor zum Herzen öffnen" (für nähere Informationen siehe: www.sallykempton.com).

Biographies

Dr. med. Brigitte Klett (Hotel Post, p. 164)

Dr. Brigitte Klett is a general practitioner, TCM physician, lecturer for Traditional Chinese Medicine, and director of the Steinbeis Institute for Asian Complementary Medicine and Management. Since 2009, she has worked at the IDA Therapy Center in Fellbach, combining Western methods with the ideas of Chinese medicine to support health and well-being.

Dr. Brigitte Klett, Fachärztin für Allgemeinmedizin, TCM-Ärztin, Dozentin für Traditionelle Chinesische Medizin und Direktorin am Steinbeis-Institut für Asian Complementary Medicine and Management. Sie arbeitet seit 2009 am IDA-Therapiezentrum Fellbach ganzheitlich im Sinne von westlicher Gesundheitsentstehung und dem Gedankengut der chinesischen Medizin.

Alcide Leali Jr. (Lefay Resort & Spa Lago di Garda, p. 230)

Alcide Leali Jr. graduated with a Bachelor's degree in Business Administration in 2006 at Bocconi University in Milan, where he also earned his Master of Science in International Management in the following years. In 2008, Leali joined Lefay Resorts as marketing director in charge of the corporate sales and marketing strategy, and in 2011 he was appointed managing director of the company, thereby contributing to the new entrepreneurial project of the Leali family in luxury and wellness first-class tourism.

Alcide Leali Jr. schloss im Jahr 2006 den Bachelor-Studiengang Business Administration an der Universität Bocconi in Mailand ab, wo er in den darauffolgenden Jahren auch den Master of Science in International Management erwarb. Im Jahr 2008 begann Alcide Leali als Marketingdirektor seine Arbeit für Lefay Resorts und war für die Bereiche Corporate Sales und Marketingstrategie zuständig. 2011 wurde er zum Geschäftsführer des Unternehmens ernannt und gibt seitdem Impulse für das neue Unternehmensprojekt der Familie Leali im Luxus- und Wellness-Tourismus erster Klasse.

Olivia Newton-John (Gaia Retreat & Spa, p. 16)

Within her career spanning more than four decades, Olivia Newton-John has sold 100 million albums. Her successes include four Grammys, numerous Country Music, American Music, and People's Choice Awards, an Emmy Award, and ten number one hits. Twenty years after her diagnosis with breast cancer, the Olivia Newton-John Cancer & Wellness Centre opened in Melbourne in June 2012. Continuing her commitment to wellness, Olivia is a co-owner of the multi award-winning Gaia Retreat & Spa. (See olivianewton-john.com for more information.)

In einer Karriere, die fast vier Jahrzehnte umfasst, hat Olivia Newton-John mehr als 100 Millionen Alben verkauft und belegte zehn Mal Platz 1 der Top-Ten-Hitliste. Olivias Erfolg wurde mit vier Grammys und mehreren Preisen gekrönt, unter anderem mit dem Country Music Award, dem American Music Award, dem People's Choice Award und dem Emmy Award. Zwanzig Jahre nach Ihrer Erkrankung an Brustkrebs wurde 2010 das Olivia Newton-John Cancer & Wellness Centre in ihrer Heimatstadt Melbourne, Australien, eröffnet. Das Wohlbefinden der Menschen stets im Auge, hat sie auch das mehrfach preisgekrönte Gaia Retreat & Spa im Hinterland von Byron Bay mitgegründet (für nähere Informationen siehe: olivianewton-john.com).

Dr. med. Petra Müller-Rupprecht (p. 248)

Dr. Petra Müller-Rupprecht is a general practitioner who also specializes in psychosomatic medicine and psychotherapy, homeopathy, and psychoanalysis. She has developed her own coaching concept, using all the tools she acquired during her intensive studies of Eastern and Western philosophy, astrology, shamanism, among others. She works as a psychological and spiritual coach for people in life-changing situations.

Dr. Petra Müller-Rupprecht ist Allgemeinmedizinerin und Fachärztin für Psychosomatische Medizin, Psychotherapie, Homöopathie und Psychoanalyse. Sie hat ihr eigenes Coaching-Konzept entwickelt, in das all ihre Erfahrungen eingeflossen sind, die sie unter anderem während ihrer intensiven Studien der Philosophie, Astrologie und des Schamanismus des Ostens und des Westens gesammelt hat. Als psychologische und spirituelle Beraterin hilft sie Menschen, deren Leben sich im Umbruch befindet.

Brigitte Preuß (Ayurveda Parkschlösschen Bad Wildstein, p. 196)

Together with her husband, Wolfgang Preuß, who taught his family about Ayurveda, Brigitte Preuß established the Ayurveda Parkschlösschen in the early 1990s. She manages the first-class hotel on the Mittelmosel and works closely with Ayurvedic physicians and therapists who have extensive experience in practicing this traditional form of medicine. Her dedication to Ayurveda, her commitment, and her expertise are largely responsible for the success of Parkschlösschen.

Zusammen mit ihrem Mann Wolfgang Preuß, der Ayurveda seiner Familie nahebrachte, baute Brigitte Preuß das Ayurveda Parkschlösschen Anfang der 90er Jahre auf. Seither leitet sie das erstklassige Hotel an der Mittelmosel und arbeitet eng mit zahlreichen erfahrenen Ayurveda-Ärzten und Therapeuten an der authentischen Umsetzung der traditionellen Heilkunst. Ihre Hingabe zum Ayurveda, ihr Engagement und ihr Know-how sind maßgeblich für den Erfolg des Parkschlösschens verantwortlich.

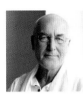

Han Shan (p. 154)

The German Han Shan, formerly Hermann Ricker, was a successful entrepreneur in a global company based in Asia. A dramatic car accident changed his outlook on life: He decided to give away his millions, become a monk, and live as a mendicant in Thailand. Today, Han Shan is an important German-speaking spiritual leader, author, and seminar leader. In addition, he shares his knowledge with others in the Nava Disa Retreat Center, which he founded in Thailand.

Der Deutsche Han Shan, vormals Hermann Ricker, war erfolgreicher Unternehmer eines global agierenden Konzerns in Asien. Ein dramatischer Autounfall veränderte seine Lebensauffassung: Er entschied sich, sein Millionenvermögen zu verschenken und ein Leben als Bettelmönch in Thailand zu führen. Heute ist Han Shan ein bedeutender deutschsprachiger spiritueller Lehrer, Autor und Seminarleiter. In dem von ihm gegründeten Nava Disa Retreat Center in Thailand gibt er sein umfassendes Wissen weiter.

Karina Stewart (Kamalaya Wellness Sanctuary & Holistic Spa, p. 74)

Karina Stewart is co-founder and concept director of Kamalaya Wellness Sanctuary & Holistic Spa in Koh Samui, Thailand. As a doctor of Traditional Chinese Medicine, Karina designed and directed medical detoxification programs in the United States before creating Kamalaya with her husband John. Karina's vision behind Kamalaya's integral wellness programs is to access the inner healing power within each individual and to support a harmonious integration of heart, body, mind, and spirit.

Karina Stewart ist Mitbegründerin und Leiterin des Konzept-Bereichs des Kamalaya Wellness Sanctuary & Holistic Spa in Koh Samui, Thailand. Als Doktor der Traditionellen Chinesischen Medizin hat Karina medizinische Entgiftungsprogramme in den Vereinigten Staaten entwickelt und geleitet, bevor sie mit ihrem Ehemann John Kamalaya ins Leben rief. Hinter den ganzheitlichen Wellness-Programmen im Kamalaya steht Karinas Vision, Zugang zu den Heilkräften im Inneren jedes Menschen zu schaffen und eine harmonische Einbindung von Herz, Körper, Geist und Seele zu fördern.

Dr. Andrew Weil, M.D. (p. 134)

Dr. Andrew Weil is the founder and director of the Arizona Center for Integrative Medicine (AzCIM) at the University of Arizona Health Sciences Center in Tucson. Here he is also a Clinical Professor of Medicine and Professor of Public Health and the Lovell-Jones Professor of Integrative Rheumatology. Dr. Weil is an internationally-recognized expert for his views on leading a healthy lifestyle, his philosophy of healthy aging, and his critique of the future of medicine. His books are bestsellers.

Dr. med. Andrew Weil ist Gründer und Leiter des Arizona Center for Integrative Medicine (AzCIM) im Health Sciences Center an der Universität Arizona in Tucson. Er ist außerdem Professor für Klinische Medizin und Professor für öffentliche Gesundheit sowie Inhaber des Lovell-Jones Stiftungslehrstuhls für Integrative Rheumatologie. Dr. Weil gilt als international anerkannter Experte aufgrund seiner Ansichten zum gesunden Lebensstil, seiner Philosophie des gesunden Alterns und seiner Kritik der Zukunft der Medizin. Seine Bücher sind Bestseller.

Editors
Herausgeberinnen

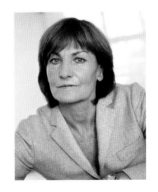
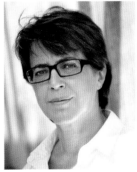

Anne Biging & Dr. Elisabeth Ixmeier
Founders and CEOs of Healing Hotels of the World.
Gründerinnen und Geschäftsführerinnen von Healing Hotels of the World.

HEALING HOTELS OF THE WORLD
Elisabeth-Treskow-Platz 6a
50678 Köln, Germany
Phone: +49 (0) 221 2053 1175
Fax: +49 (0) 221 2053 1177
meetyou@healing-hotels.com
www.healinghotelsoftheworld.com

Imprint & Credits

Editor	Anne Biging
	Dr. Elisabeth Ixmeier
Texts	Anna Löhlein
Copy Editing	Dr. Simone Bischoff
	Alexander Zajons
	Dr. Helga Schier
Editorial Management	Miriam Bischoff
	Regine Freyberg
Creative Direction	Martin Nicholas Kunz
Layout & Prepress	Sophie Franke
Photo Editing	David Burghardt
Imaging	Tridix, Berlin
Translations	WeSwitch Languages
English	Heidi Holzer
	Romina Russo
German	Romina Russo
	Bianca Dett

Published by teNeues Publishing Group

teNeues Verlag GmbH + Co. KG
Am Selder 37, 47906 Kempen, Germany
Phone: +49 (0)2152 916 0, Fax: +49 (0)2152 916 111
e-mail: books@teneues.de

Press department: Andrea Rehn
Phone: +49 (0)2152 916 202
e-mail: arehn@teneues.de

teNeues Digital Media GmbH
Kohlfurter Straße 41-43, 10999 Berlin, Germany
Phone: +49 (0)30 700 77 65 0

teNeues Publishing Company
7 West 18th Street, New York, NY 10011, USA
Phone: +1 212 627 9090, Fax: +1 212 627 9511

teNeues Publishing UK Ltd.
21 Marlowe Court, Lymer Avenue, London SE19 1LP, UK
Phone: +44 (0)20 8670 7522, Fax: +44 (0)20 8670 7523

teNeues France S.A.R.L.
39, rue des Billets, 18250 Henrichemont, France
Phone: +33 (0)2 4826 9348, Fax: +33 (0)1 7072 3482

www.teneues.com
© 2012 teNeues Verlag GmbH + Co. KG, Kempen

ISBN: 978-3-8327-9633-4
Library of Congress Control Number: 2012950719
Printed in Italy.
Picture and text rights reserved for all countries.
No part of this publication may be reproduced in any
manner whatsoever. All rights reserved.
While we strive for utmost precision in every detail,
we cannot be held responsible for any inaccuracies,
neither for any subsequent loss or damage arising.
Bibliographic information published by the Deutsche
Nationalbibliothek.
The Deutsche Nationalbibliothek lists this publication
in the Deutsche Nationalbibliografie; detailed
bibliographic data are available in the Internet at
http://dnb.d-nb.de.

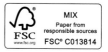

FSC MIX Paper from responsible sources FSC® C013814

Cover photo (Frégate Island Private) by Jochen Manz; Back cover photos courtesy of Saffire Freycinet, JD Marston/courtesy of Kamalaya Co. Ltd., Richard Butterfield/courtesy of Hyatt Hotels

pp 04–05 (Contents) courtesy of Post Ranch Inn; pp 08–09 (Clinton Foundation) by Gavin Jackson; pp 10–11 (Introduction) by Martin N. Kunz; pp 12–15 (Gaia Retreat & Spa) p 14 top left by David Young, all other photos courtesy of Gaia Retreat & Spa; pp 16–17 (The Power of Nature) courtesy of Gaia Retreat & Spa; pp 18–21 (Saffire Freycinet) courtesy of Saffire Freycinet; pp 22–25 (The Lyall Hotel and Spa) courtesy of The Lyall Hotel and Spa; pp 26–29 (Treetops Lodge & Estate) courtesy of Treetops Lodge & Estate; pp 30–33 (Split Apple Retreat) by Daniel Allen, Nelson, New Zealand; p 34 (Blueberry Soufflé) by Daniel Allen, New Zealand; pp 36–39 (Fivelements) by Djuna Ivereigh; pp 40–43 (MesaStila) courtesy of MesaStila; pp 44–47 (Raffles Hotel Singapore) pp 44 and 47 courtesy of Raffles Hotel Singapore, other photos by Martin N. Kunz; pp 48–51 (The Chateau Spa & Organic Wellness Resort) p 48 and 51 top by Kelvin Yeoh, 2010, other photos courtesy of The Chateau Spa & Organic Wellness Resort; pp 52–53 (Yoga) by Thomas Zerlauth/courtesy of Kamalaya Co. Ltd.; pp 54–57 (Fusion Maia Resort) by Martin N. Kunz; pp 58–61 (Mandarin Oriental Dhara Dhevi) courtesy of Mandarin Oriental Group; pp 62–63 (Energy) by Gavin Jackson; pp 64–67 (Chiva-Som) p 66 bottom left by W photography, all other photos courtesy of Chiva-Som; pp 68–69 (Banana Blossom Salad) p 68 by Songsak Paname/iStockphoto, p 69 by Le Do/both iStockphoto; pp 70–73 (Kamalaya Wellness Sanctuary & Holistic Spa) pp 71, 72, 73 top left and p 77 by JD Marston, p 73 right by

Daniel Leser, p 73 bottom right by Ingrid Rasmussen, pp 74–75 by Paul Cutter, all photos courtesy of Kamalaya Co. Ltd.; pp 78–81 (Ananda In The Himalayas) p 81 by Martin N. Kunz, all other photos courtesy of Ananda In The Himalayas; pp 82–85 (Gili Lankanfushi) courtesy of HPL Hotels & Resorts; pp 86–89 (Al Maha Desert Resort & Spa) p 87 and 89 right by Martin N. Kunz, all other photos courtesy of Al Maha Desert Resort & Spa; pp 90–93 (Park Hyatt Dubai) p 93 by Richard Butterfield, all other photos courtesy of Hyatt Hotels; pp 94–97 (Six Senses Zighy Bay) p 95 by Cat Vinton, p 97 top by Russ Kientsch, p 97 bottom by Herbert Ypma, other photos courtesy of Six Senses Zighy Bay; pp 98–99 (Meditation) courtesy of MesaStila; pp 100–103 (Frégate Island Private) p 101 by Jochen Manz, p 102 right by Martin N. Kunz, all other photos courtesy of Frégate Island Private; pp 104–107 (Entre Cielos) courtesy of Entre Cielos; pp 108–111 (Lapinha Spa) p 109 by Clóvis França, p 110 top by Gabriel Raia Carneiro, p 110 bottom and p 111 left by Felipe Pinheiro, p 111 right by Rogério Voltan; pp 112–115 (Rancho La Puerta) p 113 by Silverman 2011, all other photos courtesy of Rancho La Puerta; pp 116–117 (Healthy Sleep) by Martin N. Kunz; pp 118–121 (Jade Mountain) p 119 by Lou Metzger/www.aphotograph.com, p 120 right by Macduff Everton, all other photos courtesy of Jade Mountain; pp 122–125 (Post Ranch Inn) p 122 courtesy of Post Ranch Inn, all other photos by Gavin Jackson; pp 126–129 (Miraval Resort and Spa) p 129 right by Robin Stancliff Photography, all other photos courtesy of Miraval Resort and Spa; pp 130–133 (The Sullivan Estate & Spa Retreat) p 130 by Ansgar Freyberg, all other photos courtesy of The Sullivan Estate & Spa Retreat; pp 134–135 (Healthy Aging) by

Rogério Votran/Lapinha Spa; pp 136–139 (Lumeria Maui) courtesy of Lumeria Maui; pp 140–143 (Grail Springs) courtesy of Grail Springs Health Spa & Wellness Retreat; pp 144–145 (Yoga) courtesy of Ananda In The Himalayas; pp 146–149 (Amber Spa Boutique Hotel) by David Burghardt; pp 150–153 (Spirit Hotel) courtesy of Spirit Hotel; pp 154–155 (The Secret of Letting Go) by Rogério Votran/Lapinha Spa; pp 156–159 (Grand Park Hotel) p 157 by Foto Atelier Wolkersdorfer, p 158 bottom by Werbefotografie Gruber Michael, Gastein Tourismus, all other photos courtesy of Grand Park Hotel; pp 160–163 (Hotel Post) courtesy of Hotel Post, Bezau; pp 164–165 (What is Traditional Chinese Medicine?) by xiegenghong/iStockphoto; pp 166–169 (Lanserhof) by Hiepler & Brunier and Holger Knauf; pp 170–171 (Water is Life) by Rogério Votran/Lapinha Spa; p 172 (Grain Patties) by Pannewitz/courtesy of Lanserhof; pp 174–177 (Grand Resort Bad Ragaz) courtesy of Grand Hotel Bad Ragaz; pp 178–181 (Hubertus Alpin Lodge & Spa) by www.guenterstandl.de; pp 182–185 (Breidenbacher Hof, A Capella Hotel) pp 184 and 185 bottom by Robert Reck Photography, all other photos courtesy of Breidenbacher Hof, A Capella Hotel; pp 186–187 (Relaxing while You Travel) by Rogério Votran/Lapinha Spa; pp 188–191 (Allgäu Sonne) pp 188 and 190 top by Marcel Hagen/www.studio22.at, p 190 bottom by Gregory Anderson, p 191 courtesy of Allgäu Sonne; pp 192–195 (Ayurveda Parkschlösschen Bad Wildstein) p 190 and 192 top by Nomi Baumgartl, other photos courtesy of Ayurveda Parkschlösschen Bad Wildstein; pp 196–197 (Ayurveda) by Hajo von Keller; pp 198–201 (Le Royal Monceau, Raffles Paris) p 199 by Laurent Attias, all other photos by Philippe Garcia/both LaSociétéAnonyme; pp 202–205 (La Clairière Spa Hotel)

courtesy of La Clairière Spa Hotel; pp 206–209 (Grand Hotel Terme Trieste & Victoria) p 209 left by www.gabrielecroppi.com, all other photos courtesy of Grand Hotel Terme Trieste & Victoria; pp 210–213 (Abano Grand Hotel) courtesy of Abano Grand Hotel; pp 214–215 (Graceful Youth, Graceful Aging) by Djuna Ivereigh/courtesy of Fivelements; pp 216–219 (Borgo Egnazia) p 217 Nicola Cipriani, p 218 top left and right by Francesco Bittichesu, all photos courtesy of Borgo Egnazia; pp 220–223 (Castel Monastero) courtesy of Castel Monastero; pp 224–225 (Integrated Medicine) courtesy of Miraval Resort & Spa; pp 226–229 (Lefay Resort and Spa Lago di Garda) courtesy of Lefay Resort & Spa; pp 230–231 (Health for You and the World around You) by Rogério Votran/Lapinha Spa; pp 232–235 (Alpina Dolomites – Gardena Health Lodge & Spa) all photos by Andrea Cazzaniga; pp 236–239 (Verdura Golf & Spa Resort) courtesy of Verdura Golf & Spa Resort; pp 240–243 (AROSEA Life Balance Hotel) p 240 by Adriano Bacchella, pp 242 top left and 243 by Sören, others courtesy of AROSEA Life Balance Hotel; pp 244–247 (Adler Balance) by Manuela Prossliner; pp 248–249 (Happiness) by www.guenterstandl.de/courtesy Hubertus Alpin Lodge & Spa; pp 250–253 (Villa Padierna Thermas de Carratraca) courtesy of Villa Padierna Thermas de Carratraca; pp 254–257 (SHA Wellness Clinic) courtesy of SHA Wellness Clinic; pp 258–259 (The Power of Food) courtesy of Lumeria Maui; pp 260–263 (Villa Padierna Palace) p 261 by vision photos, all other photos courtesy of Villa Padierna Palace; pp 264–267 (Porto Elounda Golf & Spa Resort) courtesy of Porto Elounda Golf & Spa Resort; pp 268–271 (Biographies) p 271 bottom (Editors) by Boris Breuer Fotografie (2), all other photos private